The
HIPAA
Program Reference Handbook

OTHER AUERBACH PUBLICATIONS

Agent-Based Manufacturing and Control Systems: New Agile Manufacturing Solutions for Achieving Peak Performance
Massimo Paolucci and Roberto Sacile
ISBN: 1574443364

Curing the Patch Management Headache
Felicia M. Nicastro
ISBN: 0849328543

Cyber Crime Investigator's Field Guide, Second Edition
Bruce Middleton
ISBN: 0849327687

Disassembly Modeling for Assembly, Maintenance, Reuse and Recycling
A. J. D. Lambert and Surendra M. Gupta
ISBN: 1574443348

The Ethical Hack: A Framework for Business Value Penetration Testing
James S. Tiller
ISBN: 084931609X

Fundamentals of DSL Technology
Philip Golden, Herve Dedieu, and Krista Jacobsen
ISBN: 0849319137

The HIPAA Program Reference Handbook
Ross Leo
ISBN: 0849322111

Implementing the IT Balanced Scorecard: Aligning IT with Corporate Strategy
Jessica Keyes
ISBN: 0849326214

Information Security Fundamentals
Thomas R. Peltier, Justin Peltier, and John A. Blackley
ISBN: 0849319579

Information Security Management Handbook, Fifth Edition, Volume 2
Harold F. Tipton and Micki Krause
ISBN: 0849332109

Introduction to Management of Reverse Logistics and Closed Loop Supply Chain Processes
Donald F. Blumberg
ISBN: 1574443607

Maximizing ROI on Software Development
Vijay Sikka
ISBN: 0849323126

Mobile Computing Handbook
Imad Mahgoub and Mohammad Ilyas
ISBN: 0849319714

MPLS for Metropolitan Area Networks
Nam-Kee Tan
ISBN: 084932212X

Multimedia Security Handbook
Borko Furht and Darko Kirovski
ISBN: 0849327733

Network Design: Management and Technical Perspectives, Second Edition
Teresa C. Piliouras
ISBN: 0849316081

Network Security Technologies, Second Edition
Kwok T. Fung
ISBN: 0849330270

Outsourcing Software Development Offshore: Making It Work
Tandy Gold
ISBN: 0849319439

Quality Management Systems: A Handbook for Product Development Organizations
Vivek Nanda
ISBN: 1574443526

A Practical Guide to Security Assessments
Sudhanshu Kairab
ISBN: 0849317061

The Real-Time Enterprise
Dimitris N. Chorafas
ISBN: 0849327776

Software Testing and Continuous Quality Improvement, Second Edition
William E. Lewis
ISBN: 0849325242

Supply Chain Architecture: A Blueprint for Networking the Flow of Material, Information, and Cash
William T. Walker
ISBN: 1574443577

The Windows Serial Port Programming Handbook
Ying Bai
ISBN: 0849322138

AUERBACH PUBLICATIONS

www.auerbach-publications.com
To Order Call: 1-800-272-7737 • Fax: 1-800-374-3401
E-mail: orders@crcpress.com

The
HIPAA
Program Reference Handbook

Ross Leo
Editor

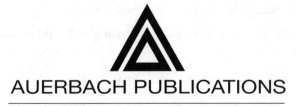

AUERBACH PUBLICATIONS

A CRC Press Company

Boca Raton   London   New York   Washington, D.C.

Library of Congress Cataloging-in-Publication Data

The HIPAA program reference handbook / Ross Leo, editor.
   p. cm.
   Includes bibliographical references and index.
   ISBN 0-8493-2211-1 (alk. paper)
     1. Medical records--Law and legislation--United States. 2. United States. Health
Insurance Portability and Accountability Act of 1996. I. Leo, Ross.

   KF3827.R4 H5652
   344.7304'1--dc22

               2004046397

Visit the Auerbach Web site at www.auerbach-publications.com

© 2005 by CRC Press
Auerbach is an imprint of CRC Press

No claim to original U.S. Government works
International Standard Book Number 0-8493-2211-1
Library of Congress Card Number 2004046397
Printed in the United States of America 1 2 3 4 5 6 7 8 9 0

CONTRIBUTORS

Oscar Boultinghouse, M.D.
Dr. Oscar Boultinghouse currently serves as the Director of Correctional Telemedicine for the University of Texas Medical Branch, Correctional Managed Care Division, which is recognized as the largest telemedicine program in the world. He is the former Director of Operations and Medical Director for the UTMB Center for Telehealth and Distance Education. He is a recognized authority in the use of telemedicine in extremely remote environments and in disaster support. Formally the Director of UTMB's Life Flight Operation, he currently serves as the Medical Director of Texas-3 DMAT. Dr. Boultinghouse is a board certified Emergency Medicine Specialist and is currently pursuing a master's degree in Health Informatics.

Mary Brown, CISSP, CISA
Mary Brown had 13 years of experience in the accounting and audit field when she developed an interest in IT and in information security in particular. For the past seven years, Mary has focused largely on network and application security. She has extensive experience in risk analysis and information security policy development. She is one of the founding members of the Healthcare Security Professional Interest Group, which meets to develop community standards for information security in health-care settings. Mary is also a member of the Computer Security Institute (CSI), the Information Systems Audit and Control Association (ISACA), and the Information Systems Security Association (ISSA). She has a B.S. in Management Information Systems from Metropolitan State University and a master's degree in Information Technology with a specialization in information security from Capella University. She has earned her CISSP and CISA, which are internationally recognized certifications for expertise in information security and IT auditing respectively. Mary works as a Senior Information Security Specialist for a large urban teaching hospital in Minnesota and has been working for Capella University teaching system

assurance and networking and on developing and refreshing information security and assurance course curriculum since 2002.

Johnathan Coleman, CISSP, CISM

Johnathan Coleman joined the ATI team in May of 2001 as a Program Manager in the Information Protection Technology Division. He brings ten years of leadership and technical project management experience in information security, distributed communications networks, information systems consulting, and technical risk management. Mr. Coleman is leading the effort in training the approximately 170 Department of Defense Medical Information Security Readiness Teams in a SEI/CERT developed approach to conducting threat and vulnerability assessments that meet HIPAA data security requirements, and has authored subject-specific training materials (instructor and train-the-trainer manuals) for use by the DOD. He is also responsible for the design and development (using proven software engineering processes) of multimedia demonstration software used to assist in the training and execution of organizational vulnerability and risk assessments.

Todd Fitzgerald, CISSP, CISA

Todd Fitzgerald is the Director of Information Systems Security and serves as the Systems Security Officer for United Government Services, LLC (part of the WellPoint Health Networks family of companies), which is the largest processor of Medicare Part A claims. Todd is a member of the Board of Directors and co-chair of the Security Taskforce for the HIPAA Collaborative of Wisconsin (www.hipaacow.org), a nonprofit corporation formed to promote sharing between Wisconsin health plans, clearinghouses, and providers. He is a participant of the Centers for Medicare and Medicaid Services/Gartner Security Best Practices Workgroup, the Blue Cross Blue Shield Association Information Security Advisory Group, a board member of the International Systems Security Association (ISSA) Milwaukee Chapter, and previously a board member for the ISSA—Delaware Valley Chapter serving Pennsylvania, Maryland, Delaware, and New Jersey. Todd has held various broad-based senior management Information Technology positions with Fortune 500 and Fortune Global 250 companies such as IMS Health, Zeneca, Syngenta, and American Airlines and prior positions with Blue Cross Blue Shield United of Wisconsin. Todd has authored articles on HIPAA security and frequently presents at conferences and association meetings to promote security awareness. Todd has earned a B.S. in Business Administration from the University of Wisconsin-LaCrosse and a M.B.A. with highest honors from Oklahoma State University.

Brian Geffert, CISSP, CISA

Brian Geffert is a senior manager for Deloitte & Touche's Security Services Practice and specializes in information systems controls and solutions.

Brian has worked on the development of HIPAA assessment tools and security services for healthcare industry clients to determine the level of security readiness with the Health Insurance Portability and Accountability Act of 1996 (HIPAA) regulations. In addition, he has implemented solutions to assist organizations addressing their HIPAA security readiness issues. Finally, Brian is a Certified Information Systems Security Professional (CISSP) and a Certified Information Systems Auditor (CISA).

Caroline Ramsey Hamilton

Caroline is the founder and president of RiskWatch, Inc., and she spends most of her time working directly with large private companies, U.S. federal agencies, and state governments to create better ways of managing their risk. Caroline is internationally recognized as an expert in security risk management. She participated as a charter member of the Risk Manager's Model Builders Workshop sponsored by the National Institute of Standards and Technology from 1989 to 1997; she was appointed as a working group member to build a working model for risk management, the Defensive Information Warfare Risk Management Model, under the auspices of the Office of the Secretary of Defense. She is currently working with the Maritime Security Council and the U.S. Coast Guard in the development of risk and vulnerability assessment guidelines for Port Security.

Ross A. Leo, CISSP, CHS-III

Ross Leo has been an information security professional for over 23 years. Most of this time was spent at NASA Mission Control, during which time Ross wrote many volumes and papers on information security policy, risk analysis, secure design standards and practices, disaster recovery, and contingency planning. A recent paper, "Single Sign-on," appeared in the fourth edition of the *Handbook of Information Security Management*. As co-chairman of the international Generally Accepted System Security Principles Committee (GASSPC), he co-authored and saw the publication of the GASSP Version 2. Ross's experience covers a broad range of enterprises. He has worked internationally as a Systems Analyst, Systems Engineer, IT Auditor, and Security Consultant. His past employers include IBM, St. Luke's Episcopal Hospital, Computer Sciences Corporation, Coopers & Lybrand, Rockwell International, and Dynegy. From 1999 to 2002, he was Director of Security Engineering and Chief Security Architect for the Mission Control Center at the Johnson Space Center. Presently, Ross is the Director of Information Systems and Chief Information Security Officer for the Correctional Managed Care Division of the University of Texas Medical Branch in Galveston, Texas.

Mark Lott

Mark Lott is an information technology professional whose primary focus is within the software quality assurance environment. He has managed successful implementations for many Fortune 100 companies while introducing and enhancing client's software testing methodologies. He has spent the last 15 years as a software tester, project manager, quality assurance manager, and consultant. Mark is currently serving as Chairman of HCCO (HIPAA Conformance Certification Organization), serving the healthcare community with practical guidelines for complying with HIPAA regulation through the use of accreditation and certification standards and services. He has effectively led the industry in the creation of a national interoperability testing process for HIPAA transactions, ensuring compliance software is accurately and thoroughly tested. A featured speaker at conferences and local industry groups Mark has shared his insights and real-world experience educating people as to the value and critical nature of incorporating proven software testing methodologies and change management within the software delivery life cycle.

Steven B. Markin

Steven B. Markin is a New York attorney and president of ComplyGuard Networks, Inc., a venture to aid covered entities in meeting the challenge of HIPAA compliance.

Kevin C. Miller

Kevin C. Miller has been a communications and journalism professional for over ten years including five years as a spokesman and journalist for the U.S. Coast Guard. He has been published in magazines and newspapers internationally and is currently the public relations coordinator for Strohl Systems, a global leader in the business continuity planning software and services market. He can be reached at kmiller@strohlsystems.com.

Uday O. Ali Pabrai, CHSS, SCNA

Creator of the first program on HIPAA skills certification and author of the number one book on HIPAA, *Getting Started with HIPAA*, Uday O. Ali Pabrai is a highly sought-after HIPAA consultant, security expert, and an exceptional speaker. Uday is an AIP Fellow and Board member, SITI member, and past chair of the Subject Matter Expert Committee for CompTIA's Internet and security certifications. Previously, as founder and CEO of Net Guru Technologies, he created the world-leading Certified Internet Webmaster (CIW) program. Uday is the co-creator of the highly successful, enterprise-centric, Security Certified Program (SCP).

Keith Pasley, CISSP

Keith Pasley is an information security professional with over 19 years of experience in the information technology field. Keith has designed and implemented security architectures for businesses in a variety of industries including healthcare and financial services. Keith is a Senior Systems Engineer. He can be reached at securityminded@comcast.net.

Ken M. Shaurette, CISSP, CISA, CISM, NSA-IAM
Ken M. Shaurette is an Information Security Solutions Manager for MPC Security Solutions located in Pewaukee, Wisconsin. Ken began gaining IT experience in 1978 and has provided managed information security professionals and programs, and provided information security and audit advice and vision, for companies building information security programs since 1985. As a frequent speaker at regional and national seminars and conferences Ken has also contributed white papers and other writing on security back to the industry. Ken is the Chairman of the Information Security Specialist Advisory Board for Milwaukee Area Technical College, President of the Western Wisconsin Chapter of InfraGard, President of ISSA-Milwaukee Chapter (International Systems Security Association), a member of the Wisconsin Association of Computer Crime Investigators (WACCI), a participant in the Cyber Security Alliance (www.staysafeonline.info), co-chair of the HIPAA-COW (Collaborative of Wisconsin) Security Workgroup, and co-chair of the annual Wisconsin InfraGard KIS (Kids Improving Security) Poster Contest.

DEDICATION

To my family, the best cheering section to be found anywhere,
and especially my wife who leads it.

DEDICATION

CONTENTS

PART II: STANDARDS AND COMPLIANCE

PART III: ECONOMICS, LEGALITY, AND LIABILITY

8 HIPAA Privacy Rules Require Security Compliance 143

Steven B. Markin

9 Legalities and Planning: The Stake Is in the Ground 149

Ken M. Shaurette, CISSP, CISA, CISM, IAM

PART IV: TRANSACTION AND INTERACTIONS

PART V: SECURITY, PRIVACY, AND CONTINUITY

FOREWORD

There are many books that deal with the various aspects of the HIPAA regulations yet very few include the pertinent facts of all three: transactions, privacy, and security. It is pleasing to read a collection of works that encompasses all three aspects of complying with HIPAA in an easy-to-understand manual of the regulations and how organizations can readily and informatively move their organizations towards HIPAA compliance. The solutions presented here for developing strategies for HIPAA transactions, privacy, and security areas are straightforward and provide detailed strategies for implementation across healthcare organizations and their business partners.

The HIPAA Program Reference Handbook has been written for several audiences. First, it is intended for high-level managers to help them more fully understand the various aspects involved in complying with the law and its implementing regulations. Second, this volume provides guidance on creating and coordinating a cohesive and enforceable policy framework, and related procedures within an organization. Third, this book provides much-needed information, based on real experience, to help individual project teams come to know the necessary requirements in other program implementation areas, thus ensuring that the teams' responses to the regulation are designed and implemented correctly to ensure compliance across the spectrum of this broad legislation.

In order for successful implementation of cohesive HIPAA policies and procedures, healthcare organizations must understand regulation requirements and responsibilities and how to effectively manage compliance and change. This compendium contains practical explanations for creating and combining the necessary work efforts and strategies for implementing successful and cost-effective solutions for organizations affected by HIPAA regulations.

Taking on HIPAA can be an extremely complex and daunting task for even the most well-prepared and organized healthcare entity. Complicating things further, with many functions being performed through business associates and third-party vendors, it is a challenge to adequately coordinate all the various policies, procedures, and technology enhancements required for such a large undertaking.

Although everyone agrees that such a program is a very large undertaking, there is a significant part of the healthcare community, in a variety of disciplines, who have dedicated themselves to ensure adequate knowledge transfer to assist all those in the industry elsewhere who need help. Management places faith that all aspects will come together in a timely manner, but usually does so without any clear idea of what exactly the completed project will produce, whether it will meet expectations, or how all the major pieces and subprojects will ultimately fit together. This volume provides these managers and teams with the information and insight that validates their faith, confirms direction and progress, and permits them to make midcourse corrections confidently when and where necessary.

This book's approach combines the best features of techniques used individually by experts in the field, yet when combined can be instrumental in the overall success of an organization in regard to their aspects of succeeding within HIPAA regulations and compliance.

Mark Lott
Chairman, HCCO

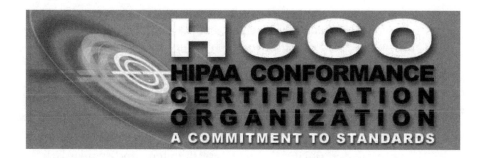

PREFACE

THE HIPAA CONFORMANCE CERTIFICATION ORGANIZATION

HCCO is a nonprofit organization serving the healthcare community with practical guidelines for complying with HIPAA regulation through a certification and accreditation process using national standards. HCCO is the industry leader in bringing interoperability of HIPAA transactions to healthcare through its CCAP testing programs. HCCO believes that all cost-effective and successful compliance strategies will require a common approach to implementation among communities of covered entities, their software vendors, and business associates. HCCO offers effective and affordable solutions for all organizations involved in HIPAA compliance initiatives.

THE VISION

To provide national leadership in the development and establishment of conformance, certification and accreditation criteria and standards, for products, services, processes and methodologies used by covered entities and their business associates to confirm their compliance with the regulations promulgated pursuant to the Health Insurance Portability and Accountability

Act (HIPAA) and the associated Standards and Implementation Guides. HCCO shall develop and maintain criteria and standards, and implement a program to certify the application of HCCO criteria and standards towards conforming products, services, processes, and methodologies.

THE HCCO MISSION

The core mission of HCCO is to establish criteria and standards for independent evaluation of the conformance of products, services, processes, and methodologies to all aspects of HIPAA Title II rules for transactions, privacy, and security. It is expected that HCCO criteria and standards will result in functional equivalency between equally certified products, services, processes, and methodologies.

COMMITTEE ORGANIZATION

HCCO has a committee for each specific area of HIPAA: transactions, security and privacy, legal issues, administrative simplification, and harmonization (of standards and or application). It is inherent in the committee's proper functioning to be inclusive, rather than exclusive. It is also inherent in the committee's composition that a balance should exist between technical and nontechnical and managerial and nonmanagerial.

COMMITTEE FOCUS

Each committee works on the adaptation (of existing and applicable) or establishment of standards and conformance criteria in the aspect of HIPAA that is its focus. The standards and criteria will include technology, policy, procedure, and professional practice. The intent is not to "reinvent the wheel," but rather to draw from the best of the work already done in the area of standards and adapt it for application to the requirements of HIPAA.

For example, the HCCO Security, Privacy, and Continuity Committee is evaluating existing standards against the requirements of the HIPAA Privacy and Security Rules to determine their applicability as potential models for industrywide standards. Examples include ISO 15408 (the common criteria), ISO 17799 (BS 7799), the Generally Accepted Systems Security Principles (GASSP), guidance issued by the National Institute of Standards and Technology (NIST), and similar organizations.

Continuing the example, the committee will take from these and other sources the best of their content, and develop a set of standards, compliance criteria, policy and procedure templates, and process frameworks that can then be generally applied in a given healthcare setting. Vendors seeking HIPAA certification against these standards will be encouraged to submit designs, specifications, templates, and product samples for evaluation and potential certification. The committee will apply its evaluation process to the vendor item, and, for those attaining certification, will issue a formal statement to the vendor to so indicate.

Given this focus, the committee must maintain independence so that it may issue credible and uncompromised opinions as to the certification status of any given vendor product or service submitted to this process. In keeping with this practice, members will not be limited in any way with respect to the committee's activities or evaluation processes except in those cases where a potential conflict of interest may exist.

Some examples of HCCO product and service offerings follow.

HCCO CCAP Interoperability Testing for HIPAA Compliance

HCCO is the industry leader in fostering interoperability in all HIPAA transactions. CCAP is a community testing effort with the nation's largest EDI translators and EDI validators to align HIPAA compliance edits with each other to promote interoperable transactions. CCAP is the only process available to vendors to test interoperability across healthcare-covered entities.

HIPAA Test File Programs

HCCO's HIPAA test file program uses various test conditions for all HIPAA transactions for organizations to test for common compliance understanding to ensure compliant transactions and interoperability with all other participants.

HCCO Free EDI Testing

HCCO invites all covered entities, business associates, and software vendors to use our free HIPAA EDI testing engine. Our testing community is guaranteed to be up to date with the latest compliance edits and is interoperable with over 90 percent of all healthcare organizations that use EDI technology certified under the CCAP Platinum Program.

HCCO HIAA Transaction Certification

HCCO offers HIPAA transaction certification for all covered entities, business associates, and software vendors. HCCO certification is definitive

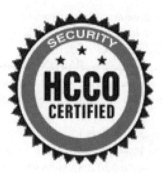

proof of your compliance capabilities and because HCCO testing is free, we have removed any obstacles from the healthcare community so they can continually test their software for HIPAA compliance.

HCCO Privacy Certification for Business Associates

The HCCO board of directors approved the HCCO Privacy Certification Program for Business Associates. The HCCO Business Associate Certification Program conforms to the HIPAA Privacy and Security Rules.

HCCO Security Certification for Vendor Products and Entity Sites

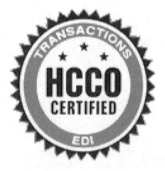

HCCO will soon offer a review and certification program for vendors of systems, software, and other technologies to covered entities and provider organizations. In addition, HCCO will soon be offering a certification program for covered entity sites which will affirm that their processes, systems, and operations conform to the requirements of the HIPAA Security standards and requirements.

HCCO HIPAA Medical Banking Certification Program

HCCO offers healthcare covered entities, financial institutions, and their business partners an industry-specific HIPAA Medical Banking Certification. This industry-leading certification is focused solely on the capability of institutions to properly handle the 835 and 820 HIPAA transaction sets.

HCCO Accreditation of Third-Party HIPAA Certifiers

HCCO is pleased to announce the establishment of our accreditation program for organizations that want to become third-party certifiers for HCCO HIPAA Transactions and Business Associate Certification Programs.

HCCO ebXML EDI Interoperability Certification

HCCO, the leader in bringing interoperability to healthcare, is proud to partner with the UCC and Drummond Group to bring ebXML interoperability testing to healthcare.

ACKNOWLEDGMENTS

I want to thank those authors who participated in the construction of this first edition of the *HIPAA Standard Reference Handbook*. It is no small task to put together a work covering something as vast as a law can be, and making the parts of it clear and accessible to those who must implement it. It is neither easy nor quick in the doing. Nor can it be done by one person. It is a team effort, and I have been very fortunate to have had the team I have had in this project. Should it be successful, it will be because of their contributions and belief in its importance and necessity.

It is hoped that this is the first in a series for this work; a work whose purpose is to bring usable information and guidance to professionals who are responsible for implementing the regulations that underlie and are the substance of the law itself. The Health Insurance Portability and Account-ability Act is rather simple in its text, but deep and wide in its effect on the healthcare industry. It is not the Act itself, but the text of the regulations found in Title 45 of the Code of Federal Regulations that are complex to understand. Much confusion and even fear of the potential impact of this legal body pervades healthcare institutions and the professionals working in them. Speaking for myself and the contributors to this volume, it is our hope that the information contained herein will dispel some of that, and add value to the efforts of those who will read it.

I also want to thank my publisher, Rich O'Hanley at CRC Press, for his belief in this project, and his support during its construction. His sharp rational mind and ready, well-tried advice to me throughout this project was sometimes funny, sometimes painful, but always important and always useful.

And finally I want to thank one individual in particular. My good friend and mentor, Hal Tipton, gave me my first "official" position in the early 1980s as ISO for the Johnson Space Centre. My career, more than twenty years hence, has found me participating in many "firsts," and working on many of the projects that produced the foundational principles and best practices of the Information Security Profession. I have had the privilege of working with Hal on several of those projects and on other occasions, including co-teaching the (ISC)^2 CISSP Review Seminar to candidates preparing for the professional certification examination. He has been a consistent and ready source of encouragement and sound counsel in all my efforts. Over the years, I have come to know him as a man of deep dedication to our profession, of great personal integrity, and a most worthy friend.

Only I know all the steps that make up the last twenty years of my professional practice, and it would take a long time to recount them. Suffice it to say that without his starting me on this path, and being a positive influence, guide, counselor, and example from then on, my professional life would have turned out very differently, and this book would ultimately not have been possible. Thanks, Hal.

INTRODUCTION

Now that HIPAA is here, a new day has dawned in healthcare. Or has it?

HIPAA is one of the most important and pervasive pieces of legislation and regulation to take flight in recent years, yet many in healthcare still don't understand what it is, and specifically, what they are expected to do about it. It is not surprising that they don't: although the law itself is fairly simple in its wording, the Code of Federal Regulations that specifies how to implement, sets standards, and so on is very thick indeed. This is to say nothing of its portent. It is this portent that concerns the authors who contributed to this body of work.

People seem to agree that electronic payment processing is an idea whose time has come. So the rules regarding transaction code sets (and all that entails) seem to be okay. No one seems to have a problem with the privacy rules; at least not in theory. Everyone has trouble with the security rules, however you look at it. According to my research, there are three reasons for these ambivalent (and stronger) feelings.

The first is that many believe that HIPAA is too big and too expensive to work; therefore it is doomed to failure. The second is that there are just as many who believe that the change required by it is too great; this is to say, the amount and type of change are more than they can manage properly over the long implementation period HIPAA will require. The third is fear: fear that the foregoing are correct, fear that they will be forced to "do HIPAA" anyway, and fear that they will suffer the legal penalties no matter what they do. Is there truth to any of this? There may well be, even if you took away the fear factor.

The greatest is fear of the unknown. They have heard so many stories: nightmare tales of the costs to implement the regulations, nightmare tales about how unwieldy the implementation is because the rules are some-what vague, standards do not provide enough information to implement, and on and on. The most pernicious fear among these is that those responsible know a lot of what needs doing, but they have not the foggiest notion about whether, after all the dust settles, their programs and systems do in fact comply with the Act and how that will be tested and measured. No one seems to be able to tell them clearly either. This brings me to the purpose for this book.

The concept embodied here is clarity. The contributors to this volume are seasoned veterans who have spent time in the trenches working out the issues and problems associated with implementing programs to become compliant with the HIPAA requirements, as specified in Title 45 of the Federal Code of Regulations, Sections 160 to 164. Some of them are consultants, some are full-time employees of covered entities, and some work for the standards bodies. All of them have worked first-hand with the standards and requirements, and are sharing from that experience in these pages.

The book is organized into five parts. The first part covers "Programs and Processes." This section discusses topics such as due diligence; program design and implementation; workforce education; human dynamics; issues analysis; a review of the legislation, policy, and procedure development; internal control structures and requirements; the chief privacy officer role; chief security officer role; and other foundational matters.

The second part, "Standards and Compliance," covers topics related to product, policy, technology, and process standards, all of which are focused on helping an organization achieve compliance with the legislation's mandates and requirements. The compliance portion addresses what standards of performance, execution, and due care must be met to actually establish organizational compliance. An additional chapter, "HIPAA Programs: Design and Implementation" by Chris Brown, CISSP, CISA, will appear in the March/April 2005 issue of *Information Systems Security,* and concurrent with the publication of this book on the journal's Web site, www.infosectoday.com.

The third section, "Finance, Economics, Legality, and Liability," deals with the aspects and analysis of the law in particular, its impacts, and the issues of liability associated with senior management, specific roles (CPO, CSO, CISO, et al.), and staff within the organization.

Section Four, "Transactions and Interactions," discusses the nature and intricacies of the transaction types, standards, methods, and implementations required by the Act. The authors cover the flow of payments and patient information within the organization, and between it, payers, government agencies, and other entities.

Section Five, "Security and Privacy," discusses the security and privacy requirements, standards, methods, and implementations required by the Act. Chapters in this section describe human and machine requirements, interface issues, functions, and other aspects of the technology required to successfully implement the required security and privacy measures in a compliant manner.

In this first edition, I have attempted to capture current useful information from practitioners on the leading edge, and I believe I have succeeded. The materials in these pages present different viewpoints in different venues and application areas from professionals in them. There will always be the theoretical methodology describing the ideal approach. The writers here have captured the pragmatics, and present information and experience that is valuable and applicable now.

Ross A. Leo, Editor

I

PROGRAMS AND PROCESSES

1

THE ROLES AND RESPONSIBILITIES

Ross A. Leo, CISSP, CHS–III

INTRODUCTION

Within the body of law and regulations known collectively as the Health Information Portability and Accountability Act (HIPAA), there are defined specific roles and responsibilities that accompany those roles. Although couched in somewhat general terms, these roles are generally known as chief security officer, chief information security officer, and chief privacy officer. There are others, but these are not specific enough to call out separately. Each of these roles must act in accordance with the requirements of the regulation to assure policy definition, awareness education, implementation, monitoring, and enforcement to achieve and maintain compliance in relation to Protected Health Information (PHI). They also have key roles in defining and implementing the enabling processes that facilitate compliance.

Throughout the text of the Act, various requirements are referred to as "required," or "addressable." These roles fall into the former category. These can be assigned within the workforce of the covered entity, or, alternatively, hired in the absence of sufficiently qualified employees. Those so emplaced are charged to ensure that the organization moves purposefully toward a state of compliance, and so to remain once there. The secretary of the Department of Health and Human Services (DHHS) is charged with the responsibility and authority to implement and enforce the Act itself. The official effective date for compliance with this portion of the Act has come and gone; that much is certain. That the work described here is vital and required to continue is also certain. What is not yet clear is how precisely this will be accomplished or measured: by whom, by when, and with what yardstick.

0-8493-2211-1/05/$0.00+$1.50
© 2005 by CRC Press LLC

SETTING THE RECORD STRAIGHT

The Health Insurance Portability and Accountability Act, Public Law 104-191, was signed into law on August 21, 1996 by then President Bill Clinton. Subsequently, various other activities have occurred relative to this law that amplify, clarify, and elaborate on the five titles within the law itself, including the privacy rules and the final security rules. Under Subtitle F: "Administrative Simplification," Section 261 "Purpose" of the Act reads:

> It is the purpose of this subtitle to improve the Medicare program under title XVIII of the Social Security Act, the Medicaid program under title XIX of such Act, and the efficiency and effectiveness of the health care system, by encouraging the development of a health information system through the estab-lishment of standards and requirements for the electronic trans-mission of certain health information.

It is clear from this example that seldom, if ever, can a federal law like HIPAA be enacted and enforced directly from its basic text. To do this requires a body of implementing regulations that describe the detailed mechanics and processes that make the law work. Given that Congress did not act to produce these within the timeframe specified in the law, the secretary of the Department of Health and Human Services was empowered to do so.

That regulatory framework comes under the Federal Code of Regulations (CFR), Title 45 "Public Welfare, Volume 1, Subtitle A: Department of Health and Human Services General Administration, Subchapter C: Administrative Data Standards and Related Requirements, Parts 160 through 164." The several hundred pages of text found here is what actually implements HIPAA. The discussion on security and privacy that follows derives from Title II of the law itself called "Administrative Simplification." This is not intended to be a thick legalistic piece, and so to simplify reading, when a reference is made to "the Act," the reference applies to this entire body of material.

DEFINING THE ASSET IN QUESTION

Our concern here is the asset governed by HIPAA known as "health information," as defined in Part II 45 CFR 160.103, as it relates to a specifically identifiable individual or individuals. This health information pertains to the physical or psychological status of an individual, whether past, present, or future, that is created, collected, or otherwise in the care of a functional entity such as a health plan, provider, school, university, or other entity, and relates in any way to provision of care or payment for that care, regardless of timeframe. This information can be in any form: written, oral, or electronically stored.

The essence of the "protected health information" concept is permitting those persons and business entities with a clear and reasonable "need to know" to create, collect, and maintain that information in accordance with business requirements, and preventing disclosure of it to those parties that have a murky need, or none at all. This, it is believed, will provide reasonable protection to individuals from adverse consequences, and possibly predatory or otherwise inappropriate marketing practices caused by disclosures of this information.

It is believed by most that there is a very close, intertwined relationship between privacy and security within the context of HIPAA. The basic mission of any information security program is to ensure the preservation of Confidentiality, Integrity, and Availability (C-I-A) of that information, and privacy, for all intents, equates to Confidentiality. This relationship is best described as privacy being the goal, and security, in all its forms, being the tool to achieve it. More precisely stated, security is that set of mechanisms, controls, and practices that is employed to ensure that privacy (confidentiality) of health information is gained and maintained in accordance with the statutes.

In the following sections, we discuss privacy and the roles of those directly involved with it at the program or institutional level. Following that, we discuss security, at which point I elaborate on the ideas mentioned above.

THE BEGINNING OF ALL THINGS HIPAA

It is a common and valuable practice to begin with a "gap analysis." This is a formal investigatory method to determine where strengths and weaknesses lie so that they can be correctly addressed and mitigated. These take various forms, but in the case of privacy, the gap analysis is best performed through interview and questionnaire, using a standard question set that relates directly to the specific requirements of the Act.

The questionnaires are quite often long and detailed, but some example questions would be:

1. Has someone been designated as having responsibility for addressing privacy issues, and overseeing corrective action to achieve compliance with the Act?
2. Have you established a policy or set of documents that outlines your entity's policies, procedures, controls, and training related to your patient privacy program?
3. Has your organization defined processes and controls for the handling of PHI in accordance with the Act, including uses, de-identification, releases, archival and storage, authorizations, amendments, and so on?

4. Have you designated a person to handle HIPAA privacy complaints and inquiries?
5. Have you established procedures to handle individuals' requests to amend, update, or correct their health information?

The main points of this exercise are in fact risk identification, mitigation, and establishment of a basis for compliance. It has long been assumed in medical and insurance practice that patient privacy is sacred and to be kept inviolate. Although there are laws in place governing this, adherence to this practice has been largely based on the "honor system." That said, this system, for all its apparent informality, has worked well; but not so well that a law such as HIPAA could be done without forever.

As is ever the case, reducing risk means reducing the probability that bad things will happen, or that the consequences from those that do will amount to "acceptable losses." In the case of HIPAA and privacy, this means litigation and losses stemming from unfavorable judgments pursuant to compromises of PHI and damages to the patients themselves. Not to be overlooked, however, is the value gained or maintained by being in a position to assure to your patient population that their privacy is indeed sacred, and that all possible is being done to protect it. Regardless of the respective position or message, an entity choosing not to begin with a gap-risk analysis of this general type can say neither with any degree of confidence, and that approach will place at risk patient trust, which may well be the highest probability and most costly risk of all.

As a final comment on the gap analysis, it is not a "do it once" task. Gap-risk analyses should be periodically reperformed to ensure that the gaps previously identified stay closed, and that opportunities to identify new ones are used to best advantage for timely closure of them as well.

THE PRIVACY ROLES: CHIEF PRIVACY OFFICIAL

The Act calls for the designation of two specific individuals under Subsection 164.530, "Administrative Requirements" of the privacy rule. The first of these is the privacy official. The Act itself reads as follows:

(a)(1) Standard: personnel designations.

(i) A covered entity must designate a privacy official who is responsible for the development and implementation of the policies and procedures of the entity.

This position has come to be known popularly as the "Chief Privacy Officer," or CPO. Although it can be anyone with the given entity, the person often designated to fulfill this required position usually works in the covered entity's legal office, possibly the chief counsel, assuming the entity is large enough to have one. Should that not be the case, small firms will frequently designate a senior officer as the nominal CPO, with a subordinate actually charged with performing the daily duties, all under the watchful eye of the covered entity's legal advisors. Either way is acceptable provided the designation is made, and the designee has the authority to act on behalf of the covered entity in such matters.

The official in charge of the privacy protection program must first understand the provisions and requirements of the Act itself, beginning with formal documentation of the designation of the individual or entity chosen for it:

> (2) *Implementation specification: personnel designations.* A covered entity must document the personnel designations in paragraph (a) (1) of this section as required by paragraph (j) of this section.

The section referenced above makes no statement about specific formats or forms. It simply requires that the designation be made in accordance with the standard processes for formalizing such declarations within a given organization, that the declaration may be maintained in either written or electronic form, and that the declaration must be maintained ". . . for six years from the date of its creation or the date when it last was in effect, whichever is later."

One of the more difficult aspects of this role requires the CPO to interact with the systems management function. This is difficult, not because systems people are in and of themselves difficult, but because of the systems themselves and how information is stored in and moved through them, and how it is accessed by authorized users.

The CPO, then, is the individual who must ultimately assure the program's success in all aspects and respects. In reading the details of the Act regarding what must follow the designation, and the tasks that the newly appointed CPO must oversee, interpolating those not directly stated that support providing that assurance, the role of the CPO is best characterized as being "a foot wide and a mile deep." This is to say that the focus is entirely dedicated to the assurance of privacy, but must do so at every level within the organization.

Once the designations are made, the easy part is over.

TRAINING REQUIREMENTS

It is not expected that the CPO will himself be an experienced curriculum developer, nor for that matter an experienced trainer. That notwithstanding, the writers of the Act realized that people cannot, as a practical matter, be held accountable for violations of a such complex regulation if (a) they are not informed of the contents of the Act itself; (b) they are not trained in the three "P's," policies, processes, and procedures; (c) they are not provided the criteria and process of achieving and maintaining compliance; and (d) they are not given a clear grasp of the penalties for violations.

With that in mind, the writers of the Act included training requirements for all persons that work for a given covered entity. It could be reasonably assumed that not all members of the entity's workforce are expected to come in contact with PHI, and thus further assumed that not everyone requires such training. The CEO is an obvious example, as would the chief operations and financial officers, and potentially others. Nevertheless, consideration must be given to the "chance" encounter with PHI. If the encounter involved these officers, they must know precisely what to do and whom to see about it. As the leaders, having a grasp of the Act and the risks and penalties associated with violations would seem mandatory given their fiduciary obligations to the entity and to any shareholders of it. Given the wording of the standard, the CPO should seek to have all members appropriately trained. The standard itself reads:

> (b)(1) <u>Standard: training.</u> A covered entity must train all members of its workforce on the policies and procedures with respect to protected health information required by this subpart, as necessary and appropriate for the members of the workforce to carry out their function within the covered entity.

Following that, the Act calls for three types of training to effectively implement the requirements of the standard:

> (2)(i)(A) To each member of the covered entity's workforce by no later than the compliance date for the covered entity;

> (2)(i)(B) Thereafter, to each new member of the workforce within a reasonable period of time after the person joins the covered entity's workforce; and

> (2)(i)(C) To each member of the covered entity's workforce whose functions are affected by a material change in the policies or procedures required by this subpart, within a reasonable period of time after the material change becomes effective in accordance with paragraph (i) of this section.

The first type is relatively simple in practice. It calls for organization-wide general awareness training to ensure that all workforce members are informed about the Act and its portent no later than the compliance date for that entity. Unless otherwise extended, the compliance date for the "small health plans" segment of covered entities was April 14, 2002; meaning that all workforce members across all covered entities, small health plans at the very least, should have received this training by that date.

The second type of training would normally take place during new employee orientation, and cover roughly the same material as the general awareness training. The most significant difference between the two would be the coverage given in this venue to the in-place policies, processes, and procedures used by the entity to implement and enforce the Act, and monitor personnel and institutional compliance.

The third type of training represents the "annual refresher" or update type of briefing. HIPAA, as with all legislation, is amended, enhanced, or even rewritten from time to time. This type of update briefing is intended to capture the significant points of such actions, and communicate them to the workforce members. Assuming that changes in entity policies or methods are necessary due to modifications made in the Act, the new versions would be presented during these sessions.

Working with an outside training firm or in-house staff, the CPO would provide input and draft review of the materials to ensure that all relevant points cover safeguarding PHI. At this stage, some specifics of the Act should be cited, tailored appropriately to meet the need of the audience: nursing staff, financial office personnel, medical staff, and patient advocacy, would need the same basics, but might need different emphasis due to differences in roles with respect to their handling of PHI. Also needing coverage would be the aspect of the penalties, if only to assure all workforce members that serious consequences will follow any violations, with potentially great and personal impact to all parties involved. This is often a real attention-getter as previous legislation was far more restricted and subdued in this aspect.

HIPAA in general requires substantial documentation of each activity described in the regulations. This is a vital part of the overall assurance process, as it provides the necessary basis for monitoring and auditing as substantive proof for internal and external reporting. Subparagraph (ii) of this section states the requirement. In accordance with the requirement, training should be documented by hardcopy or electronic form in the employee's file, recording at a minimum:

- Identification of the workforce member (name, number, etc.)
- Date and location of the training

- Type of training given
- Name of trainer
- Signed and dated by employee
- Signed and dated by employee's manager

Many organizations also have the trainees take an exam to indicate the level of understanding gained from the training, and to reinforce the information and its importance. The exam is also used to evaluate the effectiveness of the trainer and the training program itself. HIPAA compliance is a process, and as such must be included as part of an overall continuous quality improvement process.

TRAINING FOLLOW-THROUGH

Equally important with the initial training itself is the follow-through. This part of the process includes two basic aspects: review of personnel performance and violation reports, and review of the training itself with respect to personnel findings and the regulation. The two things used in conjunction provide evidence that the training is indeed effective (or not), and how well it assists (or does not) in personnel avoiding violations. This is part of the continuous quality improvement program for the entity because it provides feedback to strengthen and improve the training. It also provides opportunities to discuss compliance with employees, clarify directions, answer specific questions, and correct inappropriate behavior.

SAFEGUARDS

Those familiar with security practices understand the concept of safeguards against disclosure of information to those with no "need to know." This concept applies in this context as well, and in much the same way to hardcopy and electronic information forms. Many organizations have made it a practice to counsel their employees that even conversations wherein PHI is discussed must be undertaken cautiously and under private circumstances, and then only with others that have a true need to know. This practice recognizes the potential for possibly damaging information to be disclosed unintentionally through the casual but ubiquitous elevator conversation. The standard reads:

> (c)(1) <u>Standard: safeguards.</u> A covered entity must have in place appropriate administrative, technical, and physical safeguards to protect the privacy of protected health information.

(2) <u>Implementation specification: safeguards.</u> A covered entity must reasonably safeguard protected health information from any intentional or unintentional use or disclosure that is in violation of the standards, implementation specifications or other requirements of this subpart.

"Administrative safeguards" refers to the three "P's." This framework defines the basis and sets the boundaries for how the program will be conducted, what the responsibilities are, who has which ones, what procedures are to be followed under given circumstances, and so on. In terms of compliance, this is likely to be the most troublesome area as it is active at every moment, it is largely paper-based (meaning form and instructions-driven), and has the most human involvement.

As a consequence, the CPO must ensure that training is developed and provided, that only the most current version of a given "P" is in active circulation and use, that all such documents are reviewed periodically to ensure that following them all but guarantees no violations, and that routine spot checks are performed to doublecheck adherence by the workforce. Failure to do any of these will result in an exposure, which in turn will become a violation (unintentional or otherwise), and the eventual filing of a lawsuit. This may seem a leap, but in the current climate of e-mail spam, aggressive telemarketing, and other such unwanted invasions, a watchful and informed consumer taking such self-protective action in this highly litigious society seems all but assured.

"Technical safeguards" refers to electronic or mechanistic measures such as combination keypads on doors, closed circuit camera systems, password controls on system access, additional passwords or PIN numbers for sensitive files, and so on. These are the pieces of technology that support compliance with the policies and procedures in safeguarding PHI. Biometric identification systems, card readers, and badge swipe stations are further examples of technical controls.

The CPO does not necessarily have to understand their functioning at a deep level, although it is a very good thing if he does. The CPO must, however, understand completely what the particular technology or mechanism does to protect sensitive information, how effective it is at doing that, who is responsible for it, what monitoring and reporting functions it provides (if any), and what the outcome or backup plan is should the device fail to do its job correctly.

"Physical safeguards" means those measures taken with respect to the premises, storage containers, rooms, and the like, wherein the PHI is kept. Examples of this type are security guards, lockable storage containers, access control lists (paper or electronic), identification badges, and other such items that control access to the PHI or the system that stores it.

Again, the CPO need not be thoroughly versed in the details of all the measures, how they work, and so on. But again, he must understand completely the impact that having them in place (or not) and functioning correctly (or not) will have on the PHI and the potential for compromise, damage, or loss. Many such controls may appear to add great value to this part of the overall privacy protection picture. This is usually, but not always true. In performing his due diligence, the CPO must assure himself and his superiors that the controls used are effective in meeting the compliance criteria of the Act. Being cost effective never hurts either.

In conjunction with these specific safeguards is the privacy notice required by the Act that covers patient rights, the entity's legal duties, consensual and nonconsensual uses of the PHI, the complaints process with contact information, and other points. This notice must be carefully constructed to ensure all points are covered appropriately to provide the patient with vital and correct information, and to ensure that the entity itself is not exposed to any risk through failure to disclose or through providing erroneous information. It should be the CPO's duty, in concert with legal counsel, to ensure that the notice is accurate and meets both needs.

THE PRIVACY ROLES: PATIENT COMPLAINT OMBUDSMAN

Although the term is my own, the patient complaint ombudsman is that designated individual or organizational unit charged with receiving complaints regarding potential PHI privacy violations. The Act reads:

(a)(1) Standard: personnel designations.

(ii) A covered entity must designate a contact person or office who is responsible for receiving complaints under this section and who is able to provide further information about matters covered by the notice required by § 164.520.

The Act itself provides little direction as to how this job will be performed. That notwithstanding, the performance of this task will follow a formal process not unlike the complaints department at any consumer goods manufacturing company, in a general sense.

The process should, for example, follow process steps such as these:

1. Take an incoming call or letter regarding the complaint; calls should be recorded, and callers must be informed of that fact;
2. Diplomatically inquire as to the precise nature of the complaint or alleged violation of privacy, allowing the caller or writer to explain in his own words;

3. Using prepared and approved rules to guide what they are allowed to say, explain the entity's policies to the inquirer if necessary in order to clarify;
4. Answer all questions, using those same rules;
5. Allow the caller to speak to your superiors if so requested;
6. Offer to provide additional information, or provide if requested;
7. Provide guidance to other information sources such as DHHS and other official agencies;
8. Document everything.

These may sound like guidelines for a consumer affairs office. They are that, and more. This process can also serve to increase or decrease risk of litigation or other adverse consequences, even if only modestly, by the thoroughness, care, and sensitivity used by the individual performing the task. The main thrust is to gather all necessary facts as they are presented to get a complete picture of the alleged event. Questions, therefore, should be asked of the caller to ensure clarity and accuracy, and not be attempts to disprove the claim. No legal advice should be given either.

Records of all complaints submitted need to be thorough, and preferably forms based to ensure completeness and accuracy. These records must then be periodically sampled and reviewed by management and possibly legal counsel to evaluate possible trends, the level of seriousness, and the general nature of the complaints. The entire activity would participate in the quality improvement process by providing one form of source data to determine the accuracy and effectiveness of privacy notices, the appropriateness of employee behavior (adherence to policy and procedure), and the effectiveness of the office in handling complaints as judged by subsequent events.

A thankless job to be sure. Nevertheless, the complaints office is one of the faces patients will see, and one of the information sources they will use. It must therefore be staffed with trained, meticulous, diplomatic personnel that will deal effectively and positively with situations that will run the gamut from mild irritation to potentially explosive. It could in fact be considered a form of safeguard depending on how well it is managed and executes its mission. But as part of the HIPAA compliance process, it must exist, and it must record and provide the documentation necessary to substantiate its effective operation.

THE SECURITY ROLE: THE CHIEF SECURITY OFFICIAL

It has long been common to find organizations with a person or group that performs security functions for its information systems. Although not yet the norm, it is no longer uncommon to find organizations creating and filling a role called "Chief Security Officer" (CSO) or "Chief Information Security Officer" (CISO). The world of E-business and interconnected systems across the Internet and other networks has become far too hostile and unpredictable to overlook the importance of this role in ensuring that appropriate safeguards and countermeasures are developed and put into effect to preserve and protect those systems.

With this as a backdrop, HIPAA has made it a requirement that such an individual be designated to perform this role, though the Act does not provide the title. In §164.308 of the Act, the regulation states that:

> A (2) *Standard: Assigned security responsibility.* Identify the security official who is responsible for the development and implementation of the policies and procedures required by this subpart for the entity.

Given the level of authority this position requires to have the full force and effect necessary, the designee becomes the CSO/CISO almost automatically. Through the next section, the acronym CSO is used generically, and includes all security responsibilities discussed.

In his role, the CSO is the person ostensibly in charge of ensuring that the entity's security and information risk management programs are well designed, thorough, and effectively address the real operational risks and threats it faces. He may be a line manager and have a staff to carry out the tasks of the program, or he may occupy an advisory role to the CEO or other executive. Regardless, the CSO must ensure that the program is successfully accomplished and that compliance is maintained from his strategic program level.

TASKS AND ACTIONS: WHAT THE CSO MUST DO

The CSO, as nominal program head, is directly responsible for carrying out the required activities listed under §164.308. As one reads this section, one gets the impression that the writers took pages from several existing "best practices" sources: the International Information Systems Security Certification Consortium's ((ISC)2) "Common Body of Knowledge," and the Generally Accepted System Security Practices (the GASSP, or the FIPS 800-14 version of it), and very probably the International Standards Organization's (ISO) Standard 17799 (being first and best among them). There are many others, but each covers essentially the same material in essentially the same way, each serving as methodology validation for the others, and all reinforcing what professional security practitioners have done for some two decades or more. The point is that HIPAA draws from best practices and practitioner philosophy in presenting its security requirements, thus giving it a sound empirical basis.

Policy, Process, and Procedure

This is the first, and the most important of the three "P's." The security program under HIPAA, a complement and companion to the privacy program, begins with creating the policy basis to state the position of the entity on various aspects of security: the mission of the program, general philosophy, program objectives, what is acceptable and unacceptable, applicability and exceptions, actions and consequences, and the like. The general policy structure and topics can be derived very directly from §164.306 "Security standards: General rules." Assuming there are none extant within the entity, this section of the Act should be used to generate the policy tree, taking into account organizational idiosyncrasies regarding policy enactment and structure. Creation of this policy tree should be one of the, if not the actual, first steps in this program.

A great deal of emphasis should be placed on this activity and its products, and they should be constructed with care. It has been shown repeatedly that a company must have a well-founded and constructed policy basis for most actions it takes if it is to stand a chance of defending itself against legal challenges (this does not eliminate their possibility, however). These general statements of position and action should follow the standard model of a good policy, while remaining at a high level, covering purpose, applicability, authority and traceability, assignment of responsibility, statement of policy, requirements for compliance, consequences for noncompliance, or some variation of this as a minimum set.

Once the policy structure is laid out and the actual construction is underway, process definition must begin, which will include the construction of the detailed procedures necessary to perform the tasks and produce the products and outcomes of the processes. Again, the Act itself provides the basic framework for this activity as well by defining the general standards for performance and compliance.

Mapping the processes can be very time consuming, and yet very revealing in terms of actual workflow versus the ideal. Using the results of the gap analysis as points of risk to mitigate, processes will be immediately relevant to the compliance issue. Even where gaps do not currently exist, process mapping will reveal potential weaknesses, possible single points of failure, redundancies and duplications, and extra or extraneous steps. As is frequently the case in security, addressing these potential weaknesses in a preemptive manner is less costly and makes the total security program more effective and easier to manage.

Key to good process development is simplicity, clarity, and specificity. Process definition should begin at the highest, clearly identifiable point, such as the point of entry into the organization. During the process mapping, several factors must be identified, sequenced, and described in detail. These are inputs and their sources, actions performed using those inputs and who performs them, and outputs in form, content, and destination (they will be inputs to some other process). This activity must be performed for each area involved in a given process as every one is an input source, an output destination, or performs an action, or some combination.

As each point where action is taken is identified and clarified, a procedure should be created, or modified if necessary. The level of detail and complexity should match the task to ensure that all necessary steps are clearly addressed. Failure to do so increases the likelihood that important steps are missed, and runs the risk of building in future audit findings.

Once completed, the foundation has been established to implement and enforce the Act with compliance criteria, workflow, information products and their uses, and a clear definition of responsibilities throughout the workforce. It is the establishment of this foundation that the CSO must oversee and accomplish at his level. But, even as this work is in progress, the CSO should have another task running in parallel.

SECURITY MANAGEMENT PROGRAM

Section 164.306 begins by outlining the "General Rules" for the guiding philosophy the program must use, and overall objectives the program must achieve in its execution. The text of these can be found in Table 1.1, and a tabular summary of them is given in Table 1.2. Following the General Rules are the sections on administrative, physical, and technical safeguards. These are further subdivided into "required" and "addressable" safeguards.

Table 1.1   Text of HIPAA, 45 CFR 164: Security Requirements

§ 164.306 Security standards: General rules.
  (a) *General requirements.* Covered entities must do the following:
    (1) Ensure the confidentiality, integrity, and availability of all electronic protected health information the covered entity creates, receives, maintains, or transmits.
    (2) Protect against any reasonably anticipated threats or hazards to the security or integrity of such information.

Table 1.1   Text of HIPAA, 45 CFR 164: Security Requirements (continued)

(3) Protect against any reasonably anticipated uses or disclosures of such information that are not permitted or required under subpart E of this part.

(4) Ensure compliance with this subpart by its workforce.

(b) Flexibility of approach.

(1) Covered entities may use any security measures that allow the covered entity to reasonably and appropriately implement the standards and implementation specifications as specified in this subpart.

(2) In deciding which security measures to use, a covered entity must take into account the following factors:

(i)   The size, complexity, and capabilities of the covered entity.

(ii) The covered entity's technical infrastructure, hardware, and software security capabilities.

(iii) The costs of security measures.

(iv) The probability and criticality of potential risks to electronic protected health information.

(c) *Standards.* A covered entity must comply with the standards as provided in this section and in § 164.308, § 164.310, § 164.312, § 164.314, and § 164.316 with respect to all electronic protected health information.

(d) Implementation specifications.

In this subpart:

(1) Implementation specifications are required or addressable. If an implementation specification is required, the word "Required" appears in parentheses after the title of the implementation specification. If an implementation specification is addressable, the word "Addressable" appears in parentheses after the title of the implementation specification.

(2) When a standard adopted in § 164.308, § 164.310, § 164.312, § 164.314, or § 164.316 includes required implementation specifications, a covered entity must implement the implementation specifications.

(1) When a standard adopted in § 164.308, § 164.310, § 164.312, § 164.314, or § 164.316 includes addressable implementation specifications, a covered entity must —

(i) Assess whether each implementation specification is a reasonable and appropriate safeguard in its environment, when analyzed with reference to the likely contribution to protecting the entity's electronic protected health information; and

(ii) As applicable to the entity —

(A) Implement the implementation specification if reasonable and appropriate; or

(B) If implementing the implementation specification is not reasonable and appropriate —

(1) Document why it would not be reasonable and appropriate to implement the implementation specification; and

(2) Implement an equivalent alternative measure if reasonable and appropriate.

Table 1.1   Text of HIPAA, 45 CFR 164: Security Requirements (continued)

(e) *Maintenance.* Security measures implemented to comply with standards and implementation specifications adopted under § 164.105 and this subpart must be reviewed and modified as needed to continue provision of reasonable and appropriate protection of electronic protected health information as described at § 164.316.

§ 164.308 Administrative safeguards.

(a) A covered entity must, in accordance with § 164.306:

    (1) (i) *Standard: Security management process.* Implement policies and procedures to prevent, detect, contain, and correct security violations.

       (ii) Implementation specifications:

         (A) *Risk analysis* (Required). Conduct an accurate and thorough assessment of the potential risks and vulnerabilities to the confidentiality, integrity, and availability of electronic protected health information held by the covered entity.

         (B) *Risk management* (Required). Implement security measures sufficient to reduce risks and vulnerabilities to a reasonable and appropriate level to comply with § 164.306(a).

         (C) *Sanction policy* (Required). Apply appropriate sanctions against workforce members who fail to comply with the security policies and procedures of the covered entity.

         (D) *Information system activity review* (Required). Implement procedures to regularly review records of information system activity, such as audit logs, access reports, and security incident tracking reports.

    (2) *Standard: Assigned security responsibility.* Identify the security official who is responsible for the development and implementation of the policies and procedures required by this subpart for the entity.

    (3) (i) *Standard: Workforce security.* Implement policies and procedures to ensure that all members of its workforce have appropriate access to electronic protected health information, as provided under paragraph (a)(4) of this section, and to prevent those workforce members who do not have access under paragraph (a)(4) of this section from obtaining access to electronic protected health information.

       (ii) Implementation specifications:

         (A) *Authorization and/or supervision* (Addressable). Implement procedures for the authorization and/or supervision of workforce members who work with electronic protected health information or in locations where it might be accessed.

         (B) *Workforce clearance procedure* (Addressable). Implement procedures to determine that the access of a workforce member to electronic protected health information is appropriate.

         (C) *Termination procedures* (Addressable). Implement procedures for terminating access to electronic protected health information

Table 1.1   Text of HIPAA, 45 CFR 164: Security Requirements (continued)

when the employment of a workforce member ends or as required by determinations made as specified in paragraph (a)(3)(ii)(B) of this section.

(4) (i) *Standard: Information access management.* Implement policies and procedures for authorizing access to electronic protected health information that are consistent with the applicable requirements of subpart E of this part.

(ii) Implementation specifications:

(A) *Isolating health care clearinghouse functions* (Required). If a health care clearinghouse is part of a larger organization, the clearinghouse must implement policies and procedures that protect the electronic protected health information of the clearinghouse from unauthorized access by the larger organization.

(B) *Access authorization (Addressable).* Implement policies and procedures for granting access to electronic protected health information, for example, through access to a workstation, transaction, program, process, or other mechanism.

(C) *Access establishment and modification* (Addressable). Implement policies and procedures that, based upon the entity's access authorization policies, establish, document, review, and modify a user's right of access to a workstation, transaction, program, or process.

(5) (i) *Standard: Security awareness and training.* Implement a security awareness and training program for all members of its workforce (including management).

(ii) Implementation specifications. Implement:

(A) *Security reminders* (Addressable). Periodic security updates.

(B) *Protection from malicious software* (Addressable). Procedures for guarding against, detecting, and reporting malicious software.

(C) *Log-in monitoring* (Addressable). Procedures for monitoring log-in attempts and reporting discrepancies.

(D) *Password management* (Addressable). Procedures for creating, changing, and safeguarding passwords.

(6) (i) *Standard: Security incident procedures.* Implement policies and procedures to address security incidents.

(ii) *Implementation specification: Response and Reporting* (Required). Identify and respond to suspected or known security incidents; mitigate, to the extent practicable, harmful effects of security incidents that are known to the covered entity; and document security incidents and their outcomes.

(7) (i) *Standard: Contingency plan.* Establish (and implement as needed) policies and procedures for responding to an emergency or other occurrence (for example, fire, vandalism, system failure, and natural disaster) that damages systems that contain electronic protected health information.

Table 1.1   Text of HIPAA, 45 CFR 164: Security Requirements (continued)

(ii) Implementation specifications:
   (A) *Data backup plan* (Required). Establish and implement procedures to create and maintain retrievable exact copies of electronic protected health information.
   (B) *Disaster recovery plan* (Required). Establish (and implement as needed) procedures to restore any loss of data.
   (C) *Emergency mode operation plan* (Required). Establish (and implement as needed) procedures to enable continuation of critical business processes for protection of the security of electronic protected health information while operating in emergency mode.
   (D) *Testing and revision procedures* (Addressable). Implement procedures for periodic testing and revision of contingency plans.
   (E) *Applications and data criticality analysis* (Addressable). Assess the relative criticality of specific applications and data in support of other contingency plan components.
(8) *Standard: Evaluation.* Perform a periodic technical and non-technical evaluation, based initially upon the standards implemented under this rule and subsequently, in response to environmental or operational changes affecting the security of electronic protected health information, which establishes the extent to which an entity's security policies and procedures meet the requirements of this subpart.

§ 164.310 Physical safeguards.
A covered entity must, in accordance with § 164.306:
(a) (1) *Standard: Facility access controls.* Implement policies and procedures to limit physical access to its electronic information systems and the facility or facilities in which they are housed, while ensuring that properly authorized access is allowed.
   (2) Implementation specifications:
      (i) *Contingency operations* (Addressable). Establish (and implement as needed) procedures that allow facility access in support of restoration of lost data under the disaster recovery plan and emergency mode operations plan in the event of an emergency.
      (ii) *Facility security plan* (Addressable). Implement policies and procedures to safeguard the facility and the equipment therein from unauthorized physical access, tampering, and theft.
      (iii) *Access control and validation procedures* (Addressable). Implement procedures to control and validate a person's access to facilities based on their role or function, including visitor control, and control of access to software programs for testing and revision.
      (iv) *Maintenance records* (Addressable). Implement policies and procedures to document repairs and modifications to the physical components of a facility which are related to security (for example, hardware, walls, doors, and locks).

Table 1.1   Text of HIPAA, 45 CFR 164: Security Requirements (continued)

(b) *Standard: Workstation use.* Implement policies and procedures that specify the proper functions to be performed, the manner in which those functions are to be performed, and the physical attributes of the surroundings of a specific workstation or class of workstation that can access electronic protected health information.

(c) *Standard: Workstation security.* Implement physical safeguards for all workstations that access electronic protected health information, to restrict access to authorized users.

(d) (1) *Standard: Device and media controls.* Implement policies and procedures that govern the receipt and removal of hardware and electronic media that contain electronic protected health information into and out of a facility, and the movement of these items within the facility.

    (2) Implementation specifications:

        (i) *Disposal* (Required). Implement policies and procedures to address the final disposition of electronic protected health information, and/or the hardware or electronic media on which it is stored.

        (ii) *Media re-use* (Required). Implement procedures for removal of electronic protected health information from electronic media before the media are made available for re-use.

        (iii) *Accountability* (Addressable). Maintain a record of the movements of hardware and electronic media and any person responsible therefore.

        (iv) *Data backup and storage* (Addressable). Create a retrievable, exact copy of electronic protected health information, when needed, before movement of equipment.

§ 164.312 Technical safeguards.

A covered entity must, in accordance with § 164.306:

(a) (1) *Standard: Access control.* Implement technical policies and procedures for electronic information systems that maintain electronic protected health information to allow access only to those persons or software programs that have been granted access rights as specified in § 164.308(a)(4).

    (2) Implementation specifications:

        (i) *Unique user identification* (Required). Assign a unique name and/or number for identifying and tracking user identity.

        (ii) *Emergency access procedure* (Required). Establish (and implement as needed) procedures for obtaining necessary electronic protected health information during an emergency.

        (iii) *Automatic logoff* (Addressable). Implement electronic procedures that terminate an electronic session after a predetermined time of inactivity.

        (iv) *Encryption and decryption* (Addressable). Implement a mechanism to encrypt and decrypt electronic protected health information.

Table 1.1 Text of HIPAA, 45 CFR 164: Security Requirements (continued)

(b) *Standard: Audit controls.* Implement hardware, software, and/or procedural mechanisms that record and examine activity in information systems that contain or use electronic protected health information.

(c) (1) *Standard: Integrity.* Implement policies and procedures to protect electronic protected health information from improper alteration or destruction.

(2) *Implementation specification: Mechanism to authenticate electronic protected health information* (Addressable). Implement electronic mechanisms to corroborate that electronic protected health information has not been altered or destroyed in an unauthorized manner.

(d) *Standard: Person or entity authentication.* Implement procedures to verify that a person or entity seeking access to electronic protected health information is the one claimed.

(e) (1) *Standard: Transmission security.* Implement technical security measures to guard against unauthorized access to electronic protected health information that is being transmitted over an electronic communications network.

(2) Implementation specifications:

(i) *Integrity controls* (Addressable). Implement security measures to ensure that electronically transmitted electronic protected health information is not improperly modified without detection until disposed of.

(ii) *Encryption* (Addressable). Implement a mechanism to encrypt electronic protected health information whenever deemed appropriate.

§ 164.316 Policies and procedures and documentation requirements.

A covered entity must, in accordance with § 164.306:

(a) *Standard: Policies and procedures.* Implement reasonable and appropriate policies and procedures to comply with the standards, implementation specifications, or other requirements of this subpart, taking into account those factors specified in § 164.306(b)(2)(i), (ii), (iii), and (iv). This standard is not to be construed to permit or excuse an action that violates any other standard, implementation specification, or other requirements of this subpart. A covered entity may change its policies and procedures at any time, provided that the changes are documented and are implemented in accordance with this subpart.

(b) (1) Standard: Documentation.

(i) Maintain the policies and procedures implemented to comply with this subpart in written (which may be electronic) form; and

(ii) If an action, activity, or assessment is required by this subpart to be documented, maintain a written (which may be electronic) record of the action, activity, or assessment.

Table 1.1   Text of HIPAA, 45 CFR 164: Security Requirements (continued)

(2) Implementation specifications:
   (i)   *Time limit* (Required). Retain the documentation required by paragraph (b)(1) of this section for 6 years from the date of its creation or the date when it last was in effect, whichever is later.
   (ii) *Availability* (Required). Make documentation available to those persons responsible for implementing the procedures to which the documentation pertains.
   (iii) *Updates* (Required). Review documentation periodically, and update as needed, in response to environmental or operational changes affecting the security of the electronic protected health information.

Table 1.2   Tabular Compilation of the Security Requirements Shown in Subpart C of Part 164

Standards	Sections	Implementation Specifications[a]
Administrative Safeguards		
Security management process	164.308(a)(1)	Risk analysis (R) Risk management (R) Sanction policy (R) Information system activity review (R)
Assigned security responsibility	164.308(a)(2)	Designation of security official (R)
Workforce security	164.308(a)(3)	Authorization and/or supervision (A) Workforce clearance procedure (A) Termination procedures (A)
Information access management	164.308(a)(4)	Isolating healthcare clearinghouse function (R) Access authorization (A) Access establishment and modification (A)
Security awareness and training	164.308(a)(5)	Security reminders (A) Protection from malicious software (A) Log-in monitoring (A) Password management (A)
Security incident procedures	164.308(a)(6)	Response and reporting (R)

Table 1.2 Tabular Compilation of the Security Requirements Shown in Subpart C of Part 164 (continued)

Standards	Sections	Implementation Specifications[a]
Contingency plan	164.308(a)(7)	Data backup plan (R) Disaster recovery plan (R) Emergency mode operation plan (R) Testing and revision procedure (A) Applications and data criticality analysis (A)
Evaluation	164.308(a)(8)	(R)
Business associate contracts and other arrangement	164.308(b)(1)	Written contract or other arrangement (R)
Physical Safeguards		
Facility access controls	164.310(a)(1)	Contingency operations (A) Facility security plan (A) Access control and validation procedures (A) Maintenance records (A)
Workstation use	164.310(b)	(R)
Workstation security	164.310(c)	(R)
Device and media controls	164.310(d)(1)	Disposal (R) Media reuse (R) Accountability (A) Data backup and storage (A)
Technical Safeguards (see § 164.312)		
Access control	164.312(a)(1)	Unique user identification (R) Emergency access procedure (R) Automatic log-off (A) Encryption and decryption (A)
Audit controls	164.312(b)	(R)
Integrity	164.312(c)(1)	Mechanism to authenticate electronic protected health information (A)
Person or entity authentication	164.312(d)	(R)
Transmission security	164.312(e)(1)	Integrity controls (A) Encryption (A)

[a](R) = Required; (A) = Addressable.

The first means simply that it **must** be accomplished (task or plan) or implemented (device, software, or control). A review of the required standards indicates that the required items have an "on/off" character; this is to say that the test of compliance is that they are either in place or they are not. For example, either a CSO has been appointed or not; you either have log-in IDs or you do not.

The second class, addressable, means that there is some flexibility in how the standard can be accomplished to achieve compliance. As in the above, the aspects of the environment affected by the addressable standards are in many cases themselves flexible to some degree in terms of how they function or are performed. For example; workforce clearance and termination procedures vary from place to place; contingency operations must be flexible because there is not one type of contingency condition, just as there is not one type of entity.

There are also cases where, if an addressable standard were to become a required standard, a particular implementation vehicle or technology would, in all necessary detail, have to be specified. This would lock in certain technologies and devices, such as DES for encryption use, or password rules that are not inherently supported by some systems. This approach would have an impact on the cost and even the ability to comply, and might make it impossible to do so in some cases. More importantly, it could lock in a technology that may have a limited lifespan of effectiveness. Given how some technologies must be implemented in order to function, this could render it all but impossible to upgrade or replace, again raising the cost or possibly preventing continued compliance.

Wisely, the writers included a section that permits an entity to use methods and technologies of its own choosing to meet the requirements. This is very significant because it takes into account the variances in infrastructure that exist across the variety of entities, and gives them the necessary freedom to remain within their unique operational models, and implement technologies that fit them, as long as they meet the objectives of the Act and its standards of performance. It also makes the cost lower and likelihood of compliance higher by allowing this freedom.

Step One: Risk Analysis

The first step required by HIPAA, or any security program, is the risk analysis. Whether a qualitative or quantitative type of analysis, a properly conducted assessment will determine:

- Vulnerabilities and weaknesses in systems, environments, and processes that can be exploited
- Threats and agents to which these vulnerabilities are susceptible

- Quantification of potential losses through any form of compromise in confidentiality, integrity, or availability should the threat materialize and exploit a given vulnerability
- Probability of occurrence of a given threat able to act on a vulnerability
- Frequency of occurrence of the identified threats

Performing a risk analysis by purely quantitative methods is very tedious, time consuming, and expensive. It is by design a painstaking thorough process that produces a wealth of data to enable the CSO to lay out a comprehensive plan of mitigation and remediation. There are automated tools that perform these for use by the CSO or a staff member to streamline the process and create a history of these analyses and their products. Given its highly detailed output, this type of assessment may be required by insurers and others on which to base underwriting and investment decisions.

By contrast, the purely qualitative risk assessment judges the environment more experientially by using company records, insurance claim reports, subject matter experts, and possibly a lot of "walking around." This *in situ* assessment is augmented with information from local sources such as police departments, fire departments, and others. The end result is a less detailed analysis that relies largely on the current state of the environment, history, and a general but finely honed sense of the probability of adverse events occurring. As nebulous as this may sound, very practical and effective results can be produced that have a very positive impact on the risk profile of the entity and its operations.

A hybrid method, using aspects of both, is often an attractive choice. It allows for straightforward assessments where highly analytical approaches would be overkill, and more detailed analyses where qualitative methods would not be as revealing as necessary. This hybrid approach is attractive because it allows for more rapid progress and completion, is less costly to perform, and produces results that are more readily understood.

Whichever approach is used, the product of this activity is a report that describes clearly, and in sufficient detail, the risks and vulnerabilities found, identifies the threats that can exploit them, gives calculations of probability or likelihood that losses will occur through these threats materializing, and provides estimates on losses (called exposure) in dollars. This feeds the next step.

Step Two: Risk Management

Following completion of the risk analysis comes what the Act calls "risk management." Also called a "security management plan," the program of risk management deals directly with the vulnerabilities and their related threats or agents that can exploit them to cause losses. For this discussion, this part of the overall program is called the Security and Risk Management Plan (SRMP).

The SRMP begins with the results of the risk analysis, and defines a program of risk reduction through specific safeguards, controls, and countermeasures. Basic to the SRMP are two assumptions; that in some cases "acceptable levels of loss" must be established, and that risk cannot be eliminated, but only reduced to within those acceptable levels. Many security professionals have some trouble with the latter, and many executives have trouble with the former, but the reasoning behind the principles rests on the ability to affect the environment, and simple economics.

The CSO must recognize that he can have no effect on the presence of certain threats: earthquakes, hurricanes, network-borne (including the Internet) hostile code, and others. He must also recognize that no amount of money or personnel will bring about a perfect security program or system, free of all measurable risk and immune to all potential threats. Furthermore, the CSO must accept and ensure that no security measure taken will be allowed to compromise the ability of the entity to conduct its operations profitably.

He must be able to convey these facts and his appreciation of them to his fellow executives, which they must likewise accept. His objective is to build consensus regarding the necessity to take a balanced approach to achieving compliance, and that all parties concerned have a stake in its successful accomplishment. Among these parties should be a representative from the internal audit function, often known as the Office of Institutional Compliance. Achieving the consensus will be the first step in reducing the overall risk of the program, and thus also reducing the risk of the compliance effort failing.

It cannot be emphasized too strongly that those with whom consensus is achieved should by now be partners in the process, and that their review and agreement with the overall plan is key to maintaining their continued support. An informal but very real requirement upon the CSO is his ability to effectively manage the internal politics that will be associated with this program. Keeping them involved in the process and in the information loop as things progress can make a great difference in how smooth the process will be.

The SRMP should define the overall approach to initial risk reduction and continuous risk management. It should define at a minimum (topically, approximately in order):

1. The general approach to risk and its management
2. Categorization of threat types, environment and infrastructure issues, personnel issues, and the steps to be taken for both initial reduction and continuous management of them

3. Specifics regarding methodologies and technologies to reducing it
4. A section on risk acceptance, acceptable loss levels, monitoring, and compensating controls to manage the potential impacts for those risks and threats where the agents themselves cannot be directly affected
5. A section on the waiver process, conditions that warrant waiving risk mitigation in a given situation, compensating controls and other countermeasures to be used, if any, in lieu of direct mitigation, and the required documentation to be prepared for periodic compliance reviews

Once drafted, the SRMP must be vetted by other officers and appropriate senior staff. This must be done to ensure that all parties that will have responsibility under the plan become aware of their respective roles, that the plan has a logical flow, and to ensure that the program aligns with the business operations. Once all arguments have been addressed and all appropriate comments incorporated, the plan is ready for final sign-off, and implementation can go forward.

The sanction policy, wherein disciplinary measures are described for those not complying with the standards and requirements, should in actual practice be incorporated as part of the policies discussed earlier. This would normally be within the purview of the human resources department, to ensure that corporate guidelines are followed. The CSO may participate in the preparation of them, but most likely only in an advisory role and for awareness that this requirement has in fact been met.

The section called "Information System Activity Review" addresses the need for regular log reviews to assess user activity, and actually addresses two separate but similar activities. The first is essentially a daily audit activity, checking for invalid password attempts, unsuccessful file access attempts, and the like to ascertain if any inappropriate user activity is taking place, and to investigate and determine necessary corrective actions to take.

The second is a longer-term activity, and its goal is to determine patterns of behavior exhibited by users or processes run by users. This second-level review attempts to establish patterns and trends, and may make use of an internal intrusion detection system as one of the information-gathering tools. Attacks and inappropriate use or access can come from inside the entity or outside, and both sources must be reviewed. It is well understood that insiders, and especially trusted insiders with privileged information or system access, represent a potentially greater threat than outsiders. This second-level analysis may be the only way to establish the presence of such activities, and must be performed to augment the daily review activity to do so.

The next steps involve specific risk reduction measures. There will be three approaches to this, as alluded to above, that will guide the process to select and implement suitable and effective safeguards, countermeasures, controls, and monitors:

1. In the event that the threat itself can be affected, take action that will remove the threat itself;
2. In the event that the threat itself can be affected but not removed, take action that will alter the nature of the threat itself to reduce its ability to cause harm; or
3. In the event that the threat itself can neither be removed nor altered, take action to reduce the impact of the threat on the asset by altering or removing the asset, if possible.

These approaches will apply equally in each of the three categories of security requirements.

For the remainder of the requirements, the CSO will have a variable role in the preparation and implementation of the standards. The standards will, and should, come from other areas of the organization, as they apply to functions that are properly a part of those respective areas. The CSO's role in these cases will most likely be to provide input regarding specific concerns of security that must be addressed, review to ensure a proper text, and enforcement within his organization. Although the management of these other areas will be responsible for ensuring implementation and ongoing compliance with the standards, the CSO must ensure that security is accounted for and appropriately addressed in each case.

In the "Administrative" category (process and procedure oriented), procedures and workflow must be created or modified to address any identified risks and threats as well as possible. As can be seen from Table 1.2, the main specifications call for appropriate levels of authorization, supervision, and continued awareness training to ensure that the workforce members are both informed and compliant. These are "addressable" security measures, and should be scaled or configured to meet organizational and administrative needs while accomplishing the standard.

The category called "Workforce Security" sets standards for addressing security concerns directly to the authorization, supervision, clearance processing (background checks), and termination procedures of employees. In the main, such procedures should already exist as part of the human resources department's collection of procedures. The CSO should meet with the management of that department, and review the pertinent documents with them to establish their existence and relevance.

In the "Information Access Management" category, the required standard is a case of isolating nonhealthcare operations from healthcare-related information resources within a mixed business environment, a type of environment wherein healthcare is only one of the operations. This isolation can be either logical or physical, but to meet the standard the separation must be in place, tested and proven effective, and monitored to ensure no breaches occur without associated alerts.

The addressable standards in this category relate to authorization of access to information and systems. This includes the granting of access, the level of that access (e.g., privileged, nonprivileged, etc.), the process for promoting or demoting that level, and removal of all access. The CSO should define the policy that governs access and privileges, but only after careful review and research into the real data access requirements of the workforce.

A system/network test protocol will provide reliable proof of the robustness of the separation between systems. However, the CSO must satisfy himself that the process for access management is inherently sound, leaves no gaps for inadvertent granting of inappropriate access or privilege levels, is properly enforced, and is reviewed to ensure compliance with the standards.

The "Security Awareness and Training" we have already addressed. However, this category also includes standards for protection from malicious software, log-in monitoring, and password management. The first of these standards requires users to receive training about viruses and how to protect their systems from them. The second is a system function that records all valid and invalid log-in attempts. The third regards providing users with information about password construction rules, periodicity, and other aspects of good password management.

The first is fairly straightforward, and involves ensuring that users understand the ways viruses infect systems, and the means to reduce the risk or prevent this from occurring. The second function would be performed as part of the system reviews performed (described earlier). The third would educate the users on how to manage their passwords: the best mixture of characters to use (alphanumeric, mixed case, nonrepeating), avoidance of patterns (FIDO001, rover042, rover 043, etc.), avoidance of actual words (j0hnnIe), and frequency of changes (more often for privileged, less often for non-). The CSO must ensure that these standards are in place and actively enforced, taking into account the differences and limitations of the systems in which they are implemented: not all systems support the same functions identically, or in some cases, at all.

Security incidents occur in every business of every kind, and more now than ever before. These incidents are caused by attacks, viruses, criminal activity, and simple user error. Having an incident response capability is a required standard. Irrespective of source or agent, every incident must be responded to, investigated, and documented. There are guides available that describe how to build a Computer Incident Response Team (CIRT), and the Carnegie-Mellon University CERT Group provides an excellent example. The CSO must ensure that this capability exists, has clear, concise, and complete procedures on responding to a variety of incidents, and that it documents each case.

The "Contingency Plan" category is also a required standard. The composition of the "Disaster Recovery Plan," as it is commonly known, is more often the responsibility of a specific department other than the information systems department. As it relates to this activity, the information systems department must have its own plan, which should be a part of the larger institutional disaster recovery or emergency preparedness plan. What is most important about this standard is that the plan called for is in fact complete, up to date, and periodically tested to ensure that it is accurate and relevant to the operation.

The evaluation requirement calls for periodic review and documentation to the effect that the measures described remain accurate and relevant to the operation, and are effective in reducing the risk of PHI being compromised.

Change control (called "Testing and Revision procedure") is a vital process to ensure continued system integrity and correct operation, and must be controlled through appropriate procedural steps. This is normally a function of the information systems department, and involves representatives from other departments as necessary. The security concerns in this case will include, among others, separation of duties, possible compromise of integrity, version management, and access controls. This is also an addressable standard due to the fact that it will vary widely in actual process flow from one entity to the next. Again, it is the accomplishment of the standard that is required, and the methodology to do so is permitted some flexibility in implementation.

The legal officer will be the person constructing the language regarding duties and expectations of an entity's business associates with respect to PHI that the entity will share with them. The CSO should request the opportunity to review and discuss the language with the legal officer so that both are comfortable that the requirement has been satisfied.

The remaining categories, "Physical and Technical Safeguards," contain both required and addressable standards. Unless the employees that work in these areas are on his staff, the CSO will have a consultative and collaborative interaction with them. The CSO should be intimately involved in the selection process of specific safeguard technologies and methods in order to ensure that they are appropriate, compliant with the standards, and actually address the identified risks effectively.

Examples include:

- Firewalls
- Encryption technology
- CCTV systems (if applicable)
- Facility and system access controls
- Monitoring, reporting, and response procedures
- Personnel identification mechanisms and technologies (cards, bio-metrics, etc.)
- Audit objectives and procedures

In some cases, there are departments that are already responsible for developing and using these devices and processes. That being the case, the CSO must establish a working relationship with each department or area in order to ensure he becomes part of the process of development and implementation, even if only from an awareness perspective. He should also ensure that the periodic evaluation requirement is enforced so that these technology and process specifics remain compliant, relevant, and effective.

CONCLUSION

In summary, the CPO is responsible for assuring the due diligence for safeguarding the privacy of PHI has been carried out, that all reasonable risks are identified, that the system of controls and safeguards is well designed and correctly implemented, that all training relating to privacy is developed to cover the Act, and delivered as circumstances (noted above) require, that the monitoring program is effective in providing a true representation of the workforce's behavior and adherence to the requirements, and that regular monitoring and timely corrective actions are performed when and where needed. The CPO must be cognizant of any legal issues that arise out of staff and patient concerns over privacy, the provisions and limitations of the Act, and take action to resolve the matter while ensuring continued compliance and protection of PHI.

The CSO's duty is to ensure that those governing the covered entity he works for understand and act to comply with HIPAA. His role is to ensure that not only is compliance achieved, but that it is maintained. He must also ensure that the program of security and risk management aligns with (is not an impediment to) the business operations while it provides effective protection of PHI. In his role, the CSO must be both technical and business oriented. He must function at a program or corporate level despite the need to have knowledge of many technical details. He must be both technical and political as he works to achieve consensus with the various internal organizations and his fellow executives. He must strike the balance between the need for protection and the need to be operationally successful — sometimes opposing objectives.

Working in partnership, the CSO and CPO play crucial parts in the overall compliance of an entity with the Act, and as such become key participants in the overall success of the entity itself through clear understanding of his environment, well-considered decisions, creation of consensus and partnerships, and appropriate risk management.

BIBLIOGRAPHY

Beaver, K. and R. Herold, *Practical Guide to HIPAA Privacy and Security Compliance*, Boca Raton, FL: Auerbach, 2003.

Code of Federal Regulations, "Title 45, Parts 160-164," Government Printing Office.

Nebraska DHHSS, HIPAA Project Office, "Final HIPAA Rule Summary."

Public Law 104-191, "Health Insurance Portability and Accountability Act of 1996."

GLOSSARY OF DEFINITIONS APPLICABLE TO THE SECURITY FUNCTION IN 45 CFR § 164.304:

Access means the ability or the means necessary to read, write, modify, or communicate data/information or otherwise use any system resource. (This definition applies to "access" as used in this subpart, not as used in subpart E of this part.)

Administrative safeguards are administrative actions, and policies and procedures, to manage the selection, development, implementation, and maintenance of security measures to protect electronic protected health information and to manage the conduct of the covered entity's workforce in relation to the protection of that information.

Authentication means the corroboration that a person is the one claimed.

Availability means the property that data or information is accessible and usable upon demand by an authorized person.

Confidentiality means the property that data or information is not made available or disclosed to unauthorized persons or processes.

Encryption means the use of an algorithmic process to transform data into a form in which there is a low probability of assigning meaning without use of a confidential process or key.

Facility means the physical premises and the interior and exterior of a building(s).

Information system means an interconnected set of information resources under the same direct management control that shares common functionality. A system normally includes hardware, software, information, data, applications, communications, and people.

Integrity means the property that data or information have not been altered or destroyed in an unauthorized manner.

Malicious software means software, for example, a virus, designed to damage or disrupt a system.

Password means confidential authentication information composed of a string of characters.

Physical safeguards are physical measures, policies, and procedures to protect a covered entity's electronic information systems and related buildings and equipment, from natural and environmental hazards, and unauthorized intrusion.

Security or security measures encompass all of the administrative, physical, and technical safeguards in an information system.

Security incident means the attempted or successful unauthorized access, use, disclosure, modification, or destruction of information or interference with system operations in an information system.

Technical safeguards means the technology and the policy and procedures for its use that protect electronic protected health information and control access to it.

User means a person or entity with authorized access.

Workstation means an electronic computing device, for example, a laptop or desktop computer, or any other device that performs similar functions, and electronic media stored in its immediate environment.

2

THE FINAL HIPAA SECURITY RULE IS HERE! NOW WHAT?

Todd Fitzgerald, CISSP, CISA

INTRODUCTION

We are privileged to live in a society that values freedom and the individual rights of its citizens to have the opportunity to make choices that affect their own well-being. These freedoms are exercised on a daily basis without conscious thought and are many times taken for granted. For example, people make choices about where they will eat for lunch, where they will have their cars repaired, who will provide childcare for their children, where they will spend their money, the leisure activities they will participate in, and how they will use their time. One of the most important choices individuals make is the selection of healthcare. The choice of healthcare provider — be it a doctor, hospital, or an integrated clinical system with a network of doctors and treatment facilities — is a personal choice based on many factors such as professional competence, practice location, specialty of the medicine, and trust in the ability of the medical professional. Selection of someone to provide medical attention is no small matter to be taken lightly; being able to trust the medical professional is arguably of utmost importance.

In a generation where access to information is literally only seconds away, this trust is not blind. The Internet is used extensively by the patient, or concerned family members, for researching medical ailments and then suggesting treatments or questioning the physician's recommended course of action. Although a high level of "trust" may be invested in the physician, individuals still feel a need to find other sources of information that corroborate the recommended treatment. Due to this phenomenon, the patient is much more informed about treatment choices, medications, and potential outcomes. The Internet has accelerated this shift, which started as the baby-boomer generation, also known as the "sandwich generation,"

0-8493-2211-1/05/$0.00+$1.50

needed to simultaneously care for their own children and elderly parents, in addition to being concerned with the medical effects of their own aging.

Just as patients must be able to *trust* their medical professionals for their treatment, patients also *trust* that those medical professionals are using their medical health information — their *personal* medical health information — solely for the purposes of treatment, payment, or operations. They also *trust* that this information is kept private and that appropriate measures are being taken to ensure that the information is not inadvertently disclosed, destroyed, or changed in such a way that could adversely affect their treatment or create personal embarrassment. However, analogous to the trust that is placed in the medical professional, much more information is available today about privacy issues; thus, people are also much more informed. The media has communicated countless examples: for example, hackers disclosing personal medical information by posting on the Internet, company e-mails inadvertently revealing patients using a particular medication, being solicited through someone having knowledge of personal medical history, or disclosure within an organization of psychological notes of other employees. People expect that their confidentiality will be maintained and that the trust relationship between the patient and provider will not be compromised. Privacy issues address the rights of the individual with respect to this trust relationship, whereas security is the mechanism that ensures that this privacy is reasonably maintained throughout the system. True privacy of information cannot be achieved without adequate security controls. The Health Insurance Portability and Accountability Act (HIPAA) has several objectives, one of which is to ensure that the appropriate security safeguards are in place to protect the privacy of health information.

HIPAA ARRIVES ON THE SCENE

The Health Insurance Portability and Accountability Act (HIPAA) of 1996 was enacted by Congress (Public Law 104-191) with two purposes in mind: (1) to reform health insurance to protect insurance coverage for their workers and families when they changed or lost their jobs, and (2) to simplify the administrative processes by adopting standards to improve the efficiency and effectiveness of the nation's healthcare system. Title I of HIPAA contains provisions to address health insurance reform, while Title II addresses national standards for electronic transactions, unique health identifiers, privacy, and security. Title II is known as Administrative Simplification and is intended to reduce the costs of healthcare through the widespread use of electronic data interchange. Administrative simplification was added to Title XI of the Social Security Act through Subtitle F of Title II of the enacted HIPAA law.

While the initial intent of the Administrative Simplification was to reduce the administrative costs associated with processing healthcare transactions, Congress recognized that standardizing and electronically aggregating healthcare information would increase the risk of disclosure of confidential information, and the patient's privacy rights needed to be protected. Security provisions were needed not only to protect the confidentiality of information, but also to ensure that information retained the appropriate integrity. Consider the situation where the diagnosis or vital sign information is changed on a medical record, and subsequent treatment decisions are based on this (changed) information. The impact of not being able to rely on the information stored within the healthcare environment could have life-threatening consequences. Thus, privacy issues primarily focus on the confidentiality of information to ensure that only the appropriate individuals have access to the information, whereas the Security Standards take on a larger scope to ensure that the issues of integrity and availability of information are also addressed.

THE RULE-MAKING PROCESS

Each provision of the Administrative Simplification must follow a rule-making process that is designed to achieve consensus within the Department of Health and Human Services and other federal departments. When the rule is approved within the government, the public has the opportunity to comment on the proposal, and then these comments are evaluated in the determination of the final rule. Once the rules have gone through this process, they have the force of federal law. The Department of Health and Human Services implementation teams draft Notices of Proposed Rule Making (NPRMs), which are subsequently published in the *Federal Register* after being reviewed within the federal government according to the process shown in Table 2.1. Once the NPRMs are published, they are available for a 60-day public comment period that provides for input and for interested parties to influence the outcome of the final regulation. After the publication of the final rule, most large health plans, clearinghouses, and providers have 24 months to be in compliance, and smaller parties have 36 months.

The proposed Security and Electronic Signature Standards were originally published in the *Federal Register* on August 12, 1998. The Security Rule has been delayed on several occasions, as resources were committed to and focused on the proposed transaction and code set and privacy rules, both of which generated a large number of public comments. These public comments must be reviewed, and the numbers can be large. Over 17,000 public comments were received on the Transaction and Code Sets NPRM, and several thousand on the Privacy Rule and on the proposed

Table 2.1 Administrative Simplification Rule-Making Process

1. The DHHS Implementation team drafts a Notice of Proposed Rule Making (NPRM) for review.
2. The DHHS Data Council Committee on Health Data Standards reviews.
3. The advisors to the DHHS Secretary (Division Agency Heads) agree.
4. The Office of Management and Budget (OMB) reviews.
5. The proposed NPRM is published in the *Federal Register.*
6. Public comments are solicited for 60-day period.
7. Comments are open for public view.
8. Comments are analyzed and content is summarized by the Implementation Team.
9. The final rule is published, and standards become effective 24 months after adoption (36 months for small health plans).

Security Rule. The Transaction and Code Set compliance date was also delayed by one year, to October 16, 2003, as long as the covered entity filed an extension request by October 15, 2002. Additionally, the Security Rule was initiated during the Clinton administration and was carried over into the Bush administration, which created political challenges for expedient passage of the rule. As a result, the language was rewritten during 2002 to coincide with the Privacy Rule, which needed to go through the DHHS clearance process prior to final rule publication. The Centers for Medicare and Medicaid Services provided their best estimates several times during 2002 of publication of the final rule, which passed through the clearance process and was submitted to the Office of Management and Budget (OMB) in early 2003 and published in the *Federal Register* as 45 CFR Parts 160, 162, and 164 on February 20, 2003. The regulations became effective on April 21, 2003, and covered entities must comply with the requirements by April 21, 2005. Small health plans have until April 21, 2006, to comply with the rule.

THE SECURITY OBJECTIVES OF THE FINAL RULE DID NOT CHANGE SUBSTANTIALLY

Many organizations had been "waiting" for the final rule to be published before seriously embarking on security issues. Some started HIPAA security gap analysis efforts, but many were reluctant to invest large sums of money when there was the potential that the rules might change. The reality is that the rule embodies security practices that should be performed during the normal course of business to protect the information assets and should be initiated regardless of the rule. Waiting only shortens the time available to dedicate to reasonable security and can also have the negative effect of driving up costs at a later date. For example, if a new Web-based application is in the process of being designed and adequate attention to security is not taking place during early phases of the system development cycle, the costs of retrofitting security after implementation will be 10 to 20 times the cost. Reanalysis, rewriting of the applications, integrating technical security mechanisms, and retesting and implementing the system a second time all drive up the cost. There is also the business opportunity cost of deploying scarce IT and business resources toward retrofitting the application versus building new functionality.

Many of the security constructs remained in the rule, as these constructs are generally industry security practices necessary to secure information that have been successfully applied in other arenas requiring higher levels of security, such as the Department of Defense, financial institutions, and companies heavily engaged in E-commerce. The final HIPAA Security Rule recognizes the need to protect electronic health information with the appropriate Administrative, Physical, and Technical Safeguards that have been applied to other industries.

The final Security Rule was reoriented to support the final Privacy Rule, which was issued on December 28, 2000, and was last modified on August 14, 2002. The Privacy Rule compliance date for most covered entities was April 14, 2003. The proposed Security Rule focused on information maintained or transmitted by a covered entity in electronic form. The scope of the information now covered by the final Security Rule has been narrowed to health information addressed by the Privacy Rule. The Privacy Rule addresses individually identifiable health information known as Protected Health Information (PHI) in all forms, including electronic and paper. The final Security Rule focuses only on the PHI that is in electronic form (electronic protected health information or e-PHI), in transit or in storage (data at rest), otherwise the scope is the same as the Privacy Rule. This eliminates some of the confusion surrounding what information needed to be addressed by the Security Rule, which seemed to be in conflict with the Privacy Rule in the Security Rule Notice of Proposed Rule Making.

In addition to the reorientation with the Privacy Rule, the final Security Rule changed the nomenclature of the "requirements" and "implementation features" and replaced these with "standards" and "implementation specifications," respectively. The implementation specifications were also categorized as "required" or "addressable." This was done to provide consistency with the Privacy Rule and the Transactions Rule, as well as to provide a common terminology. The new approach is much cleaner, more manageable, and easier to interpret. In making this change, the original 69 implementation features were reduced to 14 required Implementation Specifications to support the requirements, or now referred to as the "Security Standards."

There also appeared to be a change from a prescriptive approach to one that requires a covered entity to look at the risks and vulnerabilities to the protected health information that they transmit or maintain in electronic form and determine the reasonable and appropriate security measures to provide adequate protection of this information. The Administrative Simplification revisions to the Social Security Act required that that Secretary of the Department of Health and Human Services adopt standards that consider (1) the technical capabilities of the record systems used to maintain the information, (2) costs of the security measures, (3) training needs for those who have access to health information, (4) the value of audit trails in computerized record systems, and (5) the needs and capabilities of small health and rural health providers. Whereas these requirements apply to the broader topic of "health information," the final Security Rule has taken this approach with respect to electronic protected health information. Therefore, each organization must make the judgments as to what is "reasonable and appropriate," based on their size, complexity of systems, capabilities, cost of security measures, and the probability and criticality of potential risks to e-PHI. Larger organizations are expected to provide more resources and have the financial ability to introduce more complex solutions.

Approximately 2350 comments were received on the initial Security Rule. These comments were assessed and taken into account with keeping the underlying goals of information protection in mind. Some of the proposed implementation specification changes were seen as resulting in standards that would be too difficult to understand or apply. Some comments proposed the expansion of applicability for all entities involved in healthcare; others sought clarification of their particular entity's requirements. Some comments demonstrated the confusion with regard to understanding the requirements, or felt that the requirements were too granular, restrictive, or that the definitions needed further explanation. These comments were reviewed and considered in the final rule, with the Department of Health and Human Services providing changes to the rule based on industry practices, government regulations, and a mandate to produce a set of security standards.

PRIVACY RULE REQUIREMENTS FOR SECURITY

Even in the absence of the final Security Rule being available for most of the period that organizations were addressing Privacy Rule issues, the references in the Privacy Rule (which was originally published for public

Table 2.2 Notice of Proposed Rule Making (NPRM) Dates

Proposed Rule	NPRM Date	Final Date	Compliance Date
Transaction and Code Sets	5/07/1998	8/17/2000[a]	10/16/2003[a]
Privacy	11/11/1999	3/2001[b]	4/14/2003[c]
Security	8/12/1998	2/20/2003	4/21/2005[d]
Employer ID	6/16/1998	3/31/2002	7/30/2004[e]

[a] Compliance date for transaction and code sets was extended through legislation enacted on 12/27/01, entitled the Administrative Simplification Compliance Act, as long as providers submitted a request for extension by October 15, 2002. Modifications were made on February 20, 2003, and corrected on March 10, 2003.

[b] Privacy Rule changes were proposed on March 27, 2002, and the final rule was published on August 14, 2002. However, the compliance date was not changed from the original date. Guidance was previously issued on July 6, 2001.

[c] Small health plans must be compliant by April 14, 2004.

[d] Small health plans must be compliant by April 21, 2006.

[e] Small health plans must be compliant by August 1, 2005.

comment on November 11, 1999, and subsequently issued with a compliance date of April 14, 2003, as shown in Table 2.2) clearly indicated the need for a reasonable level of security practices to be in place. The Safeguard Standard contained within §164.530 of the Privacy Rule states that "A covered entity must have in place appropriate administrative, technical and physical safeguards to protect the privacy of protected health information." This appears to suggest a linkage to the Security Rule requirements, which has a compliance date much further out (at least two years) from the compliance date of the Privacy Rule.

The implementation specification for safeguards in the final Privacy Rule continues this thought by stating that "A covered entity must reasonably safeguard protected health information from any intentional or unintentional use or disclosure that is in violation of the standards, implementation specifications or other requirements of this subpart. A covered entity must reasonably safeguard protected health information to limit incidental uses or disclosures made pursuant to an otherwise permitted or required use or disclosure."

It is clear from these excerpts that "reasonable" security is expected to be implemented for the Privacy Rule to protect the privacy of health information. Moreover, the proposed Security Rule only applies to electronic information, whereas the Privacy Rule applies to all forms of protected health information. This creates a situation where the Privacy

Rule assumes broader application in the form of protected information being addressed than the proposed Security Rule.

THE FINAL HIPAA SECURITY RULE

The Administrative Simplification (Part C of Title XI of the Social Security Act) provisions state that covered entities that maintain or transmit health information are required to "maintain reasonable and appropriate administrative, physical and technical safeguards to ensure the integrity and confidentiality of the information and to protect against any reasonable anticipated threats or hazards to the security or integrity of the information and unauthorized use or disclosure of the information."

Because the final Security Rule was written to be consistent with the Privacy Rule, the focus of Security Standards applied to "health information" in support of the Administrative Simplification requirements were shifted to PHI and specifically to *electronic* PHI. The applicability statement of the final Security Rule states that "A covered entity must comply with the applicable standards, implementation specifications, and requirements of this subpart with respect to electronic protected health information." Covered entities are defined as (1) a health plan, (2) a healthcare clearinghouse, or (3) a healthcare provider who transmits any health information in electronic form in connection with a transaction covered by Part 162 of Title 45 of the *Code of Federal Regulations* (*CFR*).

This is where the Security Standards become important. These standards were written to, according to the Security Rule, "define the administrative, physical, and technical safeguards to protect the confidentiality, integrity and availability of electronic protected health information." Therefore, by applying the Security Standards on electronic PHI as the scope, the objectives of Administrative Simplification will be satisfied. All of the Security Standards must be satisfied, some through Required Implementation Specifications and some through Addressable Implementation Specifications.

As shown in Figure 2.1, protecting the confidentiality, integrity, and availability of electronic protected health information is at the core of the security requirements, while reasonably anticipated threats (security), uses, and disclosures (privacy) must also be protected and compliance of the workforce with the Security Standards ensured.

LET'S JUST BE REASONABLE

The definition of "reasonable" can vary from person to person. The final assessment appears to be headed for the courts and will be determined by case law as a result of lawsuits. Consider the case where an employer

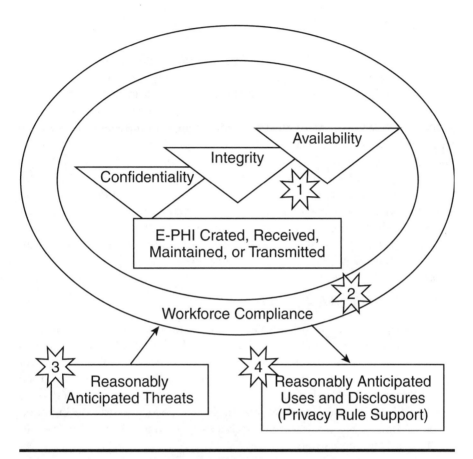

Figure 2.1 Security Rule General Requirements

has installed a proximity card reader for 500 employees at a data center containing protected health information. Assume the facility has a guard during the daytime; however, during the evening hours, the computer operators watch the surveillance cameras for suspicious activity. During one evening, while the night operator went to the restroom, someone using an unreturned visitor's badge obtained during the day enters the building and removes three laptops. Were reasonable steps taken to prevent the theft? Was the fact that the operator left his station unattended unreasonable? Was the fact that the unreturned visitor's badge still worked unreasonable? Or, would a member of the jury view this situation as one that could be reasonably expected to occur? Consider another example where patient information is discovered because a Web server was hacked into. If correct firewall configurations were set 99 percent of the time, except for one instance where the network engineer was upgrading the server and inadvertently opened some ports after a long, tiring weekend —

was the information not reasonably protected? Is "most of the time" reasonable?

Different organizations make different security decisions based on the risk they are willing to assume. Organizations take into account the costs, technical abilities, and the risk that they are willing to assume based on their business objectives. It is critical that companies assess the threats, vulnerabilities, and risks to electronic information and develop reasonable steps to address such risks. Each of these decisions and their rationale should be documented so that it can be understood at a later point in time why the decision was made. Documenting these decisions also forces the organization to really look at the decisions that are being made and whether or not they make sense. It is not uncommon to go through this process, only to find out that management team members were making different assumptions as to the level of risk and were accepting an unreasonable level of risk without being aware that they were.

THE SECURITY STANDARDS

The 1998 proposed Security Rule defined standards for the security of individual health information under the control of the covered entities (health plans, clearinghouses, and healthcare providers). The three safeguard categories of Administrative, Physical, and Technical contain a total of 18 Security Standards (versus 24 requirements in the proposed rule) that must be addressed, as shown in Table 2.3. The standards are intended to be technology-neutral so that advances in technology can be used to the best advantage as they evolve.

In support of the Security Standards, there are 14 required Implementation Specifications that address 7 of the 18 Security Standards, as some Security Standards are comprised of multiple required Implementation Specifications. For example, the Security Management Process Security Standard contains four required Implementation Specifications, including Risk Analysis, Risk Management, Sanction Policy, and Information System Activity Review.

The covered entity must decide — through executing the risk analysis, risk mitigation strategy, cost of implementation, and evaluating the security measures that are already in place — whether or not the "Addressable Implementation Specification" is reasonable and appropriate and should be implemented. If the specification is viewed as *not* reasonable and appropriate, but for the standard to be met another security safeguard is necessary to be implemented, the entity may implement the safeguard using an alternative control as long as it accomplishes the same result as the Addressable Implementation Specification. In other words, an organization could select other controls as long as the Security Standard is met.

In this case, the organization must document the decision not to implement the Addressable Implementation Specification, the rationale behind it, and the alternative control that was implemented in its place. There are 22 Addressable Implementation Specifications that address nine of the Security Standards; four of the Security Standards contain Required Implementation Specifications as well.

The six remaining Security Standards contain neither an Addressable Implementation Specification nor a Required Implementation Specification. In these cases, it was felt that the definition of the standard itself was sufficient to understand the implementation required. For example, the Assigned Security Responsibility Standard is "Identify the security official who is responsible for the development and implementation of the policies and procedures required by this subpart [Security Rule] for the entity." Additional explanation is really not necessary to understand the standard; someone needs to be designated to fulfill this role to satisfy the standard.

To "meet the Security Standards," 36 required or addressable implementation specifications must be reviewed and complied with, either through the Required Implementation Specification, the prescribed (Addressable) Implementation Specification, or an alternative control. Combined with six Security Standards without any implementation specification noted totals 42 areas that are required to be acted upon in some manner. While some of these tasks can be completed quickly, depending upon the current security profile of the organization, this still represents a significant undertaking, requiring about two of these areas to be evaluated each and every month from now until the compliance date. If someone is not "charged with the security responsibility," this would be a great time to satisfy the Assigned Security Responsibility Security Standard and draft someone. In many organizations, the need was recognized and the positions filled during the attention focused on the Privacy Rule due to the requirements to "… have in place appropriate administrative, technical and physical safeguards to protect the privacy of protected health information."

CHANGES TO THE PROPOSED STANDARDS IN THE FINAL RULE

The following is a brief summary of the intent of each Security Standard, along with the changes from the proposed Security Rule. Each of the Security Standard descriptions contains references to addressable or required implementation specifications. The reader is referred to Table 2.3 for the specific Implementation Specification designation (Required or Addressable).

Table 2.3   HIPAA Security Rule Standards and Implementation Specifications

Security Standard	Required Implementation Specification	Addressable Implementation Specification
Administrative Safeguards		
Security Management Process	Risk Analysis Risk Management Sanction Policy Information System Activity Review	
Assigned Security Responsibility	Required (no implementation specification)	
Workforce Security		Authorization and Supervision Workforce Clearance Procedure Termination Procedures
Information Access Management	Isolating Healthcare Clearinghouse Function	Access Authorization Access Establishment and Modification
Security Awareness and Training		Security Reminders Protection from Malicious Software Log-In Monitoring Password Management
Security Incident Procedures	Response and Reporting	
Contingency Plan	Data Backup Plan Disaster Recovery Plan Emergency Mode Operation Plan	Testing and Revision Procedure Applications and Data Criticality Analysis
Evaluation	Required (no implementation specification)	
Business Associate Contracts and Other Arrangements	Written Contract or Other Arrangement	

Table 2.3   HIPAA Security Rule Standards and Implementation Specifications (continued)

Security Standard	Required Implementation Specification	Addressable Implementation Specification
Physical Safeguards		
Facility Access Controls		Contingency Operations Facility Security Plan Access Control and Validation Procedures Maintenance Records
Workstation Use	Required (no implementation specification)	
Workstation Security	Required (no implementation specification)	
Device and Media Controls	Disposal Media Reuse	Accountability Data Backup and Storage
Technical Safeguards		
Access Control	Unique User Identification Emergency Access Procedure	Automatic Log-off Encryption and Decryption
Audit Controls	Required (no implementation specification)	
Integrity		Mechanism to Authenticate Electronic Protected Health Information
Person or Entity Authentication	Required (no implementation specification)	
Transmission Security		Integrity Controls Encryption

Administrative Safeguards

Administrative safeguards consist of the formal organizational practices that manage the selection and execution of security measures to protect data and the conduct of personnel in the protection of the data. It is important that these practices are documented in the form of policies, procedures, standards, or guidelines that are followed by the organization. While there may be accepted practices that are followed within the organization, without proper documentation, it is difficult to demonstrate that all employees are working from the same assumptions. Additionally, without the documented procedures, new employees may not be adequately informed as to their security responsibilities.

Much of the detail of this section was removed and the requirements were generalized to be less prescriptive. The order of the previous requirements (alphabetical) was rearranged to be more logical, with the establishment of the Security Management Process occurring first, as everything else within the security program should be built upon this. The previous requirements for system configurations and for a formal mechanism for processing records were dropped from the final rule as they were seen as redundant, unnecessary, or ambiguous in relation to the other requirements for documentation and processes.

Security Management Process

Conduct a risk analysis that assesses the vulnerabilities and risks to the confidentiality, integrity, and availability of e-PHI, that examines risk management of the implemented security measures, that applies appropriate sanctions to workforce members who fail to comply with the security policies and procedures, and that implements procedures to regularly review records of information system activity (i.e., audit logs, access reports, security incident tracking reports). The specification of "Internal Audit" was changed from the proposed rule because it was not intended to have a rigid, costly review process over the system activity related to security, but rather to ensure that appropriate attention to security continues to take place over time. Sanction Policies were seen as necessary to meet the requirement of "ensuring" compliance of the officers and employees and that the introduction of negative consequences for noncompliance increases the chances that compliance will be achieved. It is a typical result that if employees know that something is being monitored and followed, they are less likely to be in noncompliance with the expectations.

Security Management is an ongoing function with a continuous cycle of risk analysis, risk management, and issuance of security policies and their sanctions. Over time, attention to security within organizations tends to dissipate, which (unknowingly and unintentionally) increases the risk profile.

Assigned Security Responsibility

An individual must be identified who is responsible for the development and implementation of security policies and procedures. Many individuals may be involved in security for the organization, but there must be one individual named with the responsibility for protecting e-PHI. The proposed rule indicated that an individual or organization could be named, but this is no longer the case; it must be a single official. Multiple people are typically involved in the security function in larger organizations; however, someone must be named with the accountability for the function to ensure that policies and procedures are developed and implemented as required by the rule. The individual and supporting organization utilize the security management processes to carry out the mission of the information security program.

Workforce Security

Implement policies and procedures to ensure that all members of the workforce have appropriate access to e-PHI and prevent those who should not have access through authorization/supervision of workforce members, clearance procedures, and termination procedures. The specifications are all addressable because it will vary by organization as to whether or not they need to be formalized. Background checks are not required for all employees through the clearance specification; however, some form of screening needs to take place prior to permitting access to e-PHI. The detailed requirements of the termination procedures have been removed, again to be less prescriptive and allow flexibility for the specific environments. The intent is to ensure that when individuals with access to e-PHI are no longer associated with the entity, that the exposure for potential damage is mitigated by removing their access. Small offices would most likely not require the formalized procedures that large organizations would require to meet the standard.

Information Access Management

Implement policies and procedures for establishing, authorizing, reviewing, documenting, and modifying a user's right to access a workstation, transaction, program, process, or other means of accessing e-PHI. This forms the basis of acceptable information security access management practices through (1) authorizing appropriate access and then (2) establishing the access. This standard supports the minimum necessary requirements of the Privacy Rule, and as such, specific references to "role-based," "user-based," "context-based," discretionary/mandatory access control, and the distinctions between authorization and access control were omitted from the final rule. An additional Required Implementation Specification to isolate the clearinghouse functions from the larger organization through their own policies and procedures was added to this requirement.

Security Awareness and Training

Implement a security awareness and training program for all members of the workforce (including management), including training on protection from malicious software (viruses, Trojan horses, worms, scripting, etc.), log-in monitoring, password management, and periodic security reminders. The end users are the key to successful security and each member of the workforce must receive ongoing training. Flexibility is left to the organization as to how this can be implemented through techniques such as face-to-face, pamphlets, new employee orientation, Web-based, etc. Many security practitioners feel that security awareness and training is one of the most effective areas to invest in security. These individuals represent the "security front line," and education here causes individuals to support the security program through awareness and preventing larger security issues. It does little good to implement a complex technical solution, such as implementing dynamic passwords utilizing RADIUS or TACACS+ authentication and token cards, if the user tapes the PIN to the back of the token card. Similarly, having policies that deal with the handling of confidential information would be ineffective if the users are not aware as to what types of information are considered confidential and need extra measures to provide adequate protection. Training is a continuous process that should focus upon the different aspects of information security.

Security Incident Procedures

Incident response and reporting procedures are required to mitigate the potential harmful effects of the incident and provide documentation of the incident and outcome. An incident is defined as the attempted or successful unauthorized access, use, disclosure, modification, or destruction of information or interference with system operations. Each organization must define what event would be considered to be a security incident and the internal/external reporting processes necessary to support the incident.

Formal, current, accurate, and documented procedures for reporting and response to security incidents are necessary to ensure that violations are reported and handled promptly. Seemingly small incidents may be symptomatic of a larger problem and should be thoroughly investigated. Lack of attention to the small incidents also creates a culture that is desensitized to information security and creates a greater risk that a larger risk may occur. For example, if attention is not paid to the occasional laptop that is missing every few months because the information stored on those particular laptops was not seen as valuable, then the larger problem of laptop security awareness and the need for locking devices may be missed. Subsequently, a nurse's laptop containing health information or an executive's laptop containing confidential business strategic information may be compromised, when it could have been prevented.

Contingency Plan

In the aftermath of 9/11, many organizations have increased their focus on disaster recovery. The contingency plan provides the organizational readiness to respond to systems emergencies so that critical operations can continue during an emergency. To meet the requirement, applications and data criticality analysis, data backup plans, disaster recovery plans, emergency mode operation plans, and testing/revision procedures are included as required or addressable implementation specifications to support the Contingency Plan standard. Most large organizations have disaster recovery plans that cover the mainframe environments as a result of the Y2K contingency planning that had previously taken place. However, infrastructure and staffing are constantly changing; and as a result, many of these plans need to be updated. While most organizations tend to back up the network environments on a regular schedule, these environments rarely have adequate disaster recovery plans or are tested on a frequent basis. With the continuing shift to the network/server environment for mission-critical applications, increased attention will need to be paid to the contingency planning of these facilities.

Policies and procedures for responding to emergencies or other occurrences (i.e., fire, vandalism, system failure, natural disaster) that damage systems containing e-PHI are to be implemented. This is accomplished through data backups, disaster recovery plans, emergency mode operation plans (ability to continue business during the crisis), testing and revision procedures, and applications and data criticality analysis. This standard was proposed and remained in the final rule as data becomes most vulnerable during crisis events because security controls are typically bypassed to bring the systems back into operation. The e-PHI lost during these events impacts the availability and integrity of the information, while exposing the data to confidentiality issues of improper use and disclosure.

Evaluation

Perform periodic technical and nontechnical evaluations based on the standards initially and also after environmental and operational changes affecting e-PHI. These evaluations can be performed internally or externally, and replace the certification requirement of the earlier rule. It can be expected that independent certification guides, secure software listings, and compliance guidelines will emerge from private enterprise. To form a meaningful evaluation, the risk-level acceptance of the organization should be understood prior to the evaluation, because the security measures chosen should be a result of the risk assessment decisions.

Evaluation processes, whether performed internally or externally, have the positive impact of documenting the security actions taken and obtaining management sign-off, which tends to create greater accountability beyond the security department for the implementation. It also tends to ensure that the agreed-upon security parameters in the design process are carried through to implementation.

Business Associate Contracts and Other Arrangements

The final rule eliminated the chain of trust agreement and replaced it with the requirement for a covered entity to ensure that appropriate safeguards are assured by the business associate through inclusion of security requirements in written contracts. The scope is limited to e-PHI, as is the rest of the Security Rule. The business associate definitions are those that are utilized within the Privacy Rule. If a covered entity is aware of a pattern or practice that the business associate is engaged in and that pattern or practice is considered a violation of the business associate's obligation, then the covered entity would be in noncompliance if the covered entity failed to take reasonable steps to end the violation. Other arrangements specify situations such as how the rules apply to government entities, other laws, terminations of contracts, etc.

Physical Safeguards

Protecting the covered entity's electronic information systems and the buildings that contain these systems from fire, natural and environmental hazards, and unauthorized intrusion are the focus of the Physical Safeguards. These controls support many of the administrative and technical controls defined in the other safeguard sections. Consider the situation in which very tight logical access controls (Technical Safeguard Access Control Security Standard) are defined to support the administrative safeguard standards for Information Access. Assume that a computer containing these controls is located in an area where other building tenants have unrestricted access. Even with two-factor authentication, encryption of files, and properly implemented access control facilities, if the physical server can be accessed, an alternate operating system could be loaded, or worse yet, the server could be stolen, thus providing the intruder with ample time to decipher encrypted files. Unauthorized employees having physical access to the server creates unnecessary additional risk.

Two requirements of the proposed rule — (1) assigned security responsibility and (2) security awareness training — made much more sense in the Administrative Safeguards section, and they were moved to that section in the final Security Rule. The Physical Safeguard Standards and related Implementation Specifications include:

Facility Access Controls

Facility Access Controls focus on the facilities that provide physical access to the electronic information systems, and limits physical access through contingency operations (facility access in the event of an emergency), facility security plans (safeguard facility from unauthorized physical access, tampering, and theft), access control and validation procedures (validate access to facilities based on role; control access to programs for testing and revision), and maintenance records (document repairs to facility security components). The standards appear to be straightforward and permit the organization to review the risks and implement the appropriate controls, unlike the proposed rule which appeared to require all of the implementation specifications without regard to the risk analysis. It is still the covered entity's responsibility to ensure that the facilities where e-PHI is located and transmitted are secured properly, whether or not such facilities are owned by the covered entity.

Workstation Use

Implement policies and procedures specifying the proper functions and manner in which those functions are to be performed (i.e., locking workstations, logging off, invoking screen savers) and the physical attributes of the space surrounding the workstation that are allowed to access e-PHI. The "workstation" terminology is used to replace "terminal" to apply to the broad range of computing equipment with access to E-PHI (e.g., laptops, desktops, personal digital assistants, etc.) and not be limited technology-wise.

Workstation Security

Implement physical safeguards for all workstations that access e-PHI restricting access to authorized users. This is consistent with the proposed rule. Contents displayed on workstations, especially those in open areas such as nurses stations, must be secured so that private information is not viewable by unauthorized persons. Workstations should also be secured so that only authorized personnel will have access to them. In practice, some workstations need to be in open areas and approaches such as turning the monitor away from public viewing, logging off of the workstation when unattended, utilizing screen savers, and ensuring that the workstation is protected from theft would appear to be reasonable.

Device and Media Controls

Implement policies and procedures governing the receipt and removal of hardware and software in and out of a facility and movement within a facility through disposal procedures, media reuse procedures, account-ability (record of movements), and data backup and storage (in this case, this is related to the backup of e-PHI prior to the moving of equipment). Media reuse procedures were added to the rule to address the reuse and recycling. There have been news stories recently of hard drives purchased on E-bay that contained sensitive information and was subsequently able to be retrieved because they were not properly disposed of after final disposition.

Technical Safeguards

The technical security services (processes that protect, control, and monitor information access) and the technical security mechanisms (processes that prevent unauthorized access over a communications network) have been combined into the technical safeguards category. This is very logical, as many organizations viewed these all as technical requirements. "Data authentication" was renamed to the standard security terminology of "integrity." The Technical Safeguard Standards and related Implementation Specifications include:

Access Control

Implement technical policies and procedures for electronic information systems containing e-PHI to allow access only to those persons who have been granted access through the Information Access Management processes in the Administrative Safeguards. Unique user IDs are necessary to identify and track an individual's activity, emergency access procedures are required to support operations in an emergency situation, and implementation specifications of automatic log-off and the use of encryption can support the access security standards. There was much confusion surrounding the requirements for role-based, context-based, mandatory access control, discretionary access control, etc. in the proposed rule. The new specification is much clearer and affords the organization the ability to implement the appropriate rules based on the risk. For example, an organization may decide to encrypt highly sensitive e-PHI data-at-rest if there is an assessment that this information could be compromised, such as in the case of fraud investigation health information stored on a CD.

A procedure for emergency access during a crisis must be implemented. Consider the situation in which a specialist is called in to perform an emergency procedure but does not have access to needed health information from the local information system. The specialist needs a method to gain emergency access without "waiting for forms to be processed" by the security department.

Audit Controls

Recording system activity is important so that the organization can identify suspect data access activities, assess the effectiveness of the security program, and respond to potential weaknesses. Implementation of hardware, software, or procedural mechanisms that record and examine activity in information systems containing e-PHI is necessary. Some organizations have assumed that the audit trails specified under this requirement would support the Privacy Rule. Typically, the types of information dealt with are different. Whereas the Privacy Rule is concerned with tracking of uses and disclosures, the Security Rule is concerned with tracking system activity, such as log-in attempts, access, and modification to records. While similar, audit trails within the system context are typically not geared toward tracking the business-level information surrounding the use and disclosures, although some records may provide supporting information. System audit trails are also not typically turned on to monitor read access to information due to the volume of information.

Integrity (Formerly Data Authentication)

Implement policies and procedures to protect e-PHI from improper alteration or destruction through mechanisms that corroborate that the information has not been destroyed in an unauthorized manner. Techniques such as digital signatures, checksums, and error-correcting memory are all methods of ensuring data integrity. Again, the ability to assess risk, provide technology neutrality, and not be prescriptive enables the covered entity to determine the appropriate methods to ensure that the data can be relied upon.

Person or Entity Authentication (Combined Authentication Requirements)

Implement procedures to verify that the person or entity seeking access to e-PHI is really the person or entity. The proposed rule was very prescriptive in suggesting biometrics, passwords, telephone callbacks, token systems, PINs, etc., whereas the rule now allows the implementation to be determined by the entity based on the risk assessment. The requirements for "irrefutable" entity authentication were removed in the final rule.

Transmission Security

Implement technical security guarding against unauthorized access to e-PHI transmitted over an electronic communications network (versus open network in the proposed rule). Integrity controls and encryption may be applied according to the risk level of the information; for example, in cases such as dial-up lines or over a private network, encryption may not be necessary to achieve the standard's objectives; however, over the Internet, the appropriate encryption levels to thwart brute-force cracking may be necessary. This is an area where technology is constantly changing, there are interoperability issues, and the feasibility of solutions may make this prohibitive for small providers.

Documentation and Other Related Standards

In addition to the Security Standards specified in the Administrative, Technical, and Physical Safeguards, the covered entity must implement reasonable and appropriate policies and procedures to comply with the Standards, Implementation Specifications, and any other requirements of the Security Rule. These must be documented and can be changed at any time. The covered entity can take into consideration the size, complexity, and capabilities of the covered entity; the technical infrastructure; hardware and software security capabilities; the costs of the security measures; and the probability and criticality of potential risks to the e-PHI.

Documentation of policies and procedures may seem to be such a logical practice that it appears unnecessary to state it. However, many organizations operate without defined policies and procedures, and still the work gets done. The difficulty is that, many times, it is done several different ways, depending on the individual performing the activity. This increases the likelihood that inconsistencies will occur, thus increasing the potential for security incidents. While the Security Rule does not specify a requirement to adopt ISO 9000-type standard processes, implementing procedures that follow this approach would further support that a "reasonable" approach was taken. This also permits the opportunity to review and discuss the processes across organizations and work toward improving the processes, thereby increasing service delivery capabilities and reducing waste.

Consider, as an example, the practice of security configuration management changes. Security measures, practices, and procedures would need to be documented and integrated with the other system configuration practices to ensure that routine changes to system hardware and software do not contribute to compromising the overall security. Security design efforts placed into new systems could be easily compromised and resources wasted without the appropriate level of security review for what appears to be a simple change. Security management is a continuous process. Late one evening, a systems engineer was upgrading a server and unintentionally opened a security hole on the mail server that provided the capability to perform mail relays. This happened at 1:30 a.m., and the systems engineer discovered his error and closed the hole by 2:00 a.m. Unfortunately, in that brief period, a hacker discovered the open relay and used the mail server to send "get rich quick" e-mails to more than 2000 individuals. Each of the e-mail addresses included the mail header information, which showed that it was coming from the systems engineer's organization. This demonstrates that clear, documented configurations and procedures for changing these configurations are necessary.

Many times, documentation is thought of as an afterthought. The more organizations get into the practice of seeing this as an important deliverable of the development process, the more efficient and effective the organization can become because the opportunity for future improvement becomes more visible.

PRAGMATIC APPROACH

The 18 Standards and their related Implementation Specifications, at first glance, can seem like a daunting task, certainly presenting a case for the senior leadership, the IT team, and the Information Security Officer to head for the Emergency Room.

The Security Rule was meant to be scalable, such that small providers would not be burdened with excessive costs of implementation, and the large providers, health plans, and clearinghouses could take steps appropriate to their business environments. For example, backing up the data offsite of a small provider might be a simple process of rotating the information to an off-site location on a weekly basis from one server, whereas a large operation might contract with a disaster recovery company or employ electronic vaulting of the information. Decisions must be made to reasonably protect the information, and document how those decisions were determined. While earlier it was recognized that security is always a risk-based decision, it is sometimes difficult to determine what will be "reasonable" under the circumstances.

A security plan for improvement is the most pragmatic way to move toward HIPAA compliance. Stepwise improvements in the security infrastructure, beginning with an understanding of what risks are being casually accepted within the environment, then followed by targeting solutions to mitigate the critical risks, seems reasonable. Early in the process, someone needs to be assigned security responsibility to champion the security efforts. Management support should be obtained through articulation of the risks to the assets, not because "HIPAA requires that we become compliant." This approach only causes management to take a "wait-and-see" approach until it is understood what other organizations are doing with the "HIPAA issue." Squarely explaining the risks, and incrementally building support through successful delivery, is the formula that will provide for longer-term benefits for maintaining the security program. Selling the protection of assets as an ongoing activity provides the view that security is not "done" at the end of the HIPAA project. The idea should be generated that information is an asset that must be managed on an ongoing basis, just like the financial, human resource, and fixed assets of the organization. While the temptation may be even stronger now that the final Security Rule has been published to use the "HIPAA hammer" to pound the message into the organization, the value of protecting the information assets, providing reduction in long-term "hidden" costs, and the opportunities enabled through secure systems should be surfaced and promoted. A HIPAA project will have a beginning and an end, but the security program to continue protecting the information assets must survive as a fundamental business operation.

The first task in the plan should be to establish security responsibility, followed by formation of security policy and review committees, development of high-level policies, network assessments, and successive implementation of policies, procedures, and technical implementations to satisfy the various aspects of the HIPAA rule. The key is to get started, somewhere, and begin making progress. Individuals within the organization may already be working on efforts related to one of the Security Standards; use this opportunity to expand the scope and ensure that the security practices are formalized and documented and will meet the HIPAA security requirements.

RISK, RISK, RISK!

It should be very apparent at this point that much of the "prescriptive" nature of the Security Rule has been changed to an approach that places the emphasis on assessing the risk and determining the implementation choices that are "reasonable and appropriate." True, different organizations may look at the same risk information pertaining to e-PHI and evaluate it differently. This is to be expected, because management teams have different value systems, experiences, and views of criticality. As time passes, industry best practices for various sizes and types of organizations, case law, civil suits, cost-effective technology innovations, standards development, an increased focus on security, and the efforts of local and national associations focused on healthcare and HIPAA will all contribute to the emergence of "*de facto* healthcare security practices." Some of these practices/standards currently exist and others will emerge prior to the compliance date, but this will be an evolutionary refinement process over time as organizations within this industry determine what security approaches support the business of healthcare. Security practices borrowed from other industries are excellent starting points for investigation. Risk assessment and risk management activities should proactively take into account the capabilities to ensure adequate protection of e-PHI.

The change away from the prescriptive nature of the Security Rule makes the rule much easier to read and understand. It also better supports the technology neutrality and scalability principles desired. Some might view the heavy reliance on the risk assessment as the lack of ability to make a "tough" standard. The more appropriate view would be that each covered entity must meet the Security Standard, and the level to which they meet that Standard must be consistent with the risk assessment results. In the case of large organizations, with the size, capabilities, and financial ability to implement the addressable specifications, they will most likely be expected to commit the resources. Taking the view that the Standard does not need to be taken seriously because it is "addressable" would be erroneous.

In the end, it is all about the risk assessment, documenting the risks, and making good judgment calls as to the security measures that are reasonable and appropriate for the covered entity's individual situation.

CONCLUSION

HIPAA should be viewed as an opportunity to address some areas that may not have received the attention in the past due to other funding priorities. Protection of health information should be viewed as an opportunity — an opportunity to place some controls around the health information, such that new processes can be enabled. Technologies continue to emerge with new, exciting possibilities, such as wireless access, personal digital assistants, digital photography advances, cell phone proliferation, and instant messaging, to name a few. These new technologies deliver new security challenges as well as new opportunities for collaboration. Creating the proper security foundation will enable these new uses to be exploited, thus increasing the availability and quality of healthcare, such as Internet health information lookup, while reducing some overhead costs, such as reducing staffing requirements (or providing more funds for increased quality) for customer service.

In the short term, the struggle will continue to move toward compliance. By starting now, HIPAA decisions can be made with more planning and less reaction to the immediate security concern.

How can a covered entity possibly achieve compliance in less than two years (three years for small health plans)? Disney World has the answer. Anyone who has been to Disney World knows that the first thing that most likely comes to mind is that it is time away in a magical place where fun things happen and the rest of life is temporarily forgotten. The second thought is the equally magical way they hide the length of the lines to the amusements by snaking around one corner, and then the next, showing only a "manageable" line of people directly in front of you. This illusion makes the line seem shorter, as they only show it to you a little at a time.

Implementing the security standards is like Disney World in many ways. It is a very long line, with many dependencies. If we tried to look at the whole line, we might just give up in frustration and decide to try again another day. If we view each security standard as a small line along the way to meeting our goal of protecting e-PHI, the effort does not seem quite so bad!

We are now at Disney World. We have been standing in line for the past several years. Now is our chance. There will be the thrill of anticipation of getting to our destination, coupled with the fear of not getting there on time. But, we are in line now, and we need to celebrate our accomplishments... one turn at a time, and maybe, just maybe, have a little fun along the way.

BIBLIOGRAPHY

Health Insurance Reform: Security Standards; Final Rule, February 20, 2003, *Federal Register 45 CFR Parts 160, 162 and 164*, Department of Health and Human Services.

Security and Electronic Signature Standards — Proposed Rule, August 12, 1998, *Federal Register 45 CFR Part 142*, Department of Health and Human Services.

Health Insurance Portability and Accountability Act of 1996, August 21, 1996, Public Law 104-191.

The Health Insurance Portability and Accountability Act of 1996 (HIPAA), Centers for Medicare and Medicaid Services, http://cms.hhs.gov/hipaa.

HIPAA Administrative Simplification, Centers for Medicare and Medicaid Services, http://cms.hhs.gov/hipaa/hipaa2.

Standards for Privacy of Individually Identifiable Health Information; Final Rule, August 14, 2002, *Federal Register 45 CFR Parts 160 and 164*, Department of Health and Human Services.

3

INCORPORATING HIPAA SECURITY REQUIREMENTS INTO AN ENTERPRISE SECURITY PROGRAM

Brian T. Geffert, CISSP, CISA

INTRODUCTION

One of the greatest challenges in any business is protecting information — in all forms — as it moves in, out, and through an organization. Because many of today's enterprise computing environments are ensembles of heterogeneous systems to which applications have been introduced one at a time, integration of each application into a cohesive system is complex. To compound the problem, paper-driven business processes tend to have makeshift origins tailored to the needs of the individual employees implementing the processes. These factors work against effective information management and protection in an organization.

With the requirements of the Health Insurance Portability and Accountability Act (HIPAA) and the growing concerns about security and privacy of all electronic personal information, organizations are now facing the reality of quickly and significantly changing the way they manage information. Thus, the gaps between current practices and the practices required for HIPAA security and privacy compliance related to personal health information present both risks and challenges to organizations. Nevertheless, these changes must be addressed and they must be implemented to meet the HIPAA security requirements.

0-8493-2211-1/05/$0.00+$1.50
© 2005 by CRC Press LLC

MEETING HIPAA SECURITY REQUIREMENTS

For the past several years, organizations across the country have been implementing the HIPAA privacy requirements while concurrently preparing their environments in anticipation of the final HIPAA security requirements. Now that the privacy regulations have become effective and the security regulations have been finalized, organizations can begin to align their enterprises with the HIPAA requirements, both to ensure that HIPAA security requirements are incorporated into their enterprise security program and that the enterprise security program is consistent with the enterprise privacy program, privacy rules, and other regulatory compliance programs that have already been implemented.

Enforcement of the HIPAA security regulations will begin in April 2005. With this deadline looming, organizations must move quickly to develop and implement compliance plans. These plans should involve:

- Compiling an inventory of the individually identifiable electronic health information that the organization maintains, including "secondary networks" that are comprised of information kept on employees' personal computers and databases and are not necessarily supported by the organization's IT department
- Conducting risk assessments to evaluate potential threats that could exploit the vulnerabilities to access protected health information within the organization's operating environment
- Developing tactical plans for addressing identified risks
- Reviewing existing information security policies to ensure they are current, consistent, and adequate to meet compliance requirements for security and privacy
- Developing new processes and policies and assigning responsibilities related to them
- Educating employees about the security and privacy policies
- Enforcement and penalties for violations
- Reviewing existing vendor contracts to ensure HIPAA compliance
- Developing flexible, scalable, viable solutions to address the security and privacy requirements

RISKS OF NONCOMPLIANCE

The security and privacy requirements of HIPAA compliance are potentially complex and costly to implement because they are broad in scope and will require ongoing attention to ensure compliance and awareness of regulatory updates as well as incorporating the updates into your security and privacy programs. There are also significant costs, risks, and criminal penalties associated with noncompliance, including:

- *Impact on business arrangements.* Noncompliance may have an impact on business partner relationships that your organization maintains with third parties.
- *Damage to reputation.* Noncompliance can lead to bad publicity, lawsuits, and damage to your brand and your credibility.
- *Loss of employee trust.* If employees are concerned about unauthorized use of their health-related information, they are likely to be less candid in providing information and more inclined to mislead employers or health professionals seeking health information.
- *Penalties.* Penalties range from $25,000 to $250,000 and one to ten years in prison for each offense.

Entities covered by HIPAA ("covered entity") are health plans, healthcare clearinghouses and healthcare providers that conduct any of the HIPAA standard transactions. These "entities" include employers that sponsor health plans (with more than 50 covered employees), health, dental, vision, and prescription drug insurers, HMOs, Medicare, Medicaid, Medicare supplement insurers, and some long-term care insurers. Other entities that do business with a covered entity and have access to health information will be indirectly affected by HIPAA.

ENTERPRISE SECURITY AND HIPAA

HIPAA privacy regulations apply to protected health information (PHI) in any form, whereas HIPAA security regulations apply almost exclusively to electronic PHI. Any approach to enterprise security affecting this information must include both, as shown in Figure 3.1. Even though the final HIPAA security standards apply only to electronic PHI (ePHI), organizations must begin their decision-making activities with a thorough understanding of the HIPAA privacy regulations that became effective April 14, 2003.

An organization's approach to HIPAA security regulations can effectively leverage the assessment information gathered and business processes developed during the implementation of HIPAA privacy regulations to support a consistent enterprisewide approach to its enterprise security projects.

THE ROLE OF INDUSTRY STANDARDS

Although an organization may be tempted to begin its security implementation by reviewing what the regulations require, most security experts agree that the organization should look first to industry standards and generally accepted practices to develop rational security solutions based on risk for the organization, and then evaluate whether HIPAA may require

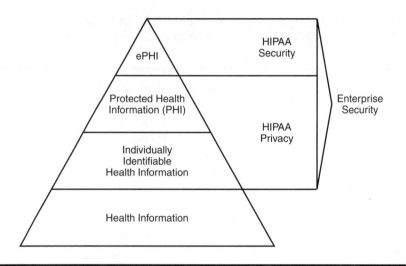

Figure 3.1   Enterprise Security

additional measures. As it turns out, the HIPAA security standards closely align with many generally accepted security standards (e.g., ISO 17799, National Institute of Standards and Technology (NIST), Common Criteria, and Centers for Medicare and Medicaid Services (CMS) standards). Moreover, organizations will be able to point to these industry standards as the basis for addressing their compliance with the HIPAA security requirements. This same risk-based approach has proven successful with other industries and regulations (e.g., GLBA in financial services) and represents an opportunity for organizations to establish and implement the best solutions for their organizations.

HIPAA security regulations allow significant flexibility as long as the organization documents through a risk analysis how its security program will meet the applicable HIPAA security requirements. This flexible, risk-based approach provides organizations with the opportunity to select and implement safeguards that will support their specific operations and environment while also meeting the HIPAA security standards. To achieve this, the organization must develop consistent, structured, and documented processes (such as decision frameworks) for ensuring that its selected security measures effectively safeguard the organization's individually identifiable health information (IIHI) as required by HIPAA.

A FLEXIBLE APPROACH: GOOD NEWS AND BAD NEWS

The final HIPAA security requirements describe what organizations should do to implement them but not how to do it, providing organizations with flexibility in addressing the individual requirements or "specifications."

This is good news for organizations because, with this flexibility, they can more easily balance the risks their particular organization faces with the costs of implementing the safeguards to address those risks.

The bad news about the flexible approach is that the regulation requires an organization to take a disciplined process-centric approach to understand and address the individual requirements.

To support this flexible and less prescriptive approach, the HIPAA security regulations introduce two new concepts: (1) required implementation specifications, and (2) addressable implementation specifications. Required implementation specifications must be implemented by all organizations subject to HIPAA security regulations. Addressable implementation specifications must be evaluated by each organization to determine whether they are reasonable and appropriate for the organization's environment, therefore allowing organizations to make implementation decisions as they relate to their operating environment. Table 3.1 summarizes the required and addressable implementation specifications included in the final HIPAA security regulations.

RISK-BASED SOLUTIONS

Organizations should choose and implement the appropriate safeguards that work in their environment based on a thorough understanding of the risks the organization faces, and selection of the appropriate safeguards should be based on the identified risks. In addition, organizations must now document the decision-making process used to select the safeguards they intend to adopt.

Addressing individual implementation specifications in an effective and efficient manner will require the development of a security decision framework for making security decisions as it relates to each organization. The framework also enables an organization to methodically and consistently review the risks it faces in its environment and to select the appropriate safeguards.

BUILDING A SECURITY DECISION FRAMEWORK

A security decision framework through which the organization can effectively and consistently review both the HIPAA security required and addressable implementation specifications can effectively be broken into a four-step process, as shown in Table 3.2.

Step 1: Business Requirements Definition

The creation of a security decision framework starts with developing a business requirements definition that addresses reasonable and practical

Table 3.1   HIPAA Security Requirements

Standard	Implementation Specifications[a]
Administrative Safeguards	
Security management process	Risk analysis (R) Risk management (R) Sanction policy (R) Information system activity review (R)
Assigned security responsibility	Security official (R)
Workforce security	Authorization and/or supervision (A) Workforce clearance procedure (A) Termination procedures (A)
Information access management	Isolating healthcare clearinghouse function (R) Access authorization (A) Access establishment and modification (A)
Security awareness and training	Security reminders (A) Protection from malicious software (A) Log-in monitoring (A) Password management (A)
Security incident procedures	Response and reporting (R)
Contingency plan	Data backup plan (R) Disaster recovery plan (R) Emergency mode operation plan (R) Testing and revision procedure (A) Applications and data criticality analysis (A)
Evaluation	Replaces "certification" (R)
Business associate contracts and other arrangements	Written contract or other arrangement (R)
Physical Safeguards	
Facility access controls	Contingency operations (A) Facility security plan (A) Access control and validation procedures (A) Maintenance records (A)
Workstation use	(R)
Workstation security	(R)

Table 3.1 HIPAA Security Requirements (continued)

Standard	Implementation Specifications[a]
Device and media controls	Disposal (R) Media reuse (R) Accountability (A) Data backup and storage (A)
Technical Safeguards	
Access control	Unique user identification (R) Emergency access procedure (R) Automatic log-off (A) Encryption and decryption (A)
Audit controls	Mechanism to record and examine ePHI systems (R)
Integrity	Mechanism to authenticate electronic PHI (A)
Person or entity authentication	(R)
Transmission security	Integrity controls (A) Encryption (A)

[a] (R) = Required; (A) = Addressable.

Table 3.2 Four-Step Process

Framework Steps	Key Activities	Key Issues
Business requirements definition	Security standards, privacy considerations	Develop reasonable and practical interpretations of HIPAA security rules
Business impact analysis	Document current environment, perform risk and safeguard analysis	Complexity, environment, risk, cost
Solution implementation	Compliance with strategy, define initiatives, define program management structure, plan projects	Develop actionable projects mapped to requirements
Compliance monitoring	Define monitoring and progress reporting, develop compliance plan, and develop management reporting process	Place projects into overall plan to report progress and compliance

interpretations of HIPAA regulations as they apply to the specific organization. Generally accepted security standards and guidelines (such as ISO 17799 and CMS), which are readily available to organizations today, can provide a context for interpreting the particular implementation specification and for understanding how certain implementation specifications have been interpreted by other groups.

For example, encrypting all of the ePHI in an organization may seem an effective way to securing information, but it is probably not practical based on current encryption methods, and it will most likely degrade the performance of the system as well as increase the costs associated with implementing such a solution.

Finally, the process of developing business requirements definitions needs to include working with both the business units and privacy program to avoid conflicts in business processes and policies. In addition, leveraging the information prepared as part of the HIPAA privacy readiness efforts (e.g., the assessment, policies, procedures, and processes) will assist most organizations with starting their efforts.

Step 2: Business Impact Analysis

The next step deals with understanding the organization's operating environment and developing a business impact analysis that addresses risks, costs, and the complexity of compliance activities in the organization's specific environment. A typical approach to HIPAA security readiness would be to apply HIPAA security requirements to the Information Technology (IT) department. This approach fails to address security as an enterprisewide function that affects all business units and all individual users alike. Also, today's Internet-driven environment is requiring ever more information sharing, even further blurring the boundaries of internal and external access. Thus, the HIPAA readiness team must segment the organization to ensure they have adequately addressed all the areas of concern for HIPAA security readiness.

The HIPAA readiness team can compartmentalize the organization in any way necessary, such as IT, strategic initiatives, key business processes, or locations; as long as they segment it in a way that makes sense to both executive management and business unit leaders who will ultimately endorse or reject the HIPAA security compliance approach.

Once the scope of the review has been defined, a risk analysis will identify the threats and the vulnerabilities faced by the organization. Gaining managerial agreement across the organization on the risks they face is important because, in the end, those managers will establish what areas are most valuable to the organization and prioritize which need to be protected. In addition, understanding what is important to the organization will help shape the enterprise security program because it will allow a focus on resources in those areas. As with any risk analysis, key stakeholders should be closely involved in the process.

Finally, based on the identified risks and using the organization's interpretations of HIPAA security regulations, the organization needs to conduct a safeguard analysis to select security measures that will account for the following factors:[1]

- The size, complexity, and capability of the organization
- The organization's technical infrastructure, hardware, and software capabilities
- The probability and criticality of the potential risk EPHI
- The cost of implementing the security measures

Once appropriate security measures are identified, they should be organized into actionable projects for implementation.

Step 3: Solution Implementation

Developing action plans mapped to the HIPAA security requirements defined in Step 1 is an essential building block in addressing HIPAA security readiness. As the organization completes the projects, executive management and key stakeholders will require periodic status reports on HIPAA readiness progress and how they link to the original plan.

Finally, due to the sheer number of projects and the amount of resources required to implement them, a formal Program Management Office (PMO) and supporting structure may be to successfully complete the projects on time and within budget. The organization does not necessarily need to create a new PMO for this purpose, but should consider leveraging an existing organizational PMO to assist them with project execution.

Step 4: Compliance Monitoring

Compliance monitoring involves ongoing measurement of the organization's conformity with HIPAA security regulations using standard monitoring and reporting templates. The compliance monitoring strategy should be incorporated into the organization's overall compliance plan that also includes the organization's existing policies, such as human resources and privacy policies.

DEPLOYING THE PEOPLE, PROCESSES, AND TECHNOLOGIES

Once the organization has developed its security decision framework for HIPAA security, the focus of its efforts should be on the components (i.e., identified risks, projects, and interpretation of requirements) within the framework and incorporating them into their overall Enterprise Security Program (ESP) and operating environment. To accomplish that, companies should develop a "road map" for prioritizing steps, creating the timeline, and developing the plan for implementing the steps. The steps in the road map are tied to specific ongoing processes involved in HIPAA security readiness. A sample of such a road map is shown below.

MERGING HIPAA INTO YOUR ENTERPRISE SECURITY PROGRAM

New solutions and modifications that enable compliance with HIPAA requirements need to be integrated into the operating environment and continuously maintained. One way to ensure this is to incorporate HIPAA security requirements and other business requirements into an overall process-oriented ESP. This approach enables the organization to shift from an IT-centric to a business-centric security focus that more effectively manages risk and more closely aligns with the HIPAA security risk-based approach.

Implementation of a program based on the proprietary Deloitte & Touche Enterprise Security Program Model shown in Figure 3.2 helps organizations develop and maintain an enterprise security program that links all necessary organizational, technical, administrative, operational controls, and physical security controls. The model incorporates a strategic combination of business drivers, legal/regulatory requirements, and acceptable risk standards to ensure they are operationally integrated with the overall IT architecture, business processes, and business culture of the organization deploying the program.

The Deloitte & Touche model enables organizations to take a bottom-up or a top-down approach, providing the flexibility to address security needs based on the maturity level of the organization's current enterprise security program and overall business priorities through five key components:

1. *Strategic Alignment.* Consensus on threats, vulnerabilities, and acceptable risks is established by leveraging ISO 17799, industry-specific standards, and strategic business drivers to create a desired risk profile to ensure that everyone is on the same page.
2. *Security Effectiveness.* A user-friendly dashboard or portal is developed to enable management to monitor and report security performance effectiveness by measuring key performance indicators of core business processes, architectures, and business management processes.

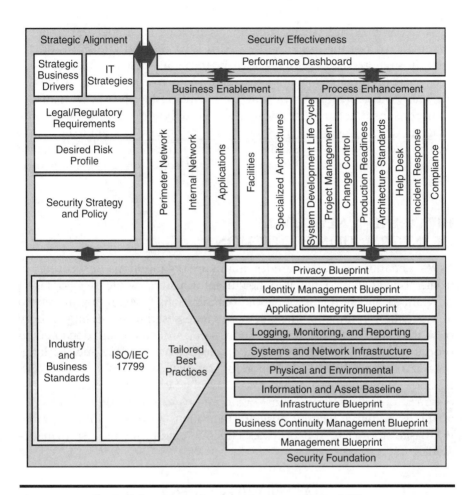

Figure 3.2   The Deloitte Enterprise Security Program Model™

3. *Business Enablement.* Core business processes and architectures are defined, developed, and deployed in concert with the core security operating model and standards-based, risk tolerance-based criteria.

4. *Process Enhancement.* Leveraging foundational blueprints, business management processes are refined and calibrated to efficiently integrate security standards and expertise throughout the system development life cycle and day-to-day operations.

5. *Security Foundation.* Standards-based, risk tolerance-based foundational blueprints are used to define, develop, and implement an enterprise-level security architecture and business operating model — a core security operating model is established.

A majority of the HIPAA security discussions fall under the strategic alignment area of the model. A desired risk profile and a business-driven security strategy are developed, in part, through facilitating management consensus on threats, vulnerabilities, and acceptable risks while maintaining links to the organization's strategic business objectives. This management consensus becomes a critical driver throughout the enterprise security program development and implementation as other important issues arise. Based on the results of these discussions and agreements, the organization can develop solutions and build the most effective implementation road map.

HIPAA AND A NEW LEVEL OF INFORMATION PROTECTION

HIPAA security regulations are forcing many organizations to secure electronic individually identifiable health information. While developing a program to protect this information, organizations have an opportunity to improve their information management processes, thus increasing security of all information. By developing a consistent, structured, and documented process to verify that HIPAA security measures are in place and working, organizations will have a foundation for compliance with other regulations. By integrating this into a process-oriented ESP that is linked with the organization's privacy programs, organizations can maintain their level of readiness within a security program that aligns with the HIPAA security risk-based approach, and provides effective enterprisewide risk management.

ACKNOWLEDGMENT

Rena Mears, Ken DeJarnette, Bill Kobel, and Terrie Kreamer also contributed their support and expertise in developing this chapter.

NOTE

1. 45 CFR Parts 160, 162 and 164; Federal Register; Vol. 68, No. 34; February 20, 2003; Page 8376; §164.306.

4

STEPS TO AN EFFECTIVE DATA CLASSIFICATION PROGRAM

Mary Brown, CISSP, CISA

INTRODUCTION

HIPAA administration simplification rules in general require that decisions about how data can be used must be made based on the sensitivity level of that data. It is important for covered entities to be able to account for all of their data and to be able to document where sensitive data exists and what controls have been put into place to protect that data. One of the ways that this can be done is by developing an effective data classification program.

Many covered entities, particularly midsized and large providers, have databases where Protected Health Information (PHI) is stored. One of the challenges to compliance with the HIPAA administrative is to identify the location of PHI so that appropriate controls can be applied. Another more daunting challenge is to develop procedures that ensure that ongoing maintenance of these controls continues on a daily basis.

An effective data classification program can be a helpful tool in ensuring that the identification of data and the development of procedures work to keep data controls up to date and well documented.

WHAT IS NEEDED PRIOR TO BEGINNING A DATA CLASSIFICATION PROGRAM?

The most essential element needed for development of a data classification program is support of senior management in general and firm sponsorship of at least one senior manager in particular. A comprehensive data classification program affects nearly all areas of a covered entity and requires resources from each of these areas to one degree or another. Data classification is not an activity that promises great rewards, although some significant ones can be realized, such as having access to a catalogue of stored data, which can often be of benefit in preventing duplication of effort across the enterprise. It is important that all stakeholders are clearly informed prior to beginning the project as to what the benefits really are in order that expectations are set at an appropriate level right off. Over-selling the benefits can result in disenchantment from stakeholders in the end. Emphasis for this project is best placed on the objective of compliance with the HIPAA security and privacy rules.

The act of classifying data is essentially only a piece of the covered entity's compliance program. Getting access to departmental resources while competing with a number of activities perceived as "more urgent" sometimes requires the intervention of the senior sponsor. Although this is a resource to be used sparingly, it can become the most critical resource in a stalled project.

Before beginning a data classification project, the decision must be made regarding the choice of technical information levels where the classification will be implemented. The two most common implementations are at the field level and at the database level. If the decision is made to classify data at the field level, the amount of resources that will be needed is much greater than if classification occurs at the database level. The advantage to classifying at the field level is that requests for data use can be expedited if the fields being requested have all been classified as public. This same request in an environment where the classification has occurred at the database level would mean that an additional analysis must occur to evaluate the fields being requested before a determination can be made as to their sensitivity levels. The advantage to classifying data at the database level is that the resources needed for classifying data can be spread over a longer period of time. The initial effort is significantly reduced and in many environments, classifying at the database level allows covered entities to begin their project in a way that allows them to make the effort at all. Many covered entities have limited resources to use and could not devote the time needed to classify data elements all at one time.

Another important element needed prior to the development of a data classification program is the existence of an enterprise policy that assigns responsibility for the safety of the information assets to specific enterprise roles. For example, in a midsized or large organization, the department head may be assigned responsibility for how the data being collected and stored as a result of the department's activities is protected from loss, damage, or inappropriate use.

Prior to implementing a data classification program, a comprehensive risk analysis of the information assets belonging to the covered entity has to occur. It is the data collected during this risk analysis that will form the foundation for the data classification program. The HIPAA security rule requires that a risk analysis be conducted as one of the first steps towards compliance with this rule.

The data gathered during the risk analysis that is integral to a data classification program includes:

- The physical and logical location of all data stores containing PHI
- Identification of the data owners, custodians, and users who depend upon this PHI to perform their jobs

Several spreadsheets or databases need to be developed to house the information being developed. This includes a metadata database that will house the inventory and data classification information, a spreadsheet that contains the department, department head, data custodians, authorized requestors, and account manager information, and finally a database of the access roles developed and the access levels assigned to each of these roles.

Data classification categories must be developed for use in assigning a level of sensitivity to each data store that is identified. The categories can be as simple as "public and private" or as complex as is needed to effectively apply the most appropriate set of controls to the data. It is recommended that the number of categories be limited as much as possible to avoid overlap and confusion in how the categories should be implemented.

Once the data and the stakeholders of the data have been identified, the enterprise information security policy has been established, approval from senior management has been obtained, the documentation systems needed to collect the information have been developed, and the classification categories have been created, the data classification project can proceed.

STEP ONE: ASSIGNMENT OF ROLES

An enterprise data classification project can be a huge undertaking and is generally being implemented for a moving target. It is impossible for a project manager, or even a project team, to control the quality of the project without enlisting the assistance of those who are closer to the data being classified.

Two important concepts within the HIPAA security and privacy rules are the need to establish accountability and to develop documentation that supports compliance with these rules. If the data classification project is to be successful long term, the need to identify those with specific responsibility for maintaining the data classification program is a crucial step to be taken, and as early in the process as possible.

In the example that charges department heads with the responsibility for the safety of the data being used within their departments, these are the stakeholders who must first be trained in the data classification process. Upon receiving their training, a large number of them will undoubtedly decide to delegate many of these activities to one or more of their subordinates. It is important to limit the number of subordinates that a department manager can use to coordinate these activities or true accountability will be lost.

Department heads will be requested to appoint from among their subordinates, the single individual who is most familiar with the data collected and used in the activities of the department. This person will be assigned the role of "data custodian" and will be the bridge between the users and the information technology and information security and privacy offices. In large departments that manage more than one major system, it may be necessary to appoint more than one data custodian.

Department heads will also be requested to identify those staff who currently request system account additions, changes, and terminations. If this activity is distributed throughout the department, the department head will be requested to centralize it among not more than three individuals within the department. These people will be assigned the role of "authorized requestor" and will be the agents of the data custodian as well as the department head.

The information technology department management will be asked to appoint from among his staff, those who are physically creating, modifying, and terminating system accounts. These individuals will be assigned the role of "account managers."

Once all of these roles have been identified, a comprehensive training program is needed to get them familiar with the HIPAA rules. They also need to understand how their roles fit in the process prior to implementation of the data classification program.

The final step is to complete the spreadsheet created for this purpose, with the departmental information and individuals assigned to fulfill each role.

STEP TWO: ASSIGNMENT OF RESPONSIBILITIES FOR EACH ROLE

As was indicated earlier, the policy that supports the data classification process assigns ultimate responsibility for the safety of PHI on a global level. In our example, the department heads are the ones responsible for this activity.

Department Heads

Department heads are busy people who therefore must be careful in their selection of appointees to the roles of data custodian and authorized requestor. The department head must be able to rely on these individuals to maintain competency in fulfilling these roles and to be consistently reliable in the discharge of these duties. Any neglect or malfeasance by any of these individuals can place the department head as well as the covered entity at risk of noncompliance with the HIPAA administrative simplification rules.

Although a number of additional controls will be implemented to ensure compliance, it is still important for department heads to take an interest in the activities of these subordinates and to develop performance measures to evaluate their performance in managing their responsibilities.

Data Custodians

Data custodians must be familiar with all of the activities occurring within their area of responsibility that pertain to the collection and use of PHI. They must also be familiar enough with the rules pertaining to the use of this data to be able to make good judgments about what activities should or should not be allowed.

Data custodians have many responsibilities in relationship to compliance with the HIPAA administrative simplification rules. Some of these responsibilities are directly related to the implementation of the data classification program and some are less directly connected but are important nonetheless. Some of these activities include providing expertise and input into data disclosure, data identification and classification, and development of appropriate access control measures.

Authorized Requestors

Also known as "trusted requestors," authorized requestors have the responsibility to process requests for access to data in a timeline that assures the access is available when it is needed. They have the responsibility to request only the access needed for the user to do the tasks for which access to data is being provided.

Authorized requestors are responsible for making sure that requests to terminate access are processed in a timeline that guarantees that access is terminated as soon as it is no longer appropriate.

Finally, authorized requestors are responsible for consulting with data custodians whenever they are unsure about a request for access they have been asked to process.

Account Managers

Account managers physically create accounts. They do not have a role in the decision as to what access is requested. They do, however, have a role in quality assurance and in seeking clarification from the security officer if a request is made that they believe to be questionable.

Account managers are responsible for processing access requests efficiently and quickly and for terminating accounts in a timely manner.

STEP THREE: DEFINE THE DATA

Before data can be classified, the data must be well defined. This activity is by far the most time-consuming and resource-intensive step in the data classification process. Most covered entities do not have well-developed data management procedures in place. Rather, databases have been developed in isolation for specific purposes with little thought to standardization or definition.

Many covered entities operate in environments where data is interfaced between systems. In this type of environment, the data should be defined at the source system and all other systems receiving this data should be pointed back to the definition at that source system.

Who defines the data can be a difficult question to answer. Information technology staff often have stewardship responsibilities for data and can play a valuable role in finding data and responding to much of the more technical documentation being gathered. They rarely are the appropriate group to define the data. This task is generally left to the users of the data. When defining enterprise-level data, the user population can be wide and diverse. It is inevitable that data elements will be found that are being used in seemingly incompatible ways. It is also inevitable that this activity will unearth a diversity of opinions as to the meaning of the data. A method for mediating disputes as to how a particular data element will be defined must be developed to avoid delays and dissention within the project.

STEP FOUR: FIND AND CLASSIFY DATA

The most efficient way of locating and classifying data is by having a project manager meet with each data custodian and collect information regarding each database being managed by his or her department.

The information that should be gathered may vary according to the needs of the organization but at a minimum should include:

- Name of the database
- Purpose of the database

- Application in which the database was written
- Operating system that the database uses
- Physical location of the database
- Logical address of the database
- Whether the database contains sensitive information
- Contact name and information of the database administrator
- Contact name and information of the data custodian

The final step is to evaluate this information, document it in the database created to house the classification data, and assign a classification category based on the information gathered.

Classification categories are ideally applied at the data element level but the amount of resources needed to implement classification in this way can be overwhelming to most organizations. It is recommended that classification categories be applied at the database level and that element classification be implemented over time as the resources can be made available.

STEP FIVE: CREATION OF ACCESS PROFILES USING ROLE-BASED ACCESS

In order to create access profiles, the project manager and data custodians must first use the database designed for collection of the role-based access data to populate all of the roles for which access is assigned within the department. This database should include the systems currently being used by these departmental users and the tasks that they are accomplishing by the use of the data.

Once all of the data custodians have completed the documentation of their existing departmental roles and the data needs of these roles, the project manager can analyze the data at the enterprise level. For example, most hospitals have a role of station clerk. By analyzing the tasks conducted within each department by the person in this role, access can be tailored for this role in such a way that only the minimal amount of information is made available, and the information available is consistent within this role.

The obvious advantage to the development of sensitivity levels and access roles is that a covered entity can demonstrate easily what systems contain PHI and what decisions were made to assign access to this sensitive information.

STEP SIX: DEVELOPMENT OF A MAINTENANCE PLAN

Now that all of the work has been done to support the data classification program, the final step is to put into place the activities needed to maintain the timeliness and accuracy of the information.

Data custodian appointments must be kept current by department heads. This role is the key role assigned the responsibility of maintaining changes to the data classification information.

Changes to systems must be kept current. For example, if a database was assigned a classification of "public" at the initial assessment but new fields are to be added that are sensitive, a review process must be put into place that will allow for the associated change in the classification of the database to be implemented and documented. For enterprises where a formal change management process is in place, this step can be incorporated into that process. The owner of the change being requested has responsibility for ensuring that this activity is included in the process. Responsibility for this activity should also be assigned to the data custodian who should also ensure that this activity has occurred prior to moving changes into production.

A procedure must be developed whereby all new development includes a classification and documentation component. For enterprises where a formal project management process is in place, this step can be incorporated into the process. Responsibility for this activity lies with the project manager but the data custodian for the department where the system is being implemented should also ensure that this classification procedure has taken place prior to implementing the new database.

An effective audit program is the final piece in a maintenance program. IT audit or information security staff are generally held responsible for conducting periodic compliance audits. It is this layering of responsibilities that provides a firm base for maintaining compliance with a data classification program.

SUMMARY

A data classification program is a powerful tool for covered entities to use in maintaining compliance with the HIPAA security and privacy rules. The initial expenditure of resources can be significant but contribute significantly to better data management for the organization as a whole, as well as providing compliance benefits. Data classification plays a role in assignment of access rights to PHI. Compliance with the data disclosure activities also is made easier by knowing what systems hold PHI and require usage tracking necessary for providing an accounting when it is requested. Finally, the data classification project provides beneficial information a covered entity needs in establishing the designated record sets by helping to locate data stores that are being used to make decisions about patients.

The initial decision to classify data at the database or system level, rather than beginning with field-level classifications, can assist organizations in offsetting some of the initial costs related to data classification and can provide a firm base for ongoing efforts to classify data elements.

An effective data classification program depends most heavily on the support of senior management and the active participation of an executive sponsor. The expectations of senior management are best expressed through the development of a formal policy that clearly assigns responsibility for data classification activities.

A data classification program routinely requires the involvement of the information technology department in development of the databases, spreadsheets, or other data storage resources needed to house all of the information being gathered through the course of the program. These data storage resources are most effective when they are housed in an area accessible by all staff; however, careful controls must be put in place to ensure that only those authorized to make changes to the information actually have the ability to do so.

The core data classification activities of locating, defining, and classifying data must be assigned to the users who really understand the meaning of the data and how it is being used. Expertise from information technology and information security staff must be made available but the activities themselves are heavily reliant on user expertise.

The nature of a data classification program is that it spans the enterprise. For organizations not accustomed to operating in a matrix environment, obtaining departmental resources can become an issue. It is at this point when the executive sponsor needs to step in and facilitate so that resources are available when needed.

Development of a maintenance program is essential to the success of a data classification program. Investing the resources needed to ensure that the classification process continues as an integral part of the organization must occur or the process will become ineffective almost immediately and the resources invested will be wasted.

Creating a data classification program in a midsized or large organization is a large undertaking and should only be attempted with the full support of senior management. The value of ensuring compliance with the HIPAA security and privacy rules makes undertaking this effort worthwhile.

II

STANDARDS AND COMPLIANCE

5

HIPAA SECURITY AND THE ISO/IEC 17799

Uday O. Ali Pabrai, S+, CHSS, SCNA

INTRODUCTION

In this chapter we examine the International Organization for Standardization (ISO)/International Electrotechnical Commission (IEC) 17799:2000 security standard and compare it to the categories established in the HIPAA security rule. Whereas HIPAA security establishes requirements across five categories (domains), the ISO/IEC 17799 standard includes ten domains that organizations must address for a secure infrastructure. There is significant overlap between these two specifications, although they are organized very differently. Also, major differences include the fact that the HIPAA security rule is closely tied into the HIPAA privacy rule and its scope is limited to electronic Protected Health Information (ePHI) only.

ISO 17799 AND HIPAA

In this section we review the ISO/IEC 17799 and British Standard (BS) 7799 security standards. ISO/IEC 17799:2000 is a detailed security standard. The standard covers ten areas and was published in December 2000. The BS 7799 and the ISO/IEC 17799 are very similar standards — the ISO/IEC 17799 standard includes two nonaction sections at the start of the document. The standards are organized into ten major sections, each covering a different topic or area. The first area covered by the standard is security policy.

ISO/IEC 17799 Standard

The ISO/IEC 17799 is a code of practice for information security management. This standard gives recommendations for information security management for use by those who are responsible for initiating, implementing, or maintaining security in their organization. The standard is based on the principle of the preservation of the confidentiality, integrity, and availability of information.

This document is formally referred to as the ISO/IEC 17799:2000 Information technology — Code of practice for information security management.

The ten domains of the ISO/IEC 17799 standard are:

1. Security Policy
2. Organizational Security
3. Asset Classification and Control
4. Personnel Security
5. Physical and Environmental Security
6. Communications and Operations Management
7. Access Control
8. Systems Development and Maintenance
9. Business Continuity Planning
10. Compliance

Information on the ISO/IEC 17799 standard is available from the American National Standards Institute (ANSI) at www.ansi.org.

ISO/IEC 17799 Web Site

To get more information on the ISO/IEC 17799:2000 security standard, visit: http://www.iso.ch/iso/en/prods-services/popstds/informationsecurity.html.

The final HIPAA security rule outlines the requirements in five major categories:

1. Physical safeguards
2. Administrative safeguards
3. Technical safeguards
4. Organizational requirements
5. Policies, procedures, and documentation requirements

Let us take a closer look at the HIPAA security rule's administrative, physical, and technical safeguard categories. These categories are then compared to the domains defined in the ISO/IEC 17799 standard.

The administrative safeguards category forms the foundation on which the other standards depend. Covered entities are required to implement administrative, physical, and technical safeguards. These entities must ensure that data is protected, to the extent feasible, from inappropriate access, modification, dissemination, and destruction.

Administrative safeguards are administrative actions, policies, and procedures to manage the selection, development, implementation, and maintenance of security measures to protect ePHI and to manage the conduct of the covered entity's workforce in relation to the protection of that information.

Physical safeguards are physical measures, policies, and procedures to protect a covered entity's electronic information systems and related buildings and equipment from natural and environmental hazards, and unauthorized intrusion.

Technical safeguards refer to the technology and the policy and procedures for its use that protect ePHI and control access to it.

The HIPAA security rule makes no distinction between internal networks and external networks — both need to be secured. Furthermore, the HIPAA security rule covers ePHI at rest (i.e., in storage) as well as during transmission. Covered entities must protect ePHI when they transmit information. The HIPAA security rule requires protection of the same scope of information as that covered by the privacy rule, except that it only covers that information if it is in electronic form. Per the HIPAA security rule, a covered entity's responsibility to implement security standards extends to the members of its workforce, whether they work at home or on site. Documentation related to the HIPAA security rule implementation must be retained for a period of six years.

In the HIPAA security rule, the implementation specification may either be a required implementation specification or an addressable implementation specification. The concept of addressable implementation specifications is to provide covered entities additional flexibility with respect to compliance with the security standards. A covered entity will do one of the following for addressable implementation specifications:

- Implement one or more of the addressable implementation specifications
- Implement one or more alternative security measures
- Implement a combination of both
- Not implement either an addressable implementation specification or an alternative security measure

After its own risk analysis, risk mitigation strategy, an assessment of what security measures may already be in place, and the cost of implementation, the covered entity must decide:

- If your organization determines that a given addressable implementation specification is reasonable and appropriate for it, then you must implement it.
- If you determine that one of the addressable implementation specifications is not inappropriate and/or is an unreasonable security measure, but the standard cannot be met without implementation of an additional security safeguard, the organization may implement an alternate measure that accomplishes the same end as the addressable implementation specification.
- An entity that meets a given standard through alternative measures must document the decision to not implement the addressable implementation specification, the rationale behind that decision, and the alternative safeguard implemented to meet the standard.
- A covered entity may also decide that a given implementation specification is simply not applicable (i.e., neither reasonable nor appropriate) to its situation and that the standard can be met without implementation of an alternative measure in place of the addressable implementation specification. In this scenario, the covered entity must document the decision not to implement the addressable specification, the rationale behind that decision, and how the standard is being met.

For example, under the information access management standard, an access establishment and modification implementation specification reads: "implement policies and procedures that, based upon the entity's access authorization policies, establish, document, review, and modify a user's right of access to a workstation, transaction, program, or process." It is possible that a small practice, with one or more individuals equally responsible for establishing and maintaining all automated patient records, will not need to establish policies and procedures for granting access to that electronic protected health information because the access rights are equal for all of the individuals.

Our advice would be to follow the HIPAA security rule requirements very closely, as that will enable your organization to become compliant with the legislation. However, our advice is also to be very aware of the ISO/IEC specifications as that may lead to a more complete implementation of security activities.

Approach and Philosophy

HIPAA requires that the security measures by all covered entities must be documented and kept current. Keep in mind that the HIPAA security standards are designed to be:

- *Comprehensive* — they cover all aspects of security safeguards including:
  - Identification
  - Authentication
  - Access control
  - Accountability and nonrepudiation
  - Integrity
  - Communications
  - Administration
- *Technology neutral* — standards can be implemented using a broad range of off-the-shelf and user-developed technologies and security solutions
- *Scalable* — the goals of the regulations can be achieved by entities of all sizes from single practitioners to large multinational healthcare organizations

The regulations explicitly recognize that very small organizations will be able to satisfy the requirements with less elaborate approaches than larger, more complex organizations.

The security rule does not address the extent to which a particular entity should implement the standards and implementation specifications. Instead, the security rule requires that each covered entity assess its own security needs and risks and devise, implement, and maintain appropriate security to address its business requirements. How individual security requirements would be satisfied and which technology to use would be business decisions that each organization would have to make.

Security Principles

Under the HIPAA security rule, security of health information is especially important when health information can be directly linked to an individual. For example, confidentiality is threatened not only by the risk of improper access to electronically stored information, but also by the risk of interception during electronic transmission of the information.

The HIPAA security rule consists of the requirements that a healthcare entity must address in order to safeguard the confidentiality, integrity, and availability of its electronic data. It also describes the implementation features that must be present in order to satisfy each requirement. The central principles of security are:

- Confidentiality
- Integrity
- Availability

Security-related impairment generally includes, but is not limited to, "damaging disclosure or the asset to unauthorized recipients (*loss of confidentiality*), damage to the asset through unauthorized modification (*loss of integrity*), or unauthorized deprivation of access to the asset (*loss of availability*)."

The HIPAA security rule requires that each healthcare entity engaged in electronic maintenance or transmission of health information assess potential risks and vulnerabilities to the individual health data in its possession in electronic form, and develop, implement, and maintain appropriate security measures. Most important, these measures must be documented and kept current.

These principles are consistent with what is in the ISO/IEC 17799 standard. The ISO/IEC 17799 standard clearly states that information security is characterized by the preservation of confidentiality, integrity, and availability of information. The scope of the HIPAA security rule is limited to ePHI whereas that of the ISO/IEC 17799 covers information in all formats including paper, electronic, or oral.

SECURITY POLICY

The objectives of this section in the ISO/IEC 17799 standard are to provide management direction and support for information security. The information security policy document is a written policy document that must be developed and made available to all employees. The security policy document must have an owner (e.g., the security officer), and this individual must be responsible for maintaining and updating the document on a regular basis.

HIPAA Security Policy

The HIPAA security rule includes the policies, procedures, and documentation requirements. This requirement includes two standards:

1. Policies and procedures standard
2. Documentation standard

HIPAA Policies and Procedures Standard

A covered entity must implement reasonable and appropriate policies and procedures to comply with the standards and implementation specifications. This standard is not to be construed to permit or excuse an action that violates any other standard, implementation specification, or other requirements of this subpart. A covered entity may change its policies and procedures at any time, provided that the changes are documented and are implemented in accordance with this subpart.

HIPAA Documentation Standard

A covered entity must maintain the policies and procedures implemented to comply with this subpart in written (which may be electronic) form. If an action, activity, or assessment is required to be documented, the covered entity must maintain a written (which may be electronic) record of the action, activity, or assessment.

The implementation specifications of the documentation standard are:

- Time limit (Required)
- Availability (Required)
- Updates (Required)

Time Limit (Required)

Retain the documentation required for six years from the date of its creation or the date when it last was in effect, whichever is later.

Availability (Required)

Make documentation available to those persons responsible for implementing the procedures to which the documentation pertains.

Updates (Required)

Review documentation periodically, and update as needed, in response to environmental or operational changes affecting the security of the electronic protected health information.

The ISO/IEC 17799 standard and HIPAA security rule are fairly consistent in emphasizing the importance of management setting a clear policy direction and commitment to information security and communicating the message in information security policies across the organization.

SECURITY ORGANIZATION

The objectives of this section in the ISO/IEC 17799 standard are:

- *Information security infrastructure:* To manage information security within the organization
- *Security of third-party access:* To maintain the security of organizational information-processing facilities and information assets accessed by third parties

The responsibility for the management of the security of the infrastructure for covered entities rests with the individual who is assigned security responsibility — this is a HIPAA security rule requirement. Also, the security of third-party access maps closely to the organizational requirements under the HIPAA security rule. The ISO/IEC 17799 objective states that the security of a third party's information-processing facilities and information assets must be maintained. Furthermore, access to the organization's information-processing facilities by third parties should be controlled.

The ISO/IEC 17799 domain also emphasizes the need for addressing the security requirements of an organization in outsourcing contracts. Outsourcing arrangements should address the risks, security controls, and procedures for processing of all sensitive business information in the contract between the entities.

HIPAA Organizational Requirements

This includes the standard business associate contracts or other arrangements. A covered entity is not in compliance with the standard if the covered entity knew of a pattern of activity or practice of the business associate that constituted a material breach or violation of the business associate's obligation under the contract or other arrangement, unless the covered entity took reasonable steps to cure the breach or end the violation, as applicable. If such steps were unsuccessful:

■ Terminate the contract or arrangement, if feasible.
■ If termination is not feasible, report the problem to the secretary (DHHS).

Table 5.1 summarizes organizational security requirements in the HIPAA security rule.

Table 5.1 Organizational Security Requirements in the HIPAA Security Rule

Standards	Implementation Specifications	R = Required A = Addressable
Administrative safeguards' assigned security responsibility		R
Administrative safeguards' business associate contracts and other arrangement	Written contract or other arrangement	R

The required implementation specifications associated with this standard are:

- Business associate contracts
- Other arrangements

Business Associate Contracts

The contract between a covered entity and a business associate must provide that the business associate will:

- Implement administrative, physical, and technical safeguards that reasonably and appropriately protect the confidentiality, integrity, and availability of the electronic protected health information that it creates, receives, maintains, or transmits on behalf of the covered entity.
- Ensure that any agent, including a subcontractor, to whom it provides such information agrees to implement reasonable and appropriate safeguards to protect it.
- Report to the covered entity any security incident of which it becomes aware.
- Authorize termination of the contract by the covered entity, if the covered entity determines that the business associate has violated a material term of the contract.

Other Arrangements

When a covered entity and its business associate are both governmental entities, the covered entity is in compliance if:

- It enters into a memorandum of understanding with the business associate.
- Other law (including regulations adopted by the covered entity or its business associate) contains requirements applicable to the business associate.

If a business associate is required by law to perform a function or activity on behalf of a covered entity or to provide a service described in the definition of business associate, the covered entity may permit the business associate to create, receive, maintain, or transmit electronic protected health information on its behalf to the extent necessary to comply with the legal mandate without meeting the requirements of this section, provided that the covered entity attempts in good faith to obtain satisfactory assurances as required and documents the attempt and the reasons that these assurances cannot be obtained.

The covered entity may omit from its other arrangements authorization of the termination of the contract by the covered entity, if such authorization is inconsistent with the statutory obligations of the covered entity or its business associate.

Group Health Plan

Except when the only electronic protected health information disclosed to a plan sponsor is disclosed as authorized, a group health plan must ensure that its plan documents provide that the plan sponsor will reasonably and appropriately safeguard electronic protected health information created, received, maintained, or transmitted to or by the plan sponsor on behalf of the group health plan.

The plan documents of the group health plan must be amended to incorporate provisions to require the plan sponsor to:

- Implement administrative, physical, and technical safeguards that reasonably and appropriately protect the confidentiality, integrity, and availability of the electronic protected health information that it creates, receives, maintains, or transmits on behalf of the group health plan.
- Ensure that the adequate separation required is supported by reasonable and appropriate security measures.
- Ensure that any agent, including a subcontractor, to whom it provides this information agrees to implement reasonable and appropriate security measures to protect the information.
- Report to the group health plan any security incident of which it becomes aware.

The ISO/IEC 17799 standard clearly establishes, as does the HIPAA security rule, that responsibility for security leadership should be formalized and assigned to an individual. This individual will coordinate the implementation of security across the organization.

ASSET CLASSIFICATION AND CONTROL

The objectives of this section in the ISO/IEC 17799 standard are:

- *Accountability of assets:* To maintain appropriate protection of corporate assets
- *Information classification:* To ensure that information assets receive an appropriate level of protection

Table 5.2 HIPAA Security Rule's Requirements Related to Asset Classification

Standards	Implementation Specifications	R = Required A = Addressable
Administrative safeguards' system management process	Risk analysis	R
	Risk management	R
	Information system activity review	R

This domain establishes the requirement that all major information assets should be accounted for and have a nominated owner. Accountability should remain with the nominated owner of the asset. Information classification as well as information labeling and handling are emphasized in this domain.

HIPAA System Management Process

This ISO/IEC 17799 domain requirement is most closely seen in the HIPAA security rule in the system management process standard requirements related to risk analysis and management as well as an information system activity review.

Table 5.2 summarizes requirements related to review of systems and processes under the HIPAA security rule.

In this domain, the ISO/IEC 17799 standard emphasizes that organizations must maintain an appropriate protection of organizational assets. This is similar to the requirements defined for risk analysis and management in the HIPAA security rule.

PERSONNEL SECURITY

The objectives of this section in the ISO/IEC 17799 standard are:

- *Security in job definition and resources:* To reduce risks of human error, theft, fraud, or misuse of facilities
- *User training:* To ensure that users are aware of information security threats and concerns, and are equipped to support the corporate security policy in the course of their normal work
- *Responding to incidents:* To minimize the damage from security incidents and malfunctions and learn from such incidents

Training as well as incident response is emphasized in this domain. The domain clearly states that users must be aware of information security threats and concerns, and must be equipped to support organizational security policy in the course of their normal work. All employees should also be made aware of the procedures for reporting security incidents that might have an impact on the security of the organizational assets. The HIPAA security rule also establishes training and incident procedures as standards in the legislation.

HIPAA Workforce Security

The HIPAA security rule has specific requirements related to workforce security in its administrative safeguards section. Administrative safeguards are administrative actions, policies, and procedures to manage the selection, development, implementation, and maintenance of security measures to protect ePHI and to manage the conduct of the covered entity's workforce in relation to the protection of that information.

Table 5.3 summarizes standards and implementation specifications related to workforce security in the HIPAA security rule.

Table 5.3   HIPAA Security's Workforce Security Requirements

Standards	Implementation Specifications	R = Required A = Addressable
Administrative safeguards' security management process	Sanction policy	R
Administrative safeguards' workforce security	Authorization and/or supervision	A
	Workforce clearance procedure	A
	Termination procedures	A
Administrative safeguards' security awareness and training	Security reminders	A
	Protection from malicious software	A
	Log-in monitoring	A
	Password management	A
Administrative safeguards' security incident procedures	Response and reporting	R

Both the ISO/IEC 17799 standard and the HIPAA security rule emphasize workforce security or personnel security extensively in the specifications.

PHYSICAL AND ENVIRONMENTAL SECURITY

The objectives of this section in the ISO/IEC 17799 standard are:

- *Secure areas:* To prevent unauthorized access, damage, and interference to business premises and information
- *Equipment inventory:* To prevent loss, damage, or compromise of assets and interruption of business activities

HIPAA Physical Safeguards

The HIPAA security rule's physical safeguards requirements address the protection of physical computer systems and related buildings and equipment from fire, other natural and environmental hazards, and intrusion. Physical safeguards include physical security access, card access solutions, paper destruction procedures, and computer room access. The use of locks, keys, and administrative measures used to control access to all computing systems and facilities management are also included.

Table 5.4 summarizes standards and implementation specifications defined in the physical safeguards category.

Table 5.4   HIPAA Security Physical Safeguards

Standards	Implementation Specifications	R = Required A = Addressable
Facility access controls	Contingency operations	A
	Facility security plan	A
	Access control and validation procedures	A
	Maintenance records	A
Workstation use		R
Workstation security		R
Device and media controls	Disposal	R
	Media reuse	R
	Accountability	A
	Data backup and storage	A

Both the ISO/IEC 17799 standard and the HIPAA security rule emphasize physical security extensively in the specifications.

COMMUNICATIONS AND OPERATIONS MANAGEMENT

The objectives of this section in the ISO/IEC 17799 standard are:

- *Operational procedures and responsibilities:* To ensure the correct and secure operation of information processing facilities
- *System planning and acceptance:* To minimize the risk of systems failures
- *Protection from malicious software:* To protect the integrity of software and information
- *Housekeeping:* To maintain the integrity and availability of information processing and communication
- *Network management:* To ensure the safeguarding of information in networks and the protection of the supporting infrastructure
- *Media handling and security:* To prevent damage to assets and interruptions to business activities
- *Data and software exchange:* To prevent loss, modification, or misuse of information exchanged between organizations

HIPAA Integrity Controls and Transmission Security

The HIPAA security rule establishes specific requirements related to transmission of information as well as integrity controls. Table 5.5 summarizes implementation specifications related to integrity and information transmission in the HIPAA security rule. This addresses both integrity controls as well as encryption.

Table 5.5   Integrity-Related HIPAA Security Rule Requirements

Standards	Implementation Specifications	R = Required A = Addressable
Technical safeguard's integrity	Mechanism to authenticate electronic PHI	A
Technical safeguard's transmission security	Integrity controls	A
	Encryption	A

Both the ISO/IEC 17799 standard and the HIPAA security rule emphasize transmission security extensively in the specifications. Both specifications clearly state the requirement for security of data at rest as well as in motion (transmission).

ACCESS CONTROL

The objectives of this section in the ISO/IEC 17799 standard are:

- *Business requirements for system access:* To control access to business information
- *User access management:* To prevent unauthorized access to information systems
- *User responsibilities:* To prevent unauthorized user access
- *Network access control:* To ensure the protection of networked services
- *Computer access control:* To prevent unauthorized computer access
- *Application access control:* To prevent unauthorized access to information held in computer systems
- *Monitoring system access and use:* To detect unauthorized activities

HIPAA Access Controls

HIPAA security rule's technical safeguards refer to the technology and the policy and procedures for its use that protect ePHI and control access to it. This category includes requirements related to access controls as shown in Table 5.6.

Both the ISO/IEC 17799 standard and the HIPAA security rule emphasize access control requirements extensively in the specifications.

SYSTEM DEVELOPMENT AND MAINTENANCE

The objectives of this section in the ISO/IEC 17799 standard are:

- *Security requirements of systems:* To ensure security is built into operational systems
- *Security in application systems:* To prevent loss, modification, or misuse of user data in application systems
- *Security of application system files:* To ensure IT projects and support activities are conducted in a secure manner
- *Security in development and support environments:* To maintain the security of application system software and data

Table 5.6   HIPAA Security's Access Control Requirements

Standards	Implementation Specifications	R = Required A = Addressable
Administrative safeguards' information access management	Isolating healthcare clearinghouse function	R
	Access authorization	A
	Access establishment and modification	A
Technical safeguards' access control	Unique user identification	R
	Emergency access procedure	R
	Automatic log-off	A
	Encryption and decryption	A
Person or entity authentication		R

This domain is not directly addressed in the HIPAA security rule, although certain areas such as encryption are addressed as implementation specification in the technical safeguards category of the HIPAA security rule.

BUSINESS CONTINUITY PLANNING

The objectives of this section in the ISO/IEC 17799 standard are to counteract interruptions to business activities and to support critical business processes from the effects of major failures or disasters. This includes:

■ Business continuity planning process
■ Business continuity planning framework
■ Testing business continuity plans
■ Updating business continuity plans

HIPAA CONTINGENCY PLAN REQUIREMENTS

HIPAA security rule's requirements for contingency planning are defined in the administrative safeguards section of the legislation. Table 5.7 summarizes implementation specifications related to contingency planning in the HIPAA security rule.

Table 5.7   HIPAA Security Rule's Contingency Plan Requirements

Standards	Implementation Specifications	R = Required A = Addressable
Contingency plan	Data backup plan	R
	Disaster recovery plan	R
	Emergency mode operation plan	R
	Testing and revision procedure	A
	Applications and data criticality analysis	A

Both the ISO/IEC 17799 standard and the HIPAA security rule emphasize business continuity extensively in the specifications. Business continuity directly relates to the security principle of availability. Both ISO/IEC 17799 and HIPAA are fairly consistent in the requirements in this area.

COMPLIANCE

The objectives of this section in the ISO/IEC 17799 standard are:

- *Compliance with legal requirements:* To avoid breaches of any criminal or civil law, statutory, regulatory, or contractual obligations, and of any security requirements
- *Security review of IT systems:* To ensure compliance of systems with organizational security policies and standards
- *System audit considerations:* To maximize the effectiveness of and to minimize interference to/from the system audit process

HIPAA Security Core Requirements

The HIPAA security rule is a United States legislative requirement that must be complied with by all covered entities. The final HIPAA security rule outlines the requirements in five major categories:

1. Administrative safeguards
2. Physical safeguards
3. Technical safeguards
4. Organizational requirements
5. Policies, procedures, and documentation requirements

Table 5.8 HIPAA Security Rule's Evaluation Requirement

Standards	Implementation Specifications	R = Required A = Addressable
Administrative safeguard's evaluation		R

Table 5.9 HIPAA Security's Audit Controls Requirement

Standards	Implementation Specifications	R = Required A = Addressable
Technical safeguard's audit controls		R

HIPAA Security Review

Table 5.8 summarizes requirements related to review of systems and processes under the HIPAA security rule.

HIPAA Audit Controls

HIPAA security rule's technical safeguards refer to the technology and the policy and procedures for its use that protect ePHI and control access to it. This category includes requirements related to audit controls as shown in Table 5.9.

Both the ISO/IEC 17799 standard and the HIPAA security rule emphasize requirements related to review and audit extensively in the specifications. You cannot protect what you do not know — this domain establishes the need to periodically review and audit the critical elements of an organization's infrastructure.

SUMMARY

The ISO/IEC 17799 is an important security standard that provides a useful reference to any HIPAA security officer's activities. We understand that the core objective of HIPAA is to protect individuals from the unapproved and unwarranted release of information related to their personal health. The objective of the HIPAA security rule is to protect the storage and transmission of ePHI. For ePHI maintained or transmitted by covered entities, the security rule addresses the steps that the covered entity must take to prevent unauthorized:

- Disclosure
- Destruction
- Corruption

The identification of solutions to meet the requirements of the security rule must take into account:

- HIPAA security rule standards and implementation specifications that must be supported by the enterprise
- Threats to the entity
- Requirements related to the privacy rule such as flow of PHI and business associates

The ISO/IEC 17799 and the HIPAA security rule consist of the requirements that an entity must address in order to safeguard the confidentiality, integrity, and availability of its sensitive information. The recommendations from the HIPAA security rule state that all organizations that handle ePHI — regardless of size — should implement and address standards and implementation specifications identified in the categories of administrative, physical, and technical safeguards.

The standard does not address the extent to which a particular entity should implement the specific features that have been defined. The HIPAA security rule requires that each healthcare entity engaged in electronic maintenance or transmission of health information assess potential risks and vulnerabilities to the individual health data in its possession in electronic form, and develop, implement, and maintain appropriate security measures.

Most important, these measures must be documented and kept current. How individual security requirements would be satisfied and which technology to use would be business decisions that each pharmacy organization would have to make.

My strong recommendation is for organizations to view the HIPAA security rule as a starting point, not an end point, and to go beyond HIPAA security requirements in defending business assets and information. This is where the information in the ISO/IEC 17799 standard can provide further guidance to activities being initiated by covered entities. At the very least, an awareness of the ISO/IEC 17799 standard can influence the scope of security activities of the organizations.

6

EXECUTION OF A SELF-DIRECTED RISK ASSESSMENT METHODOLOGY TO ADDRESS HIPAA DATA SECURITY REQUIREMENTS

Johnathan Coleman, CISSP, CISM

INTRODUCTION

This chapter analyzes the method and training of a self-directed risk assessment methodology entitled OCTAVE[sm] (Operationally Critical Threat Asset and Vulnerability Evaluation) at over 200 DOD medical treatment facilities. It focuses specifically on how OCTAVE built interdisciplinary hierarchical consensus and enhanced local capabilities to perform health information assurance. The risk assessment methodology was developed by the Software Engineering Institute at Carnegie Mellon University as part of the Defense Health Information Assurance Program (DHIAP). The basis for its success is the combination of analysis of organizational practices and technological vulnerabilities. Together, these areas address the core implications behind the HIPAA security rule and can be used to develop organizational protection strategies and technological mitigation plans. A key component of OCTAVE is the interdisciplinary composition of the analysis team (patient administration, IT staff, and clinician). It is this unique composition of analysis team members, along with organizational and technical analysis of business practices, assets, and threats, that enables facilities to create sound and effective security policies. The risk assessment is conducted in-house, and therefore the process, results, and knowledge remain within the organization, helping to build consensus in an environment of differing organizational and disciplinary perspectives on health information assurance.

Information Security Management Concepts

Krutz and Vines[1] discuss information security management concepts in terms of the security requirements: Confidentiality, Integrity, and Availability (or the "CIA triad"). When reviewing these requirements for sensitive medical information that is stored on paper (such as patients' paper medical records) it is easy to visualize some basic controls that illustrate the presence of these security requirements. For example, it is generally understood by healthcare employees that a patient's paper medical record should be physically stored in a controlled area and should only be viewed by an authorized person, an attempt to maintain confidentiality. It should only be written to or modified by an appropriately authorized person, a document integrity control. Records should be labeled and managed appropriately, thereby ensuring they can be located quickly and are available when needed, an information availability control. Procedures to implement the same three security measures of confidentiality, integrity, and availability for a patient's electronic paper record are less tangible and not so easily visualized. A network-based electronic patient record has many possible access points (e.g., computer workstations) and in some cases, where the record can be obtained remotely over the Internet, the possible access points are too numerous to quantify. In terms of data integrity, role-based access control is one method of helping to manage who can modify a record, but it is not so easy to confirm that a person's digital identity matches that of his or her actual identity (password and user-name sharing is an obvious example). We have become increasingly reliant upon the use of technology to perform our business functions, and our business practices have developed based upon a level of expectation of the availability of such technology. Technical measures to ensure availability of service are often complex, and require detailed planning and changes to organizational practices in order for a high level of redundancy to exist.

Background on HIPAA Privacy and Security

The privacy provisions of the federal law, the Health Insurance Portability and Accountability Act of 1996 (HIPAA), apply to health information created or maintained by healthcare providers who engage in certain electronic transactions, health plans, and healthcare clearinghouses. The Department of Health and Human Services (DHHS) has issued the regulation "Standards for Privacy of Individually Identifiable Health Information,"[2] applicable to entities covered by HIPAA. The Office for Civil Rights[3]

(OCR) is the departmental component responsible for implementing and enforcing the privacy regulation. The final rule was published in the *Federal Register* (65 FR 82462) on December 28, 2000 and final modifications published on August 14, 2002. The rule effective date was April 14, 2001 and covered entities (certain healthcare providers, health plans, and healthcare clearinghouses) are required to comply with the HIPAA privacy rule by the compliance date of April 14, 2003 (April 14, 2004, for small health plans). The privacy rule includes the requirement for covered entities to have in place "appropriate *administrative, technical and physical* safeguards to protect the privacy of protected health information" (45 CFR §164.530 (c)(1)) regardless of the form in which it is used—on paper, electronically, and verbally. To satisfy the HIPAA privacy rule "safeguards" requirements, sites should examine their operational practices, determine where and how patient information is used, and address circumstances that place the information at risk. The investigation should evaluate how people accomplish their work, including both their operational practices and their use of computer systems.

The final rule adopting HIPAA standards for the security of electronic health information was published in the *Federal Register* on February 20, 2003. Under the published rule, each covered entity must "*conduct an accurate and thorough assessment of the potential risks and vulnerabilities to the confidentiality, integrity and availability of electronic protected health information held by the covered entity*" (§164.308 (a,1,ii,A)). These measures must be documented and kept current. The standards are applicable to the same organizations as the privacy rule. The security standards set guidelines for developing and maintaining the security of all *electronic* individual health data. They also specify the minimum requirements and implementation features that must be included in the security measures and cite, among other items, the need for a contingency plan that incorporates data backup plans, disaster recovery plans, and business continuity plans.

The proposed security rule supports that privacy rule by specifying requirements for protecting information that is in electronic form. Because it is possible that a technical security breach in a computing system could result in an unintended disclosure of personally identifiable health information, it is possible that such a breach may also be the cause of a consequential violation of the HIPAA privacy rule.

DEVELOPMENT OF A RISK ASSESSMENT METHODOLOGY TO BE USED AS A DECENTRALIZED INFORMATION ASSURANCE DECISION-MAKING TOOL

The specific requirement under the HIPAA security rule to conduct a risk and vulnerability assessment clearly reaches into areas that are also addressed under the HIPAA privacy rule. For the most part, a "traditional" information security evaluation does not adequately address the risk assessment requirements of the proposed HIPAA security rule. Traditional information security evaluations are often executed by a team of outside experts who descend upon an organization, ask some questions of the staff and management, execute automated network scanning tools, and print an exhaustive list of so-called network vulnerabilities. This list was too often meaningless in terms of which vulnerabilities would, if exploited, have a negative impact on certain business functions within the organization. The criteria for identifying what a high, medium, or low impact actually meant to the organization were not obvious, and it was difficult to prioritize the risks associated with the vulnerabilities and subsequently to mitigate those risks. A vulnerability that appears on an automated tool report may actually be of low or acceptable risk to an organization, and the "mitigation" of that vulnerability may cause an undesirable effect in terms of the availability of services or decreased functionality.

DOD's Health Information Assurance Risk Assessment Methodology

Considering these difficulties and acknowledging their need to address the HIPAA regulatory requirements, the Office of the Assistant Secretary of Defense for Health Affairs, and the Offices of the Surgeons General of the U.S. Army, Navy, and Air Force recognized the need for a risk assessment methodology that could be readily implemented by DOD medical treatment facilities. The Advanced Technology Institute in Charleston, SC, and the Telemedicine and Advanced Technology Research Center (TATRC), U.S. Army Medical Research and Materiel Command were collaborating on the Defense Healthcare Information Assurance Program (DHIAP).[4] As a partner with that work, the Software Engineering Institute at Carnegie Mellon University was the ideal candidate to combine their work on software engineering risk management and their information protection expertise to develop and pilot such a risk assessment methodology as one of the major tasks under DHIAP.

Key Characteristics of OCTAVE

The developmental philosophy for the methodology included the need to identify and address the organizational vulnerabilities and risks to an organization, as well as the technical vulnerabilities associated with their computing and communications infrastructure. An additional developmental goal was to build a risk assessment methodology that could be self-directed, in that the method itself is transitioned to the organization, and that each of the facilities performs its own risk assessment. By using this approach it is possible to build a community of expertise that remains within the organization long after the risk assessment is deemed complete. The self-directed risk assessment is conducted by in-house staff members, so information comes from within the organization. Because senior management is involved in the process, ownership of the results is not in question, knowledge remains inside the organization, and implementation of recommendations is much more likely. The process helps to build consensus in an environment of differing organizational and disciplinary perspectives on health information assurance. Finally, the methodology was intended to advance beyond the identification of organizational risks and technological vulnerabilities; it had to incorporate the development of organizational protection strategies and mitigation plans based on the risks and threats it identified. The intent was to draw mitigation techniques from good, industry standard security practices and compile those into a catalogue of practices integrated into the risk assessment methodology. Sources for the catalogue of practices would include the Computer Emergency Response Coordination Center (CERT/CC), the British Standards Institute, the National Institute for Standards and Technology, and U.S. government regulations.

The risk assessment methodology that was ultimately developed and deployed has a number of key characteristics, some of which are alluded to in its name: Operationally Critical, Threat, Asset, and Vulnerability Evaluation (OCTAVE).[5] The basis for its success as a risk assessment methodology is the combination of analysis of organizational practices and technological vulnerabilities. Together, these areas can address the core implications behind the HIPAA data security rule and can be used to develop organizational protection strategies (based on an industry-accepted catalogue of good practices) and technological mitigation plans (to assess vulnerabilities associated with physical assets). The OCTAVE methodology is comprised of eight processes that are contained within three phases (see Figure 6.1).

Phase 1 takes an organizational view of the risk assessment process. It consists of four distinct processes. Processes one, two, and three elicit, through a series of workshops, information from different hierarchical levels of personnel in the organization. Senior managers, operational area managers (division heads), IT staff, and general staff are all asked to provide information relating to their perspective of critical assets, business practices, and associated risks. Current organizational security practices and deficiencies are identified through a comparison of these perspectives based on the catalogue of good practice previously discussed. It is as this part of the OCTAVE process that it becomes apparent if managers, IT-staff, and general staff have different perspectives on where policies are being adhered to, or in some cases if certain policies even exist. A good

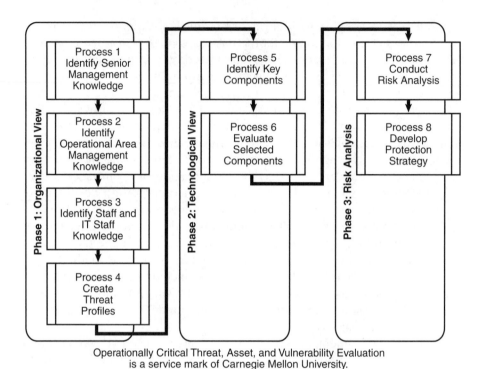

Operationally Critical Threat, Asset, and Vulnerability Evaluation
is a service mark of Carnegie Mellon University.

Figure 6.1   Octave Risk Assessment Process as Used by the Department of Defense Military Health Community

example of this is a security policy that states users must not share user identities or passwords. Although senior management may take some comfort in knowing that this policy exists, staff members on the ground who are treating patients and rapidly moving between workstations at multiple treatment locations may forget to log off as they move away from the terminal, possibly exposing the system to unauthorized use. This type of scenario would be captured and used to build protection strategies for the organization in Phase 3. The need for security awareness programs and better contingency plans also often emerges from this part of the risk assessment. Process 4, which is the last process in Phase 1 of OCTAVE, consolidates all the information obtained thus far, such as the list of critical assets and the threats to those assets as perceived by the different hierarchical and functional groups of individuals in the organization.

Phase 2 takes a technological view of the organization and consists of two predefined processes. This part of the risk assessment process may require that the interdisciplinary analysis team be augmented with network security specialists for the duration of Phase 2. The first process in Phase 2 is Process 5, which identifies any key technological components that may be an integral part of a critical asset. For example, if senior management reached consensus that their e-mail was a critical asset, related components such as routers, switches, and mail servers might be included at this time. By following logical access paths on a network topology diagram, all of the key technological components that interconnect to the critical asset are drawn into the scope of the evaluation. Various vulnerability detection tools, scripts, and manual methods are selected and used to check for known vulnerabilities in the selected components. The second process in Phase 2 is Process 6, which evaluates the results and vulnerabilities identified with the tools. It is here that the analysis team decides which of the vulnerabilities are indeed high risk, or perhaps an acceptable risk based on their business needs. For example, many network tools will identify default passwords on computer systems that may make them vulnerable to attack. This is probably an unacceptable risk and one that can often be quickly mitigated. Alternatively, certain network services or applications may show up on the report as being high risk, such as Telnet, but there may be a legitimate business case for accepting that service and leaving it running. The strength of including non-IT personnel on the analysis team and involving them in this process is often demonstrated at this stage.

Phase 3 is the risk analysis itself, which includes the development of protection strategies (to address deficiencies in organizational security practices) and mitigation plans (to address technological vulnerabilities). Once again the catalogue of practices is used to build the proposed protection strategies and mitigation plans.

RESULTS

Transitioning the OCTAVE Method to the DOD Healthcare Community

The surgeon generals' offices for the army, navy, and air force have endorsed the OCTAVE methodology as the preferred means of accomplishing a risk assessment and have requested that each DOD Medical Treatment Facility (MTF) appoint a clinician, patient administration staff member, and an information technology/information management representative to form a Medical Information Security Readiness Team (MISRT) responsible for execution of the OCTAVE risk assessment at their facility. During the spring of 2001, over 580 individuals representing MISRT from all services, lead agents, and other commands attended a series of seminars on HIPAA and health information assurance sponsored by TATRC and the U.S. Army Medical Research and Materiel Command in collaboration with the HIPAA Integrated Product Team (HIPAA IPT) of the Office of the Secretary of Defense/Health Affairs. A second series of seminars followed that focused on training MISRT from all MTFs in OCTAVE, commencing on September 5 to 7, 2001 in Washington, DC at the first DOD HIPAA Summit. OCTAVE training continued from May 2002 to August 2003 until the DHIAP team had successfully trained interdisciplinary medical information security readiness teams from over 200 DOD medical treatment facilities, at locations throughout the United States, Europe, and Asia.

Although they share common DOD policy and regulatory mandates, each MTF also has its own unique set of business circumstances and associated threats. For example, MTFs operating outside of the continental United States must rely on foreign carriers for Internet connectivity. This poses a special set of risks in terms of HIPAA data security, from a confidentiality and availability standpoint. The regional approach to training facilitated the sharing of organizational threats and protection strategies among only those facilities to which they were pertinent. This built a community of participation (regional capacity in health information assurance) among interdependent and asset-sharing facilities. Representative examples of the need for this community capability are USCG facilities that utilize army access to the Composite Health Care System (CHCS) while depending on USAF support staff.

The training itself was structured in such a way as to enact the process of conducting a complete risk assessment at a medical treatment facility, with full audience participation. Guided by two DHIAP OCTAVE instructors, attendees were required to enact the roles of workshop facilitator and scribe during each step of the OCTAVE process, while the remainder of the group was tasked with providing results as if they were conducting the process at their own facility. The results from each classroom-generated workshop activity were carried forward for analysis at subsequent stages of the two-day training class. Up to ten different treatment facilities were represented by their three-person, interdisciplinary MISRTs at each of the training seminars, allowing for the sharing of ideas and development of organizational protection strategies among services, facilities, and individual job functions.

The objectives of the OCTAVE training seminars were not only to train MISRTs in how to execute an OCTAVE at their MTFs, but also to improve attendees' understanding of the HIPAA compliance program of the Department of Defense and improve their understanding of health information assurance as a whole. After each group of analysis teams had been trained on how to conduct a risk assessment at their facility, the instructors introduced tools and support available to help them through their evaluations, including the OCTAVE Automated Tool (OAT), the OCTAVE Information Center, and the Risk Information Management Resource (RIMR).[6] To assure consistent instruction, the Defense Health Information Assurance Program developed an OCTAVE instructor's support package that all instructors used during the training seminars.

Attendees' Evaluation of the OCTAVE Training Seminars[7]

All attendees were invited to complete a detailed evaluation form at the conclusion of the training. The evaluation survey included questions designed to measure attendees' perceptions of the seminars' success in meeting their objectives. Of the 314 MISRT members who completed an evaluation at the advanced OCTAVE training seminars (September 2001 and May to August 2002), the composition of respondents by discipline included:

- 76 (24 percent) clinical staff
- 94 (30 percent) patient administration staff
- 115 (37 percent) IT staff
- 29 (9 percent) other

The results support that the seminars met their objectives. A strong majority stated that they sufficiently understand OCTAVE to participate in (89 percent) or lead (79 percent) an evaluation at their MTF. A majority (74 percent) stated that the seminar helped them better understand the DOD HIPAA compliance program. Almost all respondents stated that the seminar helped them better understand the role of risk assessment in managing a hospital's information system (94 percent) and helped them better understand health information assurance (87 percent).

With respect to their confidence in fellow MISRTs, a strong majority (84 percent) stated that they understand OCTAVE well enough to contribute to the MISRT and that the seminar increased confidence in their fellow MISRT members (80 percent). Most (59 percent) stated that the members of their MISRT were sufficiently well trained to conduct an OCTAVE evaluation. Although 67 percent stated that they could obtain sufficient resources to conduct their OCTAVE, many respondents commented that obtaining senior command support and adequate time constituted major barriers to beginning their OCTAVE evaluations.

CONCLUSION

The offices of the surgeons general for the army, navy, and air force have adopted OCTAVE as their preferred risk assessment methodology. They have requested that each DOD medical treatment facility appoint a clinician, patient administration staff member, and an information technology/information management representative to form an interdisciplinary medical information security readiness team to be responsible for execution of the OCTAVE risk assessment at their facility. After three rounds of training, over 1000 military personnel from over 200 medical treatment facilities have been trained on OCTAVE. The significant local knowledge provided by this unique composition of analysis team members, along with organizational and technical analysis of business practices, assets, and threats, is enabling DOD medical treatment facilities to create sound and effective security policies at their local level while remaining in conformance with DOD and other regulations. Although OCTAVE is being used as the preferred method to ensure that results are obtained in a sound and auditable manner, analysis team members are empowered by their commanders to tailor the process and develop policies and strategies that make information security workable at their local site. This represents a major milestone in execution of the DOD's HIPAA compliance program, promoting a culture of defense health information assurance at all levels of every military medical treatment facility and helping to support and enhance decentralized decision making on health information assurance throughout the military health system.

ACKNOWLEDGMENTS

This work was supported by the U.S. Army Medical Research and Materiel Command, Fort Detrick, MD, under the Defense Healthcare Information Assurance Program (DHIAP), Contract No.: DAMD17-010C-0048.

Carnegie Mellon, CERT, and CERT Coordination Center are registered in the U.S. Patent and Trademark Office.

OCTAVE; Operationally Critical Threat, Asset, and Vulnerability Evaluation are service marks of Carnegie Mellon University.

REFERENCES

1. R. L. Krutz and R. D Vines, *The CISSP Prep Guide—Mastering the Ten Domains of Computer Security*. New York: Wiley, 2001.
2. Department of Health and Human Services, Office of the Secretary, 45 CFR Parts 160 and 164: *Standards for Privacy of Individually Identifiable Health Information*, p. 82462 *Federal Register*, Vol. 65, No. 250, December 28, 2000/Rules and Regulations.
3. U.S. Department of Health and Human Services—Office of Civil Rights: http://www.hhs.gov/ocr/hipaa.
4. A. Andrews, L. Crane, J. Stinson, S. Pellissier, S. Packard, C. Alberts, D. Fisher, R. Rosenstein, T. White, K. McCall, and P. Wise, *Defense Healthcare Information Assurance Program (DHIAP) Final Report: Phases I and II*, Fort Detrick, MD, 30 June 2001.
5. C. Alberts and A. Dorofee, *Managing Information Security Risks—The OCTAVEsm Approach*, Boston: Addison-Wesley, 2002.
6. W. Wright, *Risk Information Management Resource (RIMR): Modeling an Approach to Defending Against Military Medical Information Assurance Brain Drain*, Telemedicine and Advanced Technology Research Center, February 2003.

7. J. Coleman, *Medical Information Security Readiness Teams, A Report on Advanced OCTAVEsm Training*, Telemedicine and Advanced Technology Research Center, 7 October 2002.

8. J. Coleman, "Execution of a self-directed risk assessment methodology to address HIPAA data security requirements," in Proceedings of SPIE Vol. 5033 *Medical Imaging 2003: PACS and Integrated Medical Information Systems: Design and Evaluation,* edited by H. K. Huang and O. M. Ratib, Bellingham, WA: SPIE. 2003.

7

TEN STEPS TO EFFECTIVE WEB-BASED SECURITY POLICY DEVELOPMENT AND DISTRIBUTION

Todd Fitzgerald, CISSP, CISA

INTRODUCTION

Paper, dust, obsolescence: affectionately known as shelfware, are the magnificent binders filled with reams of outdated policies, procedures, standards, and guidelines. Many times the only contribution to effective security these binders have is to increase the security risk by having more to burn during a fire! Many times these documents are the proud creations of the security department, but have little impact on the end user who is posting her password on her terminal or leaving confidential documents lying on his desk. The documents are typically voluminous and who will take the time to read them? Simple answer — the same people who read their complete car owner's manual before they put the first key into the ignition — definitely a small segment of the population (not sure we want these individuals driving either!).

So where does this leave us? Granted, documented procedures require a level of specificity to truly become a repeatable process. It is through the process of documentation that consensus is reached on the policies and procedures required for an organization. Without going through this process, many practices may be assumed, with different interpretations between the parties. Organizational members from the different business units, human resources, legal, and information technology need the opportunity to provide input to the documents as well. However, does this mean that the end product must be a dusty set of binders that no one looks at, except on the annual update cycle? This appears to be a great waste of resources and results in limited effectiveness of the deliverable.

ENTER THE ELECTRONIC AGE

Beginning in the mid to late '90s large organizations were beginning to realize the efficiencies of the intranet for distributing information internally to employees. External Web presence (Internet) obtained most of the budget dollars, as these were seen as competitive and worthwhile investments due to their potential for revenue generation and increased cost efficiencies to those areas such as customer service, order entry, and creating self-service mechanisms. After this functionality was largely in place, the same technology was reviewed for potential savings within the internal environment to support employees. Organizations seem to start and stop these initiatives causing intranet content to be rich for some areas and nonexistent for others. The level of existing documented procedures as well as their use of technology also contributed to the maturity level of the intranet, Web-based applications. Debates among who should distribute policies — compliance? human resources? legal? information technology? individual business units? — can also slow down the decision process in selecting the proper tool. At some point, organizations need to "dip their toe in the water" and get started versus trying to plan out the entire approach prior to swimming! If there is an existing intranet, security departments would be wise to integrate within the existing process for delivering policies, or influence changing the environment to accommodate the security policy considerations versus creating a new separate environment.

It is unrealistic to believe that we will ever move completely away from paper; however, the "source of record" can be online, managed, and expected to be the most current version. How many times have you looked at a document that was printed, only to guess whether there was a later version? Many times we print documents without the proper data classification specified (internal use, public, confidential, restricted) and date–time stamped, making it difficult to determine the applicability of the document. In addition, if the documents are online and housed on personal folders and various network drives, determining the proper version is equally difficult.

FUNCTIONALITY PROVIDED BY WEB-BASED DEPLOYMENT

Deploying security policies electronically can provide several advantages, depending upon the deployment mechanism. In the simplest form, policies can be placed on the intranet for users to view. This should be regarded as an "entry level" deployment of security policies. In the remaining sections we discuss the approach and delivery of implementing security policies that are created through a workflow process, deployment to the intranet, notification of new policies, tracking for compliance, limiting distribution to those who need them, informing management of noncompliance, and planning the release of the policies. Placing the policies "on the Web" without managing the process is insufficient in today's regulatory environment of controls with such influences as the Health Insurance Portability and Accountability Act (HIPAA), Graham–Leach–Bliley (GLBA), Sarbanes–Oxley, California Senate Bill 1386, and so on. Verification that users have received the policies and can refer to them at a future point is essential for security.

A PRAGMATIC APPROACH TO SUCCESSFUL E-POLICY DEPLOYMENT

Deploying policies in a Web-based environment has many similarities to developing paper-based policies; however, there are some additional considerations that must be appropriately planned. The following ten-step approach for the development and distribution of policies will reduce the risk that the electronic policies will become the digitized version of shelfware of the future. (In the security profession we never completely solve problems, but instead reduce risk!)

Step 1: Issue Request for Proposal

Issuing a Request for Proposal (RFP) to multiple vendors serves several purposes. First, it forces the organization to think about what the business requirements are for the product. A list of considerations for selecting a tool is listed in Table 7.1. Second, it causes vendors to move beyond the sales pitch of the product and answer specific questions of functionality. It is very useful to include a statement within the RFP stating that the RFP will become part of the final contract. For example, vendors may indicate that they "support e-mail notification of policies" in their glossy brochures, while at the same time omitting the fact that the e-mail address has to conform to their standard format for an e-mail address, thus requiring an extra step of establishing aliases for all the e-mail accounts. Third, pricing can be compared across multiple vendors prior to entering into pricing negotiations without having to respond to the sales pressure of "end of the sales quarter" deals. Fourth, a team can be formed to review the responses objectively based upon the organizational needs. And finally, more information on the financial stability and existing customer references can be obtained.

Table 7.1 Considerations in Selecting a Policy Tool Vendor

Subscription versus perpetual license pricing
Process for creating security policies
Workflow approval process within tool
Methods for setting up users (NT groups, LDAP, individually maintained)
Pass-thru authentication with browser
E-mail notification of new policies capability
Construction of e-mail address
Import/export capabilities
Ability to change policy after distribution
Quizzing capability
Role-based administration access (to permit departments other than
  security to manage policies in their areas)
Levels of administrative access
Intranet/Internet hosting requirements
Vendor customer base using the tool in production
Annual revenues
Application service provider, intranet- or Internet-based model
Protection of information if not hosted locally
HIPAA/GLBA policy content included with tool or add-on pricing
Reporting capabilities to track compliance
Policy formats supported (Word, PDF, HTML, XML) and limitations of using
  each
Context searching capability
Linkage to external documents from the policy (such as standards,
  procedures)
Test server instances — additional pricing
Two- to three-year price protection on maintenance, mergers, acquisitions
Predeveloped content available
Number of staff dedicated to product development versus committed to
  sales and administration
Mechanism for distributing policies to different user groups

There are several players in the policy development and deployment market space, albeit the market is relatively immature and the players change. As of this writing, there are several vendors promoting solutions, such as NetIQ's VigilEnt Policy Center (formerly Pentasafe), Bindview Policy Center, NetVision Policy Resource Center, PriceWaterhouseCooper's Enterprise Security Architecture System (ESAS), PoliVec 3 Security Policy Automation System, Symantec, and others. There are also the E-learning companies that overlap this space, such as QuickCompliance, Eduneering, Mindspan, and Plateau systems to name a few. Articulating the pros and cons of each of these products is beyond the scope of this chapter; however, the information provided should provide a reasonable method to start raising knowledgeable questions with the vendors.

To move toward a product that would support the business requirements, an organization could build the product itself. However, there are advantages in purchasing a product to perform these capabilities. From a cost perspective, most organizations would spend more in resources developing these tools than on their purchase price. There is also the issue of time-to-market. The tools are already available and can be deployed within a few months, depending upon the match with the technical infrastructure of the organization. Vendors also provide starting policy content that can jump-start the creation of security policies. This content is updated according to the changing requirements of the regulatory bodies.

A cross-functional team made up of representatives from Human Resources, Legal, Information Technology, Institutional Compliance, and other key business units should be formed to review the requirements and responses from the proposals. These are the individuals that will have to support the policy tool once implemented, therefore, bringing them into the process early on is essential. The tool may be extended beyond the needs of the security department to deliver other organizationwide policies once the basic infrastructure is in place.

Prior to issuing the request for proposal, a scoring matrix should be prepared that will allow the team to evaluate the vendors independently. The matrix does not have to be complicated and should be driven from the business and technical requirements, the criticality of the requirement, and the level to which the requirement was met (3 = exceeds requirements, 2 = meets requirements, 1 = does not meet requirements). Once the matrices are scored individually by team members, group discussion focusing on the differences between the products narrows down the selection. The duration of the RFP process can be as little as six to eight weeks to select the appropriate product and is time well spent.

It is beneficial to include the company's software purchasing contract within the RFP so that the appropriate terms and conditions can be reviewed by the vendor. This saves time in contract negotiations as the legal departments will typically review the contract as part of the RFP process. Considerations for the contracting phase include the following:

- Standard vendor contracts include "no-warranty" type language — add escape clauses if the product does not function within 90 days of the start of testing.
- Subscription versus perpetual licenses — evaluate two- to three-year product cost.
- Secure two- to three-year price increase protection, especially on "new to market tools."
- Obtain protection in the event either company merges or is acquired by another company.

- Place source code in escrow, and terms and conditions for obtaining it in the event of vendor company failure.
- Be aware of future "unbundling" of previously purchased items; ensure functionality is covered in the RFP.
- Establish how a "user" is counted for licensing.

The "security policy tool" market is being entered by vendors with different product beginnings. Attempt to understand the company and whether this is an "add-on" market for them, or the product was specifically developed for this market space. Add-on products typically have limited investment by the vendor, and functionality enhancements are subject to the product's origins and the direction the product (being added on to) is headed.

The RFP is a critical step providing focus for the team in clarifying the requirements expected of the product, engaging the stakeholders earlier in the process, and providing the means to compare company and technical product information quickly between the vendors.

Step 2: Establish Security Organization Structure for Policy Review

If a security council or committee has not already been established, this is an excellent time to form one. The security council becomes the "sounding board" for policies that are introduced into the organization. One of the largest challenges within any information security program is establishing and maintaining support from management for information security practices, many times referred to as "lack of management commitment." The first question is to ask why there is a lack of commitment. What steps have been taken to build the management commitment? Think of an organization being like a large skyscraper. Each successive floor depends upon the preceding floor for support. The walls, bricks, concrete, and steel all have to work together to form the needed support to prevent the building from collapsing. It also must be strong enough to withstand high winds, rainstorms, and earthquakes. If we envision our organizations as skyscrapers, with senior management occupying the top floors (they seem to always get the best views!), with middle management just below (translating senior management vision into operational actions to accomplish the vision), and the co-workers below that (where the real mission is carried out), we see that the true organizational commitment is built from the bottom up. This occurs brick by brick, wall by wall, and floor by floor. The "reality check" occurs by each level in the organization querying their subordinates to see if they are in agreement. Obviously it would take a significant amount of time to engage all users and all management levels in the process of policy development. Granted, someone in the organization below the senior executive leadership must have the security vision to get started, but it is the support of the middle management and the co-workers that is essential to maintain long-term senior management support.

The individual typically having the security vision is the director, manager of information security, chief security officer, or chief information security officer. This individual has typically reported through the information technology department to the CIO or head of information systems. A good indication of success of the security vision being accepted by senior leadership is if positions such as chief security officer, chief information security officer, or information security officer positions have been established, with a communication path through the organization's audit and compliance committees or board of directors. The establishment of these roles and development of the communication lines typically indicates that security has moved out of an operational, data center type function and into a strategic function necessary to carry out the business objectives of the organization. Some organizations are fortunate to have the CEO, CFO, or COO already with a good understanding and strong belief in information security; however, this is the exception. Security has a long history of being viewed as an expense to the organization that was necessary and that did not contribute to top-line revenues, and thus the suggestion to spend more in this area to a C-level management individual should not be immediately expected to be readily embraced. The business case for enabling new products, attaining regulatory compliance, providing cost savings, or creating a competitive advantage must be demonstrated.

The security council should be made up of representatives from multiple organizational units that are necessary to support the policies in the long term. Human Resources is essential to provide knowledge of the existing code of conduct, employment and labor relations, and termination and disciplinary action policies and practices that are in place. The Legal department is needed to ensure that the language of the policies is stating what is intended, and that applicable local, state, and federal laws are appropriately followed. The Information Technology department provides technical input and information on current initiatives and the development of procedures and technical implementations to support the policies. The individual business unit representation is essential to understand how practical the policies may be in carrying out the mission of the business. The Compliance department representation provides insight on ethics, contractual obligations, and investigations that may require policy creation. And finally, the Information Security department (if one exists) should be represented by the security officer, who typically chairs the council, and members of the security team for specialized technical expertise.

Step 3: Define What Makes a Good Security Policy

Electronically distributed policies must be written differently if they are to be absorbed quickly, as the medium is different. People have different expectations of reading information on a Web site than what would be expected in relaxing in an easy chair to read a novel or reviewing technical documentation. People want the information fast and seconds feel like hours on a Web site. Therefore, policies should be no longer than two typewritten pages as a general rule. Any longer than this will lose their attention and should be broken into more policies. Hyperlinks were designed to provide immediate access only to the information necessary, making it quick to navigate sites. Individuals may not have time to review a long policy in one sitting, but two pages? No problem, especially if that is communicated to them ahead of time.

Organizations typically do not have a common understanding of what a "policy" is. It seems like such a simple concept, why the difficulty? The reason is not the lack of understanding that a policy is meant to govern the behavior within the organization, but rather that in an effort to reduce time, organizations combine policies, procedures, standards, and guidelines into one document and refer to the whole as "the policy." This is not really a time saver because it introduces inflexibility into the policy each time a procedure or standard has to change. For example, if the password "standards" are written into the password policy for a primarily Windows-based (NT, 2000, XP, 98) environment, what happens when a UNIX server with an Oracle data warehouse project is initiated? Will the password "policy" have to be updated and distributed to all end users again, even though a small percentage of the organization will actually be using the new data warehouse? Consider an alternative approach whereby the password standards are placed in standards documents specific to the individual platform and hyperlinked from the high-level password policy. In this case, the high-level policy stating that "passwords appropriate for the platforms are determined by the security department and the information technology departments are expected to be adhered to in an effort to maintain the confidentiality, integrity, and availability of information..." will not be required to change with the addition of the new platform. Republishing policies in a Web-based environment is a key concern and should be avoided, especially when they are broken into "many" two-page policies.

At this point, some definitions are in order.

■ *Policy* — Defines "what" the organization needs to accomplish and serves as management's intentions to control the operation of the organization to meet business objectives. The "why" should also be stated here in the form of a policy summary statement or policy purpose. If the end users understand the why, they are more apt to follow the policy. As children, we were told what to do by our parents and we just did it. As we grew older, we challenged those beliefs (as four- to five-year-olds and again as teenagers!) and needed to understand the reasoning. Our organizations are no different, people need to understand the why before they will really commit.

■ *Procedure* — Defines "how" the policy is to be supported and "who" does what to accomplish this task. These are typically drafted by the departments having the largest operational piece of the procedure. There may be many procedures to support a particular policy. It is important that all departments with a role in executing the procedure have a chance to review the procedure or that it has been reviewed by a designate (possibly the security council representative for that business area). Ownership of the procedure is retained within the individual department.

■ *Standard* — Standards are a cross between the "what" and "how" to implement the policy. The standard is written to support the policy and further defines the specifics required to support the policy. In the previous UNIX/Oracle data warehouse example the standard would be written to include specific services (Telnet, FTP, SNMP, etc.) that would be turned on and off and hardening standards such as methods for remote administration authentication (TACACs, RADIUS, etc.). These do not belong in the policy, as technology changes too frequently and would create an unnecessary approval/review burden (involving extra management levels for detail review) to introduce new standards.

■ *Guideline* — Similar to standards, but different in focus and intent. A good exercise is to replace the word "guideline" with the word "optional." If by doing so, the statements contained in the "optional" are what is desired to happen at the user's discretion, then it is a great guideline! Anything else, such as required activities, must be contained within the standard. Guidelines are more than suggestions, but have limited enforceability. Guidelines should be rare within policy architecture and the presence of many guidelines is usually indicative of a weak security organization and failure to obtain the appropriate management commitment through the processes discussed in Step 2.

These definitions should provide insight into what makes a good policy. Each of the items above (with the exception of guidelines) is necessary to having a good policy. Without procedures, the policy can't be executed. Without standards, the policy is at too high a level to be effective. Having the policy alone does not support the organization in complying with the policy.

So, the implications are for electronic policies:

- Policies should be written to "live" for two to three years without change.
- Policies are written with "must," "shall," or "will" language or they are not a policy, but rather a guideline containing "should," "can," and "may" language (exceptions to the policy are best dealt with through an exception process with formal approvals by senior management).
- Technical implementation details belong in the standards.
- Policies should be no more than two typewritten (no less than ten-point font, please!) online pages.
- Policies, procedures, standards, and guidelines should by hyper-linked to the policy (the best way to do this is to link one static Web page off the policy and then jump to specific standards, procedures, and guidelines to eliminate need to change the policy with each addition of a standard).
- Review, review, review before publishing.
- Provide online printing capability; however, stress that current source is always on the intranet.

Time spent up front defining a standard format for policies, procedures, standards, and guidelines is time well spent. These formats do not have to be complex, and simpler is better. For example, a simple online policy approach may be to define four areas:

1. *Policy Summary* — brief one-paragraph description of the intent of the policy
2. *Policy Scope* — defining to whom the policy applies
3. *Policy Purpose* — defining the "why" of the policy
4. *Policy Statement* — brief reiteration of the policy summary and the actual policy

These four areas provide all that is needed for the policy. Judge the policy not on the weight of the printed document, but rather on the clarity of purpose, communication of the benefits to the organization, and clearness of what people are expected to do. With the advantage of electronically posting the policies on the intranet, the ability of users to navigate to the information they need is also a measure of effectiveness of the policy.

Step 4: Establish Security Policy Review Process

Now that the organization has identified an individual responsible for the development and implementation of security policies, the security council has been created, and an understanding of what makes a good policy has been communicated, there needs to be a process for reviewing the policies. This process may be developed during the creation of the security council; what is important is that the policy development process is thought out ahead of time to determine who will (1) create the policy, (2) review and recommend, (3) approve the final policy, (4) publish, and (5) read and accept the policies. The time spent in this process, up front, will provide many dividends down the road. Many organizations jump right in and someone in the security department or information technology department will draft a policy and e-mail it out, without taking these steps. Proceeding along that path ends up with a policy that is not accepted by the organization's management and thus will not be accepted by the organization's end users. Why? Because the necessary discussion, debate, and acceptance of the policies by the leaders of the organization never took place. In the end, the question of management commitment again surfaces, when there was never a process in place to obtain the commitment.

The process could be depicted in a swim-lane type chart showing the parties responsible, activities, records created through each activity, and decision boxes. Senior management will want this presented at a high level, typically no more than one to two pages of process diagram. The process will vary by organizational structure, geographic location, size, and culture of decision making; however, a successful process for review should contain these steps.

A. Policy Need Determined

Anyone can request the need for a policy to the information security department. Business units may have new situations that are not covered by an existing security policy. If no security policies exist in the organization, the information security department needs to take the lead and establish a prioritization of policies that are necessary.

B. Create, Modify Existing Policy

The information security department creates an initial draft for a new policy. Many Internet sources are available to obtain existing policies (perform a Google search on security policy as a starting point), and other model policies are available through organizations such as www.sans.org and vendors such as NetIQ through the publication of books and CDs including *Information Security Policies Made Easy*. Caution must be taken not to copy and distribute these policies "as-is" as they may not be completely appropriate, enforceable, or supported by procedures within the organization. The level of detail and grade level (shouldn't exceed grade level 8) need to be assessed to determine how acceptable these will be to the organization.

C. Internal Review by Security Department

People within the security department will have varying levels of technical expertise, business acumen, and understanding of the organizational culture. By reviewing within the team first, many obvious errors or misunderstandings of the policy can be avoided before engaging management's limited review time. This also increases the credibility of the information systems' security department by bringing a quality product for review. It also saves time on minor grammatical reviews and focuses the management review on substantive policy issues.

D. Security Council Reviews and Recommends Policy

This is arguably the most critical step in the process. This is where the policy begins the acceptance step within the organization. The policies are read, line by line, during these meetings and discussed to ensure that everyone understands the intent and rationale for the policy. The management commitment begins here. Why? Because they feel part of the process and have a chance to provide input, as well as thinking about how the policy would affect their own departments. Contrast this method with just sending out the policy and saying, "This is it" and the difference becomes readily apparent. These are the same management people that are being counted on to continue to support the policy once it is distributed to the rest of the workforce. Failing in this step will guarantee failure in having a real policy.

Okay, if we buy into the notion that a security council is a good practice, logical, practical, and appears to get the job done, what is the downside? Some may argue that it is a slow process, especially when senior management may be pushing to "get something out there to address security" to reduce the risks. It is a slower process while the policies are being debated, however, the benefits of having a real policy that the organization can support, buy-in from the management on a continuing basis, reduced need to rework the policies later, and increased understanding by management of their meaning and why they are important outweigh the benefits of blasting out an e-mail containing policies that were copied from another source, the name of the company changed, and distributed without prior collaboration. Policies created in the latter context rarely become "real" and followed within the organization as they were not developed with thorough analysis of how they would be supported by the business in their creation.

E. Information Technology Steering Committee Approves Policy

A committee made up of the senior leadership of the organization is typically formed to oversee the strategic investments in information technology. Many times these committees struggle with balancing decisions on tactical "fire-fighting" one- to three-month concerns versus dealing with strategic issues and this perspective needs to be understood when addressing this type of committee. The important element in the membership of this committee is that it involves the decision leaders of the organization. These are the individuals whom the employees will be watching to see if they support the policies that were initially generated from the security department. Their review and endorsement of the policies is critical to obtain support in implementing the policies. Also, they may be aware of strategic plans or further operational issues not identified by middle management (through the security council) that may make a policy untenable.

Because time availability of the senior leadership is typically limited, these committees meet at most on a monthly basis and, more typically, on a quarterly basis. Therefore, sufficient time for planning policy approval is necessary. This may seem to run counter to the speed at which electronic policies are distributed, however, as in the case with the security council review, the time delay is essential in obtaining long-term commitment.

F. Publish Policy

Organizations that go directly from Step 2 to this step end up with shelfware, or if e-mailed, "electronic dust." By the time the policy gets to this step, the security department should feel very confident that the policy will be understood by the users and supported by management. They may agree or disagree with the policy, but will understand the need to follow it because it will be clear how the policy was created and reviewed. Care must be taken when publishing policies electronically, as it is not desirable to publish the same policy over and over with minor changes to grammar and terminology. Quality reviews need to be performed early in the development process so that the security council and information technology steering committee can devote their time to substantive issues of the policy versus pointing out the typos and correcting spelling. End users should be given the same respect and should expect to be reviewing a document free from error. The medium may be electronic, but that does not change the way people want to manage their work lives — with the amount of e-mail already in our lives, we should try to limit the amount of extra work that is placed upon the readers of the policies.

The Web-based policy management tools provide the facilities to publish the policies very quickly. Because tracking on reading the policies is a key feature of these products, once the policy is published, they typically cannot be changed unless a new policy is created! This has major implications for the distribution of the policy. This means that any change made will require the republishing of the policy. Imagine thousands of users in the organization that now have to reread the policy due to a minor change. This situation should be avoided with the review process in place in the preceding steps. The electronic compliance tracking software is usually built this way (and rightly so), so that it is clear on which policy version the user actually signed off.

It should be clear by now that even though some of the policy development tools support a workflow process within the tool to facilitate approvals of the policies through the various stages (such as draft, interim reviews, and final publishing), there is no substitute for the oral collaboration of the policies. Electronic communications are very "flat" and do not provide expression of the meaning behind the words. Through the discussions within the various committees the documented text becomes clearer beyond just those with technical skills. The purpose is more apt to be appropriately represented in the final policies through the collaborative process.

Step 5: Installation and Configuration of Web-Based Policy Distribution Application

Although this is noted as Step 5 in the process, the actual installation may occur earlier and in parallel with the prior steps. There are usually technical issues that are specific to the company's own operating environment and previous implementation decisions that were made. Vendor products must be written to adapt to a majority of the environments and there may be one technical "gotcha" that takes up 90 percent of the implementation time to work through the particular issue. Some vendors offer a training class or consulting to get the product up and running, each lasting on average two to three days. These are worth taking advantage of and can save time in understanding the product.

Some configuration options made during this step in the process are not easily changed in the future, so attention should be paid to the impact of each option, asking questions about the impact of the decisions. Although the following list will vary product by product, these are some considerations to probe beyond the vendor's glossy brochures and sales claims to understand the specific technical answers to the questions.

A. How Are the Individual Users Set Up with the Product?

The users could be set up within the tool itself, which means that every new employee added, terminated, or changing job roles (if policies are published to different groups based upon job function) would have to be updated manually within the tool. This could result in many hours of maintenance just keeping up with the changes. As an alternative, the product may offer using the existing NT groups or using Lightweight Directory Access Protocol (LDAP) to retrieve the previously established members. By using the NT group approach, accounts are assigned to an NT group outside the policy tool (within NT), and these groups are then referenced to ensure that the appropriate departments have access to the policies (i.e., a management group, all users, information technology, remote users, temporary employees, contractors, etc.). Organizations usually do not have these groups predefined by department areas and thus need to be constructed and maintained with the implementation and ongoing support of the product. The question becomes — who is going to take on this "extra" administrative task? If the information security department takes on this role, there needs to be extra communication with the human resources and information technology departments to ensure that changes in membership between these groups are kept current. These added processes are usually not communicated by the vendors of the policy products, but rather the inference that "policies can be published using your existing NT groups!" In practice, there will be additional NT groups that will need to be defined with this approach.

If LDAP is used, this simplifies the process as the existing distribution groups set up on a Microsoft Exchange Server can be utilized as the groups. Maintenance processes should already be in place with distribution list update owners specified, making adoption of the process easier. There can still be gotchas here depending upon the product. In the installation of the NetIQ product, delays were experienced because a special character (comma) in the distinguished name on the exchange server caused the vendor's software to crash. After working with the vendor, it was indicated that the implementation had to be changed to use NT groups to function within our environment. Subsequently, the vendor product has been fixed, but not until we had to change directions, implement the product, and spend the resources investigating and trying to resolve the issue. Other vendor products will have their own gotchas in different areas. The lesson here? Always build test cases utilizing your environment early in the process to uncover the major gotchas. The product needs to work in your installation and whether it works in 100 percent of the other implementations becomes irrelevant.

B. Is E-Mail Supported?

Users are very busy individuals and the last thing they need to be instructed to do is check a Web site daily to see if there are any new policies. In support of this, e-mail notification of new policies is essential so that the policies can be pushed to the individual. How the e-mail address is constructed becomes an important integration issue. Is there flexibility in the construction of the e-mail address, or is it always composed of first name followed by last name? If this is the case, aliases may need to be created and maintained, adding to the administrative burden. In addition, if NT groups are used, do all the users across all domains defined have unique NT IDs? If not, this will cause problems when the product constructs the e-mail address according to the predefined methods, as different individuals in different domains will equate to one e-mail address. Again, the products are written to be generic and ignore any company standards that are in use. A thorough examination of the IDs and e-mail addresses will lead to a discussion as to what changes need to be made to support the implementation, either through workarounds (adding aliases) or changing the existing setups (eliminating duplicates). Some implementations may support Simple Mail Transfer Protocol (SMTP) e-mail addresses and do not support the creation of Messaging Application Programming Interface (MAPI). If there are users who do not have external (Internet, SMTP) e-mail addresses due to business restrictions, e-mail addresses with a different SMTP domain name that is nonroutable to the Internet would need to be established to support the internal notification of e-mail. This would permit the users to receive the "new policies are available" notifications while at the same time continuing to support the business restrictions preventing their ability to send and receive Internet e-mail.

C. How Easy Is It to Produce Accurate Compliance Reports?

Running compliance reports against domains containing large numbers of users can be very time consuming and may time out before the reports complete. What is the threshold, or number of users that can be reported on? Do these reports have to be run on each policy and each domain separately? For example, if six policies are published with users in ten NT domains, do 60 separate reports have to be run or just one? If there are users with multiple accounts in different domains, are they viewed as different users by the tool? Can the policy reports be run only for a specific NT group (i.e., management, all users, information technology)? If NT groups are used, how does the product handle disabled versus deleted accounts; in other words, will these show up in the reports as users? If exporting to Microsoft Excel or Word, are there any gotchas with the export, such as the handling of double quotes within the results? The compliance reporting can be a very time-consuming process and may not be the click of a button action that is typically reported.

D. How Do Users Authenticate to the Tool?

If Microsoft NT Network IDs are utilized, the policy product may provide for pass-thru authentication integrated with IIS. Through this method, the user would be automatically logged into the policy deployment tool after selecting the URL for the site in the Web browser. Alternatively, IDs could be set up within the tool, with log-ins and passwords to control access. Because the average corporate user today has at least eight userID/password combinations to keep track of, this approach should be avoided.

Step 6: Pilot Test Policy Deployment Tool with Users

Once the infrastructure has been established and some test cases have been run through it, the product is ready for pilot testing. A few "draft policies" with the new format should be created and distributed through the tool to a small set of users. It is important to recruit users from different departments, levels of experience, education, and familiarity with computer technology. Selecting a sample made up only of information technology individuals may not surface common user questions. The purpose of the pilot testing is to collect feedback on the ease of use of the product, establish a base of individuals who will support (get behind) the product during the rollout phase, and most important, anticipate the questions that need to be addressed to formulate the appropriate training materials.

The process should be scripted to have the users perform different functions such as reading a policy, providing comments to a policy, accepting the policy, locating the policy documents after they have been accepted, taking a quiz, searching policies for terms, reporting an incident, and so forth according to the functionality provided within the tool.

Step 7: Provide Training on the Tool

Why would training be important? After all, this is a Web-based application and should be intuitive, right? Surely much of the workforce will be able to navigate the tool correctly, provided the tool was designed with usability in mind. The key reason for providing the training is to gain the ongoing support for using the tool in the future! Just as individuals need to understand the "why" of a policy, they also need to understand "why" they should take time to read the policies presented in the tool! This is a great opportunity to get middle management and line management involved in supporting the security program — use the opportunity to "train the trainer" by training management on the use of the tool. By doing so, management will be paying more attention to the training themselves, knowing that they will in turn have to train their staff. (Who wants to look foolish in front of their staff members?)

Recognizing that management is also very busy and information security is one more thing on their list, there needs to be structure around the training, expected due dates, and provided training materials. Some management may feel comfortable creating their own training materials to shape their own message, but most will prefer to have something canned to which they can add specifics. Using this approach allows them to cover the material in a staff meeting without much preparation. The managers are also in the best position to tailor the "why this is important to us" message to their specific departmental needs. It also demonstrates their support for security versus having it always come from the information security officer.

There are several training materials that should be constructed in advance of the training by the information security department and should be posted to the intranet to be made available for the management to download, reducing the time necessary for the information security department to distribute the information and make it available to the management when they need it. It is also more efficient for the information security department to create one set of materials than to have each individual manager spend time creating his or her own. The essential training materials to roll out the policy deployment tool include:

- *PowerPoint Presentation* — Slides showing how policies are created, who is involved, screen shots of the policy tool showing specific functionality, due dates for reading and accepting the policies, and future plans for deployment of policies.
- *Pamphlet* — A three-fold pamphlet as a handy reference for using the tool. This is also useful for showing contact information of the security department(s) to call for information security questions, password resets, and policy tool questions.
- *Acknowledgment Form* — A form stating that the training was received and that they acknowledge that clicking on an acceptance button within the tool has the same effect as if they were to affix their written signature to the policy. These forms should be filed with human resources in their personnel file in the event that there is subsequent disciplinary action or termination resulting from violation of a security policy.

- *Training Roster* — A sheet that the manager can have each employee sign to confirm that he or she has received the training. This information should be captured centrally within human resources to keep track of the security awareness training that the individual has received.
- *Give-Aways* — What would security awareness training be without chocolate and a give-away? Mouse pads, pens, monitor mirrors, mugs and other tokens can be very useful, especially if the intranet Web address of the policy tool is imprinted on the token.
- *Notes* — A separate PowerPoint presentation setup to print the notes pages can be provided to help managers fill in the graphics and words on the slides.

By providing these tools, the individual users have the benefit of receiving a consistent message and having it communicated from their own manager! Even though the medium is electronic, training is still essential for the first rollout of the policies. This may very well be the first application with the organization that is distributed to all users and as such, will represent change that needs to be appropriately managed.

Step 8: Rollout Policies in Phases

The first phase rollout of policies to the end users will be the policies used in the pilot phase. A limited number of policies should be rolled out at this time, such as a password policy and policies indicating the roles of the various departments involved in creating the policies. For example, there could be a separate policy indicating the responsibility and authority of the overall security program and the executive sponsorship behind the policies. The roles of the information security department, security council, information technology steering committee, management, and the end users could be spelled out in separate policies. By having these as the first set of policies, it sets up the organizational and control structure for issuing future policies. It also sends the message that management is involved and behind the policies and they are not solely products of the information security department.

The primary goal of the first phase is to lay this foundation for future policy rollouts and also to provide users with the opportunity to use the new tool. Users will have many questions using the technology itself during this phase that should not be underestimated. They may be unable to get to the Web site due to problems with their log-in setup, they may have read the policy but not clicked the appropriate checkbox to accept the policy, or they may not understand a specific policy. It is hoped that these questions can be reduced through the train-the-trainer approach;

however, there will still be questions on usability. By keeping the policy content "simple" at this stage, more attention can be given to helping users become familiar with the tool.

A six- to nine-month plan for the rollout of policies should be established so that they are not receiving all the policies at once. There is much information to be absorbed in the information security policies due to the breadth of organizational impact. Delivering these in bite-size pieces is more conducive to really having these understood within the organization. Sometimes this may be unavoidable, especially if they are the result of a focused-policy project. Policies should be grouped into these "phases" so that users are not receiving a policy too frequently (remember, they do have other work to do). Users will appreciate the grouping and after a few phases, will come to understand that this is a normal ongoing process.

When the policies are issued, an e-mail containing a link to the Web site and, if possible, directly to the specific policy should be included. Expectations of "compliance" of the policy should be stated, with a 30- to 45-day period to read, understand, and provide acceptance of the policy through the policy deployment tool. At least 30 days are necessary as people may be on vacation, traveling, involved in some key time-sensitive projects, and so forth. As security professionals, we need to be sensitive to the fact that we think about security all the time, but end users have other jobs to perform. The timeframes are dependent upon the culture of each organization.

Step 9: Monitor Compliance

This is arguably the key difference between utilizing a Web-based policy development tool versus placing the policies on a Web site with hyperlinks to each policy. The vendors of the products promote this capability as a key feature and rightly so. When policies are simply placed on a Web site, e-mailed to new users, or distributed in paper binders, it becomes a very difficult job to ascertain who has read the policies, let alone received them! If the distributions are sent out by e-mail, many organizations still require that a signed document confirming that the documents have been read and accepted be sent back to the policy originator!

The policy deployment tools provide a much better way of tracking compliance by tracking the acceptance of the users in a database. Users are provided with assignments, provided a timeframe to complete, and then the tracking is housed within one integrated system. In addition, because the information is being captured in a database, the tools also provide functionality to report on the current status of policy acceptance. This is useful after a rollout to see how fast the adoption rate is; in other words are people reviewing the policies right away or are there a large number waiting until the last few days of the period? This can assist in future training to educate users that waiting until the final days of the period may cause unavailability problems of the Web site.

The compliance tracking process is not completely automatic as there will be differences between the vendor product (generic) and the organizational structure (specific). For example, if there are multiple geographic locations within the company, an extra step may be needed to produce reports by geographic location and manager responsible by relating the ID used in the policy tool to the human resources system (which contains the department/manager information). Alternatively, if the tool supports a data feed from the human resources system, and was set up with the department and a user role (supporting distribution of policies to only those users within that role), it may be necessary to relate the department to a manager outside the tool to produce the reports by manager. Depending upon the management reporting needs, the out-of-the-box tool may not provide all the compliance reporting functionality needed. Fortunately, many of the products have an export option to pull the information in another product such as Microsoft Access or Excel to manipulate the information.

There are other considerations in the compliance tracking as well, such as disabled accounts showing up in the user reporting lists, system accounts, and if distribution lists were used to distribute the policies, how accurate are they and how are they maintained? The completeness of the user population being reported on must receive periodic verification to ensure that the policies are reaching everyone. If there are users within the organization that do not have access to computers, then kiosks where they can log into the system need to be made available or their manager needs to take the responsibility of printing the policies for their signature as a workaround. For compliance tracking to be complete, it would need to be known which users fall under the paper-based exception.

After the 30- to 45-day "acceptance period" has been completed for the policies, the initial compliance reports are run. It is a good practice to provide the compliance reports within one week of the end of the period to the management responsible. Management can then follow up with their employees on the lack of compliance. Reports can be run again after providing management a one-week turnaround to correct the situation. At this point, a second set of compliance reports is run and organizational escalation procedures should take place by elevating the issue to senior management.

Some users may object to the policies as published, so the tool should provide the capability of providing these comments. Provided that the previous steps of management approval were followed prior to publishing the policy, it should be clear that adherence to and compliance with the distributed policies is expected. Therefore, compliance tracking should expect 100 percent acceptance by the users of the policy (hence, again stressing the importance of the management review before publishing). Compliance tracking should not have to be concerned with disagreements with the policy.

Once a few phases of policy rollouts have been completed the process becomes a very effective and efficient way to track compliance to policies.

Step 10: Manage Ongoing Process for Policy Violations

The Web-based tool should support a mechanism for users to report security incidents so that as they become aware of violations of the policy, they have the capability to report the incident. This process can be very helpful in understanding where the exceptions to the policy are occurring, gaps in training, or missing procedures to support the policy. New procedures or changes to the policies can occur as a result of receiving information directly from those required to implement the policy. Even though rigorous reviews may be done by management prior to publication, there still may be unanticipated circumstances which, upon further analysis, may require revision and republication of the policy.

Tracking numbers should be assigned within the tool to each reported incident with follow-ups occurring within a reasonable period of time (24 to 48 hours for first response). It may be necessary to supplement the Web-based tool with external tracking spreadsheets; however, if a tracking number is assigned, these items can be manageable. To some extent, this process could be considered as a "security effectiveness monitoring" process for the policies themselves. The reporting of incidents provides a means to monitor whether people are following the policies with a greatly expanded number of people monitoring (the entire workforce!).

WHEW ... TEN STEPS AND WE ARE DONE, RIGHT?

One thing that is very clear in policy development is that it is never done. However, once an organization has moved from "no policies" to a base set of security policies, procedures, standards, and guidelines and has executed the ten steps above, with multiple phased rollouts, the organization is 90 percent there in terms of policy development. It is a mistake to put the policies on the shelf creating paper, dust, and obsolescence by creating the digital world equivalent on the intranet. Policies can get stale and may get out of synch with reality. Organizations go through many changes such as mergers and acquisitions, connections with third-party business partners, outsourced services, adoption of new technologies, upgrades to existing technologies, new methods of security awareness training, new regulations that must be addressed, and so forth. Policies should be reviewed minimally annually to ensure that they are still appropriate for the organization. Upon each major organizational or technological change, policies that could be affected should be identified and reviewed.

FINAL THOUGHTS

Paper will not be going away anytime soon. Dust is optional, and obsolescence can be replaced by a mechanism that provides current, relevant, updated information on which the organization can rely. The key word here is "can," as moving the paper to an electronic format takes care of the dust problem, but does little to change the obsolescence problem if policy creation is seen as a one-time thing to "get them out there quickly."

The Web-based policy deployment tools of the past few years have done a great job of providing an infrastructure for the communication and management of the policies. If we think of the tool as a hammer, we need to remember that the hammer itself performs no work and makes no progress in building things unless there is a person using it to pound nails. People utilizing the review and approval processes are critical in the development of policy, whether the policies are paper-based or electronically deployed. Using the tools does provide great benefit in deployment of the policies as discussed in the prior sections, such as providing support to large user bases, keeping the policies fresh, enabling periodic quizzing of the content, tracking compliance, controlling the timing of the review, and ensuring that users are seeing policies appropriate to their job functions. The tools also provide great benefit to the end users by providing a mechanism for them to view up-to-date policies, submit security incidents, perform context searches, and follow the linkage to procedures, standards, and guidelines through navigating the Web site.

So it's time to enter the dust-free environment, build the infrastructure, and never return to the binders with the nice tabs that few people see. Start small, start somewhere, just start. It is well worth the effort.

III

ECONOMICS, LEGALITY, AND LIABILITY

8

HIPAA PRIVACY RULES REQUIRE SECURITY COMPLIANCE

Steven B. Markin, Esq.

INTRODUCTION

There's no escaping it. There's just no privacy without security. At least according to HIPAA:

> As many commenters recognized, security and privacy are inextricably linked. The protection of the privacy of information depends in large part on the existence of security measures to protect that information.[1]

From this and other language found in the privacy and security rules we'll see the privacy rule, compliance effective April 13, 2003, actually requires compliance with the security rule, which isn't effective until April 13, 2005.

If we realize the diverse but interconnected purposes of the two rules, this is not as strange as it seems. The privacy rule sets standards for how protected health information in all forms, paper and electronic, should be controlled by setting forth what uses and disclosures are authorized or required and what rights patients have with respect to their health information. The security rule sets forth standards on safeguarding the confidentiality, integrity, and availability of electronic protected health.

The privacy rule requires: ". . . appropriate administrative, technical, and physical safeguards to protect the privacy of protected health information."[2] Indeed, the privacy rule's implementation specification for safeguards requires that a covered entity ". . . must reasonably safeguard protected health information from any intentional or unintentional use or disclosure."[3]

WHAT IS "REASONABLE" UNDER THE PRIVACY RULES?

In the absence of specific technical safeguards implementation specifications in the privacy rule, we must look to the standards set forth in HIPAA's security rule. Not only is this a logical safe bet for a safe harbor[4] but it is the intention of the rules. Answering the question of how a covered entity could comply with technical and physical safeguards in the then absence of final security rules, the rule-makers stated, in part, that the security and privacy rules work "hand in glove."[5] In fact, the rules are peppered with reference to the interdependence of privacy and security rules.

RISK ANALYSIS, RISK MANAGEMENT, AND A SANCTION POLICY ARE THE FOUNDATION OF SECURITY MANAGEMENT

The rules state that risk analysis, risk management, and sanction policy

> . . . form the foundation upon which an entity's necessary security activities are built...An entity must identify the risks to and vulnerabilities of the information in its care before it can take effective steps to eliminate or minimize those risks and vulnerabilities. Some form of sanction or punishment activity must be instituted for noncompliance.
>
> Response of HHC, 68 FR 8346 (February 20, 2003)

So the evaluation of the technical and physical risks is the first step in complying with the security rule. It's also required by the privacy rule. When reviewing the risk analysis and assessment to arrive at a security plan, the implementations must be reasonable and appropriate to its environment.[6]

> It should be noted that the implementation of reasonable and appropriate security measures also supports compliance with the privacy standards, *just as the lack of adequate security can increase the risk of violation of the privacy standards. If, for example, a particular safeguard is inadequate because it routinely permits reasonably anticipated uses or disclosures of electronic*

protected health information that are not permitted by the Privacy Rule, and that could have been prevented by implementation of one or more security measures appropriate to the scale of the covered entity, the covered entity would not only be violating the Privacy Rule, but would also not be in compliance with § 164.306(a)(3) of this [Security] rule.[7]

(68 FR 8341-2 (February 20, 2003, last column, emphasis added))

VULNERABILITY TESTING IS REQUIRED

Risk assessment and management, of which vulnerability testing is the foundation, is required to ascertain not only what the reasonable and appropriate risk management measures and security management processes will be but to prevent the reasonably anticipated invasion of privacy rights by hackers. The cost is so low that it is hard to think of a covered entity for which vulnerability testing would not be "reasonable and appropriate." 45 CFR 164.308(a) (ii) (B) requires " . . . *implementing security measures sufficient to reduce risks and vulnerabilities to a reasonable and appropriate level to comply with Section 164.306(a)."*

Vulnerability testing is further required as covered entities must conduct an accurate and thorough assessment of the potential risks and vulnerabilities to the confidentiality, integrity, and availability of electronic protected health information held by the covered entity.[8]

Data integrity is another reason for vulnerability testing. The risk assessment and management studies will yield a security management process. Pursuant to 45 CFR 164.306 and 308, any such security management plan must comply with the following required implementation standard:

- *Standard: Security management process.* Implement policies and procedures to prevent, detect, contain and correct violations. [308 (a) (1) (i)].

See also, 45 CFR 164.312(c) (1) of the privacy rule which states in relevant part:

- *Standard: Integrity.* Implement policies and procedures to protect electronic protected health information from improper alteration or destruction.

Vulnerability testing reveals vulnerabilities to expose what hackers can see and helps prevent, contain, and correct these violations, protecting the data from improper alteration or destruction.

HOW FREQUENTLY DO I NEED TO PERFORM VULNERABILITY TESTING?

Although HIPAA doesn't give a magic number as to the frequency of testing it does provide criteria. As seen above, all of HIPAA's implementations consider what is reasonable and appropriate to the environment. A larger hospital, an insurer, or a clearinghouse would be well served to test some portions of their systems and processes daily, weekly, or monthly. A small doctor's office or clinic could test less frequently.

68 FR 8346 (February 20, 2003) subheading 1, Security Management Process (section 164.308(a) (1) (i)) states:

> We note that the implementation specification for a risk analysis at § 164.308(a) (1) (ii) (A) does not specifically require that a covered entity perform a risk analysis often enough to ensure that its security measures are adequate to provide the level of security required by § 164.306(a). In the proposed rule, an assurance of adequate security was framed as a requirement to keep security measures "current." We continue to believe that security measures must remain current, and have added regulatory language in § 164.306(e)[9] as a more precise way of communicating that security measures **[8347]** in general that must be periodically reassessed and updated as needed.[10]

IN CONCLUSION

Vulnerability testing is a reasonable and appropriate security measure for all covered entities and is therefore required to be performed on a regular basis. How frequently the tests should be performed is largely a function of the size of the covered entity. Given the cost/benefit ratio of testing to risk to protected health information and the rules' stated policy towards testing as needed, a good rule of thumb might be: clearinghouses, sizeable hospitals, and insurers should consider daily testing, smaller hospitals and other covered entities should consider testing at least twice a week, and all covered entities should consider testing at least once each month. Of course testing should be done much more frequently if vulnerabilities are discovered until remediation is effected. Afterward, testing should again be performed to confirm the remediation was effective.

8356 Federal Register/Vol. 68, No. 34/Thursday, February 20, 2003/Rules and Regulations individual upon request. There has been a tendency to assume that this privacy rule requirement would be satisfied via some sort of process involving audit trails. We caution against assuming that the security rule's requirement for an audit capability will satisfy the

privacy rule's requirement regarding accounting for disclosures of protected health information. The two rules cover overlapping, but not
identical, information. Furthermore, audit trails are typically used to record
uses within an electronic information system, whereas the privacy rule
requirement for accounting applies to certain disclosures outside the
covered entity (e.g., to public health authorities).

REFERENCES

1. Security Rule (Final), 68 FR 8335 (February 20, 2003, III. Analysis of and
   Responses to, Public Comments on the Proposed Rule).
2. See 45 CFR 164.530 Administrative requirements.
   (c)(1) *Standard: safeguards.* A covered entity must have in place appropriate
   administrative, technical, and physical safeguards to protect the privacy of
   protected health information.
   (2) Implementation specification: safeguards.
   (i) A covered entity must reasonably safeguard protected health information
   from any intentional or unintentional use or disclosure that is in violation of
   the standards, implementation specifications or other requirements of this
   subpart.
   (ii) A covered entity must reasonably safeguard protected health information
   to limit incidental uses or disclosures made pursuant to an otherwise permitted
   or required use or disclosure.
3. See 45 CFR 164.530 (c)(2).
4. In this context, a "safe harbor" is a method of complying that will be recognized
   by HIPAA.
5. Including the requirement of 164.530 (67 FR 53194, August 14, 2002, The
   Privacy Rule amendment).
6. Not only must the implementation be reasonable and appropriate to its environment, but the rules grant flexibility in selecting the security measures based
   upon the Covered Entities, size, technical infrastructure, cost of the measure
   and probability of risk. Please see, 45 CFR.306 (b): *Flexibility of approach.*
   (1) Covered entities may use any security measures that allow the covered
   entity to reasonably and appropriately implement the standards and implementation specifications as specified in this subpart.
   (2) In deciding which security measures to use, a covered entity must take
   into account the following factors:
   (i) The size, complexity, and capabilities of the covered entity.
   (ii) The covered entity's technical infrastructure, hardware, and software security capabilities.
   (iii) The costs of security measures.
   (iv) The probability and criticality of potential risks to electronic protected
   health information.
7. The Security Rule addresses two types of Implementation Standards: "Paragraph
   (d) of § 164.306 establishes two types of implementation specifications, required
   and addressable. It provides that required implementation specifications must be
   met. However, with respect to implementation specifications that are addressable,

§ 164.306(d)(3) specifies that covered entities must assess whether an implementation specification is a reasonable and appropriate safeguard in its environment, which may include consideration of factors such as the size and capability of the organization as well as the risk. If the organization determines it is a reasonable and appropriate safeguard, it must implement the specification. If an addressable implementation specification is determined not to be a reasonable and appropriate answer to a covered entity's security needs, the covered entity must do one of two things: implement another equivalent measure if reasonable and appropriate; or if the standard can otherwise be met, the covered entity may choose to not implement the implementation specification or any equivalent alternative measure at all. The covered entity must document the rationale behind not implementing the implementation specification. See the detailed discussion in section II.A.3. Paragraph (e) of § 164.306 addresses the requirement for covered entities to maintain the security measures implemented by reviewing and modifying the measures as needed to continue the provision of reasonable and appropriate protections, for example, as technology moves forward, and as new threats or vulnerabilities are discovered (68FR 8341-2 need security for privacy (February 20, 2003).

8. More specifically, section 308 (a)(ii) states:

   45 CFR 164.308 (a) (ii) (A) Risk Analysis and Risk Management. (A) *Risk analysis (Required)*. Conduct an accurate and thorough assessment of the potential risks and vulnerabilities to the confidentiality, integrity, and availability of electronic protected health information held by the covered entity.

   (B) *Risk management (Required)*. Implement security measures sufficient to reduce risks and vulnerabilities to a reasonable and appropriate level to comply with Section 164.306(a).

9. (e) *Maintenance.* Security measures implemented to comply with standards and implementation specifications adopted under § 164.105 and this subpart must be reviewed and modified as needed to continue provision of reasonable and appropriate protection of electronic protected health information as described at § 164.316.

10. The text continues: "The risk analysis implementation specification contains other terms that merit explanation. Under § 164.308(a) (1) (ii) (A), the risk analysis must look at risks to the covered entity's electronic protected health information. A thorough and accurate risk analysis would consider 'all relevant losses' that would be expected if the security measures were not in place. 'Relevant losses' would include losses caused by unauthorized uses and disclosures and loss of data integrity that would be expected to occur absent the security measures.

9

LEGALITIES AND PLANNING: THE STAKE IS IN THE GROUND

Ken M. Shaurette, CISSP, CISA, CISM, IAM

INTRODUCTION

This chapter consists of observations and opinions that have been formulated from several years of practicing information security. The opinions are based on experience from seeing the computer industry grow and change since 1978. The chapter is intended to bring together ideas and questions that will help readers formulate some ideas on the state of their own organization's information security program. Much of the information is based on certification in the NSA's InfoSec Assessment Methodology, knowledge and practice of the ISO17799 Information Technology — Code of Practice for Information Security Management, along with research of signed and pending legislation.

TAKE MY ADVICE AT YOUR OWN RISK

Before getting too deep into my story, I have to first provide a disclaimer: I am not a lawyer, nor do I play one on TV, therefore I am not providing legal advice, or presenting in any form or fashion a legal opinion on any matter, covered or uncovered by the title; nor do I want to give you an impression that I am engaging in the unauthorized practice of law, or lead you to believe that I have any opinions one way or the other about lawyers who do practice law.

The information contained in this chapter is not intended to be legal advice. The intention is to inform, to educate, and if not answer, create a few questions that you will want to research. Michael Rasmussen of the Forrester Group noted in a recent presentation that "Security is like water, you can't survive without either one." The challenge is to think about

0-8493-2211-1/05/$0.00+$1.50
© 2005 by CRC Press LLC

"reasonable" and "diligence." Do you need Perrier or Evian, or can you survive with basic tap water? Maybe you need to add chlorine to improve the quality of the water you use. Worse yet, is your current security equivalent to a polluted river, exposed to the nasty run-off of numerous undesirable entities? It is important to identify whether your organization might be susceptible to potential liability. It is hoped that the following discussion provides some thought-provoking ideas regarding liability in relationship to the HIPAA security regulations as well as various other regulations.

If you are a lawyer, play one on TV, or are considering practicing law, you are still welcome; so read on.

HIPAA RULES

HIPAA requires that three general sets of security areas be considered consisting of: (1)administrative procedures, (2) physical safeguards, and (3) technical security.

The proposed rules are in response to issues from both inside and outside the healthcare industry. Entities covered by the rules include healthcare providers that transmit health information in electronic form, health plans, and healthcare clearing houses. Similar regulations such as GLBA (Gramm–Leach–Bliley Act) have been enacted for the financial industry and FERPA (Family Educational Rights and Privacy Act) to address security/privacy concerns of student data (including health information) in educational environments.

Many covered healthcare entities officially have 26 months after the final rule was signed to comply and others have 38 months. The security rule was finalized in 2003, meaning compliance with the security regulation has a deadline of April 2005 for most entities. The final rules also identified that the security only needs to address ePHI (Electronic Protected Health Information). In any case there is no time to wait as many observers feel that these timeframes are minimum timelines for companies to be able to meet some compliance requirements. The cost of getting in compliance will certainly rise if all organizations put off the necessary work until the final months.

The penalties for violation of the regulations are very severe and covered entities can even be liable for violations committed by their business partners. The penalties are: $100 per violation or a $25,000 cap per year per violation for violating any standard; for knowingly violating, fines are $50,000 and imprisonment for one year; violations under false pretenses carry fines of $100,000 and imprisonment for five years; and a violation with a malicious intent or intent involving personal gain carries a fine of $250,000 and ten-year prison terms.

It is important to note that the regulation states "knowingly violating." I ask you this question: Is ignoring the state of your security a version of "knowing violation?" A manager may state: "We can afford the risk and pay the penalty should something happen, but who is the management representative who will step forward to give part of his life and spend time in jail? Jail time often is quick to change people's attitudes. It is easy to sit around a table and agree to pay the penalty if caught, but no one is very fast to step forward and become the potential jailbird.

Does it take the compliance date to arrive for penalties to be incurred? Several years have already passed since the proposed rule was available; is there potential that when an incident occurs at a covered entity the legal system would already expect organizations to show that they have taken "reasonable" measures to improve security of ePHI? Even before the date for official compliance is here? Is it possible that even though an item in the regulation is listed as addressable, certain types or sizes of organizations would be expected to implement a solution? Because the final rule is not much different than what was proposed in 1998 and many could argue that protecting confidential information with reasonable measures is nothing more than common sense, could organizations already be liable? It is my opinion that in this regard organizations should already be implementing the commonsense measures of "reasonable" security. For example, any organization not using passwords, not changing them regularly, or using very short and easy to guess passwords to authenticate users may already be negligent of reasonable "commonsense" security. It could be argued that the organization has not taken reasonable security measures, and therefore they might find themselves staring at case law and severe penalties imposed by the court. This comes from the simple fact that they have known about the proposed security recommendations for several years and are unable to show that they have taken "reasonable" security measures, or even at minimum created an information security operational plan to illustrate how they will reach compliance by 2005.

HIPAA AND DUE DILIGENCE

As we all now remember, the drafted security regulations, proposed in 1998, did not name a specific technology for compliance, but they did outline the functions that any chosen security solution(s) must provide. The now released and signed regulation hasn't changed much. It now identifies components as "required" versus "addressable," but still does not eliminate the questions of what solutions must be implemented to meet compliance. For example, the regulations simply state "unique user identification"; they don't tell us whether simple user accounts and four-character passwords are acceptable or if there needs to be an eight-character password or maybe biometrics. Even though the regulations don't outline a specific security solution, every covered entity is required to select and implement a "reasonable" solution or in my opinion as an alternative, document why a control is not being implemented or is potentially unnecessary in the environment because of other compensating controls. The security controls that might be acceptable today might not be an acceptable practice in the future because of the changing landscape of technology and every organization is looking for continuous improvement to protect information. Remember that security is not a product or technology, but an ongoing process. Compliance is not a destination, but a journey. Passwords may one day be acceptable practice, but as technology improves and costs change, that requirement may become smart cards, biometrics, or some other form of two-factor authentication in order to access confidential information.

Although the final security rule clearly establishes the specific components that are "required" and those that are "addressable," it doesn't establish the specifics of how, and just because a component is identified as "addressable" does not mean that it is "ignorable!" Unique authentication, for example, could be handled by anything from passwords to password-generating tokens or biometrics. Depending on the organization and the accepted practices of like organizations, an addressable item may become a "required" practice based on what has become accepted practices (best practices) in similar organizations. I call it THEE-DOITRULE, "THe Everyone Else is DOing IT RULE." What I mean is that if similar organizations of your size (small, medium, or large) and type (payer, provider, or clearinghouse, etc.) are consistently implementing a control and it is commonly accepted as the best solution, then like organizations must follow suit. If an organization doesn't and an incident should occur, would the victim of the breach in security have just cause to claim that the organization had inadequate security controls? Could they claim that the controls implemented in a majority of other similar organizations are the accepted practice that should be followed? To provide an example, let's use the simple example of passwords again. If a majority of large organizations are implementing multiple-factor authentication (biometrics or smart cards), it would be wise to assume that implementing only a five-character password scheme for authentication might be considered inadequate to meet "due diligence" compared to accepted practices in like organizations for protecting the confidentiality, integrity, or availability of ePHI.

PENALTIES AND LIABILITY

In a May 9, 2002 report entitled "Security Negligence: Real Threat of Legal Liability," the GIGA analysts point out

. . . managers may incorrectly think that directors and officers (D&O) insurance [will] protect them from potential liability, or that if a situation arose, the company itself would be liable, not the individual manager. Knowingly making a business decision that places the company or its customers at risk could be named in legal actions that sought damages. D&O policies may not offer protection, since many of them ignore this vital area of a company's infrastructure. Ultimately, lawsuits arise because of poor business decisions, or lack of them.

Management cannot shift the liability for making poor decisions regarding security architecture. Ignorance of the need for security is no longer a defense; performing a security assessment then not acting on the findings can be considered negligent, but not performing the security assessment in the first place is just as negligent.

WHAT IS COMPLIANCE?

There has been a lot of discussion about what prescribing to the regulation means. The official compliance clock began ticking in the spring of 2003; for most covered entities, compliance is by 2005. The regulations are quite complex and because they don't name specific solutions for compliance they are open to interpretation. It has been said that the original authors of the security rule wanted to define "reasonable" in the rule, but it was determined that the definition could not be included. Case law and accepted practices would need to establish that as time passes.

In the United States tort law consists of four fundamental components: (1) duty, (2) negligence, (3) damage, and (4) cause. This taken in the context of information security and specifically ePHI essentially identifies that organizations and more directly, an organization's management, have a "duty," a responsibility to provide appropriate security and "reasonable" protection of ePHI and even other confidential information. An effective information security policy can help to assign various responsibilities to positions and even people in the organization. Be sure to define responsibilities in policy, including such as areas as management, security, audit, and user. An organization or manager that is negligent in supporting security policy, proper planning, or even the most basic (reasonable) implementation of security measures is susceptible to penalty, especially should "damage" occur. Damage is the quantifiable harm, such as a person having his identity stolen, or a person being denied insurance or a job because her ePHI was compromised. Duty plus negligence plus damage brings us to cause. Together this all would indicate that even without the HIPAA security rule officially in place organizations need to manage their risk, reduce their liability, and begin to implement "reasonable" security programs.

Is it possible that patients will feel that information about them is already being secured (or should be) and that reasonable security measures already protect access to and the privacy of their personal data? Is it also possible that when a patient finds out an organization has not begun to take security seriously and thus implemented reasonable controls that they could file suit based on tort law expecting that more security should be in place based on the information contained in the rule that has been proposed for several years?

What does defining "reasonable" mean? It means that case law will slowly define the required minimums and industry standard requirements for properly managing risk to ePHI data. It means that organizations will establish accepted practices based on size and type. That means reasonable may also be defined by what the majority of like organizations are doing for security in each of the HIPAA defined security areas: administrative, technical, and physical. The definition of reasonable will certainly not be totally understood or concretely established until cases of violation go before a judge or a jury, penalties are levied, and the court establishes controls that should have been in place to reduce or eliminate liability, hence affecting any penalty enforced. Case law will define compliance requirements and the actions that must be taken to comply. Case law will begin to define what is "reasonable" and the levels of proper diligence that an organization must adhere to in order to be considered compliant. It may be very difficult until reasonable is more clearly defined to completely avoid being called into court to settle the issues. There are already enacted federal guidelines that may provide some insight such as the Federal Organizational Sentencing Guidelines. These guidelines provide some insight into how to reduce and avoid potential liability.

Federal Organizational Sentencing Guidelines stiffen the penalties imposed on corporations when federal statutes are violated. The guidelines substantially increase the penalties for businesses that do not make any effort to deter or detect crime. The penalties are significantly reduced for businesses that implement basic security measures. I hold that planning and documentation will be how organizations reduce or eliminate any penalty when an incident does occur. Think of the definition of a jury. It is 12 men and women (your peers) who determine who has the best lawyer. I'm going to arm my lawyer with sufficient documentation showing what I'm doing, showing what I have done, and what I plan to do towards improving my organization's protection of ePHI so that my lawyer can argue that I've done my diligence and I'm planning reasonable measures to protect ePHI. I want to convince my peers that I have the best lawyer, and with proper documentation and planning I believe I will be able to do that.

PLANNING SECURITY COMPLIANCE?

One of the most important pieces of documentation to reduce my liability is a plan. Creating a plan by which an organization can base its security decisions is an important step to prioritizing the efforts that will be expended when improving the security for the organization's environment. It is also a necessity identified by the proposed HIPAA Security Standard, 45 CFR Part 142.314(2). In this author's opinion two of the most important tasks to become HIPAA compliant consist of planning and documentation.

Establishing an Information Security Operational Plan (ISOP) is an important baseline that helps with budgeting and leadership awareness regarding security management. It is an excellent tool to present to governing boards and decision makers to gauge the progress of the security program, compliance status, or to solicit additional budget dollars. It also can provide a good measure of covering your butt, by informing management what needs to be done. If it isn't done, or budgeted for, how much more could you do?

The plan maximizes a company's resources and organizes them so that they can be concentrated where they are most needed while not forgetting other equally important aspects of an overall information protection program. As ISO 17799 defines a code of practice for information security management, the ISOP does the same as the plan to define security management and the overall security program, because it doesn't happen overnight. The plan provides a philosophy for information security guided by vision, a mission, and quality statement. A tactical plan establishes an organized way to build on the basic mechanisms and foundation that make up the information security infrastructure. It focuses on the "required" elements of compliance and documents the items that are "addressable" and how they are prioritized within other activities. Your ISOP can also be incorporated or integrated into your corporate technology plan. Be sure not to allow security to be deemphasized in comparison to technology goals or other corporate goals.

The purpose of the information security program is to provide for the Confidentiality, Integrity, and Availability (CIA) of vital information assets. A properly constructed information security program provides for the reasonable measures, required or addressable, that will meet HIPAA security compliance and CIA. The purpose of the information security operational plan is to organize technical, organizational (in HIPAA terms, administrative), physical, and the other security program components into a plan that delivers the right combination of controls, putting into place a holistic approach providing for confidentiality, integrity, and availability of ePHI.

Performing security assessments to determine an organization's vulnerabilities will identify risk to ePHI allowing reasonable security measures to be implemented. Determining which security technologies and administrative and physical controls need priority attention is where a plan becomes critically important. It provides a covered entity the direction necessary to implement reasonable security measures in an organized manner to meet the regulations and, equally important, to reduce liability. It helps prevent an organization from assuming more risk than it can afford.

To get the overall compliance efforts kick-started, it is critical for an organization to assign internal responsibility for following through with the ISOP and managing the overall success of the security and compliance program. Assigning a person or position to be responsible for security is a necessary compliance step as identified by 45 CFR Part 142.308(b)(1).

An ISOP can be broken into eight categories. At the top level an executive summary outlines the foundation of the plan along with assumptions, any prerequisites, and requirements to execution of the plan. Each year (more frequently if desirable) updates to the tactical plan outline the status, goals, and plans for the coming year in each category and document any progress from the last report. By maintaining a planning document the status of compliance can be identified and any issues resolved. It provides management a point-in-time perspective of where their compliance measures are. It will help management remain aware of the need to continue supporting the security program. As any security professional knows, security is not a destination — it is a continuous journey. Even after meeting compliance security continues to require attention in order to remain compliant, and in order to keep reasonable controls implemented based on case law or commonly accepted practices.

A brief explanation of each of the categories that can make up an ISOP follows.

- *Baseline:* This is a baseline study, establishing where the security program is at and updated annually to establish the status of the compliance "reasonable" security measures. It provides an understanding of the current status of all company information security efforts. Where is security at and where does it need to be?
- *Policies, Standards, and Procedures:* Policy is the road map; it sets the current state of company security and where a company wants to or needs to go. Standards usually provide the technical foundation from which the business will work. Procedures provide the directions on how to comply with policy and meet standards deployment. All of these together define the business environment to ensure proper handling of information.

- *Architecture and Processes:* This area is the infrastructure and processes that provide a secure and stable operating environment. Included are approval and implementation methodologies such as change management. It addresses the need for security to be part of development and design as well as testing and deployment.
- *Awareness and Training:* Users and customers must be aware of their personal responsibilities relating to information security. Technology alone will not eliminate all vulnerability or make an organization compliant. Proper education and awareness by information handlers is critical. They must know what policy exists and what the procedures are that can help compliance.
- *Technologies and Products:* Security-related products are necessary to support policy and provide the security architecture, which protects the business processes. The technologies can range from simple logging of user activity (audit logs) to complex public key encryption systems.
- *Assessment and Monitoring:* The right information must be collected and distributed to the appropriate personnel including management reporting. Network connections, overall system performance, access to ePHI, and host activity must be monitored for anomalies or suspicious activity, even tracking of routine access.
- *Contingency:* This is the preparation for out of the ordinary events or preparing for the unexpected. This includes incidents that affect the availability of ePHI, as simple as the minor loss of access to information or business processing functions to catastrophic losses caused by disasters, human or natural.
- *Compliance:* This is the health check for the information security program. It establishes methodologies for feedback that provide the cornerstone of continuous improvement for the information security efforts. It establishes ways for management, technical staff, and end users to assess the impact of implementing components of the security program on the computing environment and business processes that may adversely affect the company's ability to remain compliant with regulations or even simply do its job.

What Can Be Done?

In the author's opinion if any individual working in a healthcare covered entity were simply to treat all ePHI as if it were information about himself, he would be meeting reasonableness for compliance. Most people would tend to be very protective and take precautionary and at least reasonable measures to protect their own personal health information. For example, consider a health insurance payments department. A payment is being processed for coverage that was performed on you; is there a need for the payments clerk to have access to all of the patient's information, such as what was covered by insurance and what was not, essentially describing what procedures were performed? Would simple billing information such as name, address, and dollar amount to be billed be sufficient? Is access to your phone number even necessary?

These are some of the kinds of questions that can help determine how best to meet the "minimum necessary" components of the privacy rule and identify how to apply security. Covered entities must basically identify what data is needed to perform each business function and who performs those functions and from that determine who needs access to it. Essentially in the information security industry this is considered the concept of "least privilege" or "need to know." Do you need to know the information to do your job? At minimum it will be necessary for covered entities to identify data flow and specific requirements of various data elements by job category. By doing that it will be possible to show that the "minimum necessary" requirements for the amount of data were disclosed for a transaction. If questions arise documentation would show justification of why data may have been identified as necessary or "reasonable" for access by this user. It provides the evidence that proper diligence was taken in an attempt to comply with the rule. This may be an extremely important factor should a situation escalate to the court system and need to be proved in front of a judge and a jury.

The kinds of things that health organizations should do to address privacy and security rules are:

- Define organizational responsibilities. Assign a person or position to be responsible for compliance activities. Who will be responsible to ensure proper planning for security and that security projects are being properly prioritized and implemented? A requirement for compliance is this kind of position, at least a proxy or consultant taking on the responsibilities. It does not necessarily mean a full-time position, but a role for someone with proper responsibility and authority to help ensure compliance.
- Begin to explore with legal counsel the extent to which the rules, proposed or final, will affect your institution. Only legal advice can fully scope the potential liability of inaction. It may be necessary to find legal counsel that specifically deals in this kind of work.
- Evaluate existing security technology and patient information systems. Assess your risks.
- Develop an ISOP that will account for the efforts to comply with privacy and security rules. Basically define the organization's security

framework and infrastructure and its status. The ISOP will provide planning, prioritization, and proper allocation of personnel and financial resources. It can then be used at least annually to communicate the status and is an excellent document to show compliance efforts. It can be used as a place to show from year to year that proper diligence is being given to the activities to remain compliant and that when issues of risk management come up there is a method of handling them appropriately.

■ Identify business partners and discuss how to evaluate their data handling. Find out if they are making compliance considerations. They may need to begin taking some of the same considerations that are listed here, especially the planning for security.

■ Put in motion an awareness program to inform end users, customers, and business partners. End users are generally the weak link and a major component of compliance. It is not a technology, hardware, or software that can be purchased to meet compliance here. It is all about making them aware of their responsibility to protect privacy, the measures they can take to improve security, and being aware of the organization security policy.

■ Don't let the hype send you out to the first hardware, software, or consulting company who proclaims to be "HIPAA compliant!" Remember, being compliant with the security regulations is about common sense.

■ Security measures are not anything new or miraculous. Remember the hysteria of the year 2000, Y2K? Organizations that claimed to specialize in Y2K services were all over the place preying on the hype. COBOL programmers were leaving organizations to join consulting firms to get sizable salaries. It will not be possible to proclaim compliance until accreditation agencies or some assigned government entity begins to review or examine the organization's information security programs.

CERTIFICATION OF COMPLIANCE

How will compliance with the new standards be evaluated? Currently, no federal agency or other organization has officially been tasked or funded to conduct compliance surveys for security. Although this may change with future regulations, initially, healthcare organizations will be expected to monitor their own compliance.

The Department of Health and Human Services' (DHHS) Office for Civil Rights (OCR) is responsible for enforcement of the privacy standards. A person who believes that a covered entity is not in compliance may file a complaint with the secretary of Health and Human Services, who may investigate.

A good possibility is that DHHS may also conduct compliance reviews to the security regulations. Will they end up with funding to proactively perform compliance audits? Will there one day be agencies similar to the financial industry (i.e., FDIC, OCC, OTS) that annually examine (audit) covered entities to be sure they remain proactive in protecting ePHI?

The JCAHO (Joint Commission on Accreditation of Healthcare Organizations) may become an entity that performs reviews of compliance for hospitals during accreditation surveys. However, it is not likely that they will not certify organizations as HIPAA compliant.

An organization titled the Security Health Care Certification and Accreditation Workgroup has formed to facilitate the identification and implementation of accepted practices in healthcare. The workgroup is sponsored by URAC (Utilization Review Accreditation Commission) and NIST (National Institute Standards and Technology). This organization consists of numerous interested healthcare organizations and standards-setting people. They may be able to begin delivering reference material and accepted practices to help covered entities of every size and type determine what must be implemented and how.

OTHER LEGISLATION'S POTENTIAL IMPACT

Sarbanes–Oxley Act (SOX)

Even though it is currently limited to financial services organizations, the natural next step will be to broaden the Sarbanes–Oxley Act to other business entities. The Federal Trade Commission (FTC) is already prosecuting and investigating violations. There are also several legislators who are looking to expand these operational risk framework requirements into new legislation that goes beyond simply the financial industry. An important component of Sarbanes–Oxley is the acknowledgment by management of the accuracy of financial statements. The impact on security becomes that there are expectations that management will also be held accountable for the controls and security that ensure the accuracy and protect the data associated with the financial statements, essentially what assurances there are of the integrity of the information. Rules would seem to indicate that as this expands it will be important for management to ensure that adequate security is being implemented.

Corporate Information Security Accountability Act

The Corporate Information Security Accountability Act of 2003 is a bill being sponsored by the chairman of the House Subcommittee on Technology,

Information Policy, Intergovernmental Relations, and the Census. Based on the initial drafts of the act it would require companies to hire an independent auditor to assess existing information security controls and ensure that they meet basic standards that the SEC has yet to determine. The SEC would have about 60 days after the bill has been signed into law to come up with specific standards for the audits.

California's SB1386

SB1386 stands for "Security Breach" (actually "Senate Bill"). Although this is a law signed in California, it affects other organizations by the fact that the information of California residents may be gathered as a result of healthcare coverage outside the state. The law dictates that organizations must inform any California resident if there is ever suspicion that any data stored about him or her may have been compromised. This could mean any compromise of your environment might need to be reported if you have data about a resident of California. This law was used as a model and submitted for federal consideration to create a similar federal requirement. Are you able to detect an incident that might have compromised data? How would you know? Can you define an incident? Do you have a process that allows you to notify the appropriate parties should an incident occur? How do you escalate to the point of notification?

Future

Until organizations begin to make changes that protect information of customers and employees as a matter of normal business the legal system will continue to find ways that will strongly encourage improvement in controls. Laws that today may only cover a very specific industry or type of business are very likely to end up being adopted to address others. For example, the laws that are requiring public companies to improve will eventually look to protect information regardless of whether it is with private or public organizations. Staff and students in colleges and universities as an example will no longer be able to argue that their environment needs to be very open and insecure for "academic freedom," because a regulation similar to HIPAA security will address implementation of a "reasonable" information security program to protect the administrative data that schools handle. Whether the data needs to include ePHI will make no difference. People everywhere increasingly have an expectation that information about them stored in electronic or even hardcopy will have reasonable security controls allowing only authorized and appropriate people to have access.

CONCLUSION

If your organization is one of the entities covered by HIPAA you need to consider how you will meet the regulations, and it doesn't pay to wait. If you don't know where to start, contacting a consulting organization with security experience and knowledge of HIPAA regulations or a law firm with specialization in HIPAA regulations are considerations you may want to make.

The proposed HIPAA security regulation has been published for several years and the signed regulation is not all that different. It could be argued that covered entities should already be taking actions to be compliant with statements in the regulation. There may already be some liability if an organization has not taken proper diligence to protect ePHI or other confidential information in the organization. Other already adopted legislation could provide insight into protections that should already be occurring before the final date for compliance with HIPAA. New legislation is being considered by government entities all the time.

The court system will end up defining what is reasonable to meet compliance with the letter of the regulations. It will be determined by what is presented in court cases and how the court cases are settled. By the courts' actions organizations will begin to know if their information security program will sufficiently reduce their liability or maybe even keep them out of court. The most important thing that every organization will need is: *documentation*. Documentation will provide evidence so a judge or jury chooses my lawyer to be the best. Evidence of "due diligence," evidence of "reasonable," evidence of "compliance," evidence to reduce civil liability, evidence to stay out of jail, and, simply enough, evidence that your organization is taking the confidentiality, integrity, and availability of information it maintains and processes seriously. "Security is like water, you can't survive without it." It is as serious as running a profitable business and you can't take either for granted.

IV

TRANSACTION AND INTERACTIONS

10

HIPAA FROM THE PATIENT'S POINT OF VIEW

Oscar Boultinghouse, M.D.

INTRODUCTION

With the enactment of Public Law 104-191, commonly known as the Health Insurance Portability Accountability Act of 1996 (HIPAA), Congress radically changed how healthcare management operates. These regulations, and their impact on modern day health delivery, are examined in detail from multiple perspectives throughout this book. In this chapter, discussion focuses on those areas of the HIPAA legislation that most directly affect the healthcare consumer's access to care and protection of personal health information.

During the years prior to 1996, Congress and other patient advocacy groups recognized that many employees were facing difficulty in obtaining health insurance when they changed jobs. As a result, Congress enacted the Health Insurance Portability and Accountability Act of 1996. HIPAA's stated function was to enable employees to remain insured when they changed employers.[1] Additionally, HIPAA assured the privacy of Personal Health Information (PHI). Prior to HIPAA, the 1974 Federal Privacy Act had established a broad standard of fair information practices, but the standard was applicable only to government agencies, and was not healthcare specific. The government itself, in its annual summary of the Privacy Act, acknowledged that "even after 20 years of administrative and judicial analysis, numerous Privacy Act issues remain unresolved or unexplored."[2] At the time that HIPAA legislation was being created, personal information privacy protections were a patchwork of state laws and regulations coupled with this weak 1974 Federal Privacy Act.[3] Although lawmakers recognized the need to deal with the limitations and ambiguities of the 1974 Federal Privacy Act, the methods and magnitude of the required changes could not be agreed upon. Despite the acknowledged necessity of improving the manner in which personal health information was protected, Congress failed to enact health privacy laws by the 1999 deadline mandated by the 1996 HIPAA legislation. The HIPAA legislation stipulated that if Congress had failed to enact privacy laws by 1999, the secretary of Health and Human Services (DHHS) would have the authority to develop the mandated regulations. The DHHS secretary subsequently exercised his authority to promulgate the final health information privacy regulations. After an extended comment period, the DHHS secretary's rules were finalized on April 14, 2001. Covered entities that would be affected by the new legislation were given a compliance date of October 16, 2002. The deadline for compliance was subsequently extended for one additional year for those covered entities that filed a "Compliance Plan."[4]

As HIPAA has begun to take hold in the healthcare workflow in the United States, most healthcare workers and consumers alike are most knowledgeable with that portion of the legislation dealing with the protection of personal health information. This consumer familiarity is in part due to the emphasis that has been placed on this HIPAA component by healthcare organizations and individual providers. This emphasis is in part due to the substantial financial penalties that can be assessed for breach of patient privacy standards. These privacy standards and how they affect the typical healthcare encounter are examined in detail below. In addition, the challenges and benefits of resolving health information to an electronic form are explored. Initially, however, the discussion examines how the HIPAA legislation enables employees to remain insured when they change employers.

OVERVIEW OF HIPAA INSURABILITY PROTECTIONS

Each year millions of Americans face a variety of life events that may affect the type of health insurance coverage that they require or that is available to them. These events may include the birth of a child, the onset of a chronic medical condition or debilitating disease, business closings, staff reductions, or divorce. Any one of these everyday occurrences could have a profound impact on a family's or individual's health insurance coverage. HIPAA provides limited protections for the employee and his family members during these disruptive events. Should a life event require a change in the employee's health coverage, understanding these HIPAA protections, as well as laws in the state of residence, will permit the affected employee to understand all available health insurance options. Although the statutory language of HIPAA can be difficult to navigate, it is worth the effort to become familiar with HIPAA's basic constructs. The following guidelines are offered as a starting point to understand how

HIPAA may help protect or provide health coverage when an employee's health or employment status undergoes sudden change.

Understand the Various Types of Health Coverage

Before the employee can understand how HIPAA may help protect health coverage, it is important to understand what the various types of health coverage are. This is important because the law provides different protections depending on the type of health coverage the employee may have or for which she may wish to apply.

Types of Coverage

HIPAA generally applies to the following three types of coverage:

1. *Group Health Plans.* A group health plan is health coverage sponsored by an employer or union for a group of employees, and possibly for dependents and retirees as well.
2. *Individual Health Insurance.* Individual health insurance coverage is insurance coverage that is sold by HMOs or other health insurance issuers to individuals who are not part of a group health plan. Even though health coverage might be provided through an association or other group, such as groups of college students or self-employed individuals, it is still considered to be "individual" health insurance if it is not provided through a group health plan.
3. *Comparable Coverage through a High-Risk Pool.* Some states have set up high-risk pools to provide health coverage for people who cannot otherwise obtain health insurance coverage in the individual market.

Eligibility for HIPAA Protections

If the employee is *not* currently covered by a particular type of plan or insurance, the employee will need to determine for what he may be eligible.

- The eligibility to enroll in a group health plan is determined by the rules of the group health plan and the contract terms of any insurance purchased by an insured plan.
- The eligibility to have HIPAA guarantee the employee the right to purchase individual health insurance coverage (which, in some states, will be through a high-risk pool) depends on the employee's ability to meet ALL of the following requirements.

- The employee must have at least 18 months of creditable coverage without a significant break in coverage — a period of 63 or more days during all of which the employee had no coverage. If the employee obtains coverage by midnight of the 63rd day, the employee has not incurred a significant break.
- The employee's most recent coverage must have been through a group health plan (through the employee's or a family member's employer or union).
- The employee is not eligible for coverage under any other group health plan.
- The employee is not eligible for Medicare or Medicaid.
- The employee does not have other health insurance.
- The employee did not lose insurance coverage for not paying the premiums or for committing fraud.
- The employee accepted and used up available COBRA continuation coverage or similar state coverage if it was offered.

If these requirements are met, then the employee becomes HIPAA eligible.

When the Employee Is Hired for a New Job

If the employee finds a new job that offers a group health plan, or, if the employee is eligible under another family member's group health plan, the employee must first determine whether HIPAA applies to the group health plan. For example, if the job is with a church, or with a state or local governmental employer, or with a very small employer, HIPAA protections may be more limited. The employee should ask the new employer or the state insurance department for information about HIPAA.

When an Employee Leaves a Job or Otherwise Loses Group Health Plan Coverage

If the employee is a HIPAA eligible individual, and applies for individual health coverage within 63 days after losing group health plan coverage, HIPAA:

- Guarantees that the employee will have a choice of at least two coverage options
- Guarantees that the employee will be eligible, regardless of any medical conditions, to purchase some type of individual coverage, whether from a health insurance issuer, high-risk pool, or other source designated by the state

■ Guarantees that the employee will not be subject to any preexisting condition exclusions

HIPAA does not limit the amount that the employee can be charged for the policy. However, state laws may set limits.

Determine the Impact of Any Preexisting Condition

Traditionally, many employer-sponsored group health plans and health insurance issuers in both the group and individual markets limited or denied coverage of health conditions that an individual had prior to the person's enrollment in the plan. These types of exclusions are known as preexisting condition exclusions.

Although such exclusions were problematic for those trying to secure health coverage in the past, HIPAA and other recent federal laws bring some relief to this problem in certain situations.

Eligibility to Minimize the Length of the Preexisting Condition Exclusion

Under HIPAA's group market rules, creditable coverage can be used to reduce or eliminate preexisting condition exclusions that might be applied to the employee under a future plan or policy. In general, if the employee has other health coverage — for example, under another group health plan or under an individual health insurance policy, Medicare, Medicaid, an HMO, or a state high-risk pool — the employee's new plan preexisting condition exclusion period must be reduced by the period of the other coverage. This earned credit for previous coverage that can help the employee reduce the exclusion period is called *creditable coverage.*

The exclusion period must be shortened by one day for each day of creditable coverage that the employee has. If the amount of creditable coverage is equal to or longer than the exclusion period, no exclusion period can be imposed on the employee. When figuring out how much creditable coverage the applicant has, however, the applicant receives no credit for previous coverage that has been followed by a significant break in coverage — a period of 63 or more full days in a row during which there was no creditable coverage.

Know the State's Law on Coverage

If an employee is in an insured plan, his state law may allow a longer break in coverage. If so, the employee may be able to count creditable coverage even if it is followed by a break of 63 days or more in a row.

An individual state may also require a shorter exclusion period, or shorter look-back period. State law requirements for preexisting condition exclusions do not affect those imposed by self-insured plans. For more information contact the state insurance department.

Understand Other Coverage Protections

Understanding how the employee can best protect her health coverage is not easy. It is complicated because the rules are different depending on each individual's special situation. The final step in understanding HIPAA and the employee's protections under the law involves knowing some general information about:

- Special enrollment rights to other group coverage
- How the employee's health status can affect access to care
- Other coverage choices that may help the employee take advantage of HIPAA protections
- The individual's rights to renew group and individual coverage

Special Enrollment Rights to Other Group Coverage

Group health plans and health insurance issuers are required to provide special enrollment periods during which individuals who previously declined coverage for themselves and their dependents may be allowed to enroll. It is important to note that individuals will be able to enroll without having to wait until the plan's next open enrollment period, but in most situations a special enrollment must be requested within 30 days.

A special enrollment period can occur if a person with other health coverage loses that coverage or if a person becomes a new dependent through marriage, birth, adoption, or placement for adoption. Special enrollment is not late enrollment, which can trigger an 18-month preexisting condition exclusion period.

In summary, the Health Insurance Portability and Accountability Act of 1996 provides important new but limited protections for employees and their families. Specifically, it increases the employee's ability to access individual and family health coverage. HIPAA reduces the probability of losing existing health coverage whether that coverage is through a job or through individual health insurance. HIPAA legislation also helps an employee avoid disruption in individual and family health coverage with job change. And finally, HIPAA helps an individual purchase health insurance coverage if coverage under an employer's group health plan is lost and no other health coverage is available.

OVERVIEW OF HIPAA PRIVACY AND SECURITY RULES

In 1996, Congress changed the way medical practices deal with patients' medical records or Personal Health Information (PHI). The Health Insurance Portability and Accountability Act of 1996 makes it mandatory to comply with privacy and security rules. Prior federal privacy protections had been established by the federal Privacy Act of 1974. Despite the ambiguity and non-healthcare focus of the 1974 legislation, the Privacy Act had established principles for fair information practices that exerted a strong influence on crafting the HIPAA privacy act. These included an individual's right of access and amendment of personal health information, and the principle that, unless specifically exempted by law or rule, consent should be obtained before an individual's protected information can be disclosed to a third party.[5]

The passage of HIPAA gave the federal government the ability to mandate how healthcare plans, providers, and clearinghouses store and transmit individuals' personal information as it relates to the administration, provision, and payment of healthcare. These regulations cover both paper-based and electronic patient information.

One of the greatest challenges faced by Congress in implementing the HIPAA legislation was developing a set of health information privacy rules to execute the standards embodied in the Act. Congressional consensus agreed that the standards were needed, but the development of a road map to implementation proved to be a very divisive undertaking. When Congress failed to meet the deadline specified in the Act, the Department of Health and Human Services stepped in and created its own set of rules. The proposed rules were released in November 1999, with the final rules published in December 2000. Theoretically, the final rules were intended to become mandatory two years and 60 days after the publication. However, initial protests from providers and public interest groups seemed to put the implementation timetable in jeopardy. In April 2001, President Bush announced that there would be no delay in the implementation of HIPAA and that the rules would not be substantially changed.[6]

The need for improved regulations for maintaining the privacy and security of personal health information was well recognized by the consumer. A 1999 survey by the California Healthcare Foundation found that two thirds of U.S. consumers didn't trust health plans or the government to maintain confidentiality of their personal health information "all or most of the time." The same survey reported that one in five Americans believes that a healthcare provider plan, government agency, or employer had improperly disclosed personal medical information.

Unfortunately, the consumer's perceptions about the lack of security surrounding personal health information were not unfounded. Prior to the HIPAA legislation, of all personal records maintained by third-party recordkeepers including financial, insurance, educational, and so on, medical records were the most widely shared. Personal health information was available to office staff, hospital support staff, lawyers, service providers, managers, benefits overseers, the inspector general, law enforcement agencies, and multiple others. Such access to this most personal information was frequently without the patient's knowledge or permission. To better understand how personal health information could be subject to misuse prior to HIPAA, consider the traditional information flow.

1. A patient visits a *medical provider* with a medical problem.
2. The provider sends samples to the *laboratory* for analysis.
3. The provider phones a prescription to the *pharmacy*.
4. The pharmacy sends prescription information to the pharmacy *benefit manager.*
5. The provider and laboratory send bills to *clearinghouses.*
6. Clearinghouses send bill to the *payer.* (It should be noted that, prior to the HIPAA legislation, the payer was not restricted in the amount of information that could be shared with the employer.)

In evaluating the traditional patient medical information flow above, only the provider and the pharmacist are bound by professional standards to assure the confidentiality of patients' medical information. Other entities that previously had access to patients' health information were not bound to protect confidentiality or security. HIPAA sets minimum standards to protect the confidentiality of patient health information by all of the entities represented in the pathway above. HIPAA also defines sanctions that can be utilized if these standards are breached. These standards are of increasing importance as the healthcare industry begins its transition from paper-based medical records to electronic medical records. This transition will result in large relational databases containing vast quantities of patient information. Information in this electronic form offers many advantages, which are briefly discussed below. Conversely, information in electronic form can be more easily pirated and misused for nefarious purposes if not adequately protected. For patients, healthcare providers, and healthcare payers to benefit from the new efficiencies and benefits that medical information in electronic form can produce, personal health information must be secured.[7,8]

As a result of the HIPAA regulations, multiple layers of user authentication, privacy, security, and data standardization now permeate all aspects of healthcare. Each of these specific regulations is discussed in greater detail in other sections of this book. They are briefly presented here primarily for the benefit of the non-HIPAA professional.

The Privacy Rule

The privacy rule essentially controls the use and disclosure of what is known as protected health information. Many of its applications are just common sense. Others are more complex, giving patients a great deal of flexibility in the knowledge of what is in their medical record and how that content is used. Patients can now control the disclosure of their protected health information to certain entities.

The Security Rule

The security rule focuses on the ability of covered entities (including medical practices) to protect and safeguard the confidentiality of medical information. It is similar to the privacy rule but more complex in its impact on medical practices in areas specific to the transmission, storage, and receipt of data. Make no mistake; your practice's computer network, who has access to it, and the methods you use to store and handle data will come under close scrutiny.

Electronic Transactions

The Transaction and Code Sets standards (TCS) deal primarily with electronic transactions. Claims submitted electronically must comply with these regulations. Failure to comply can result in substantial financial penalty.

This heightened protection of health information mandated by the above rules has resulted in significant change in how health information is gathered and managed. In the traditional world of medicine and healthcare, these necessary changes have been predictably disruptive. In contrast to the traditional health information flow presented earlier, consider how these new regulations affect the health information flow when a patient presents to his local emergency department to be evaluated for an acute medical problem.

1. Patient is registered by the admitting clerk into the hospital's information database.

- The admitting clerk must have received privacy and security training developed by the hospital.
- The clerk needs to have been granted permission to use only those functions of the information system relevant to her duties. Her authority must be confirmed by the system each time she uses the system.
- The information system must create and maintain an audit of the information viewed and modified by the clerk.

- If the patient is a new patient to the hospital, the admitting clerk must provide the patient with notice of the hospital's privacy practice no later than the date of the first service delivery, and must obtain general consent for use and disclosure of protected health information "as soon as is reasonably practical."
- If the patient has been treated at the hospital before, no action is required because both the notice of privacy practice and the consent remain valid unless privacy practices have changed or the consent is rescinded.

2. The admitting clerk prints the most recent health information about the patient on the emergency department printer.

- The printer must be protected from access and view of unauthorized personnel.
- The printed health information document is covered by HIPAA regardless of the storage or transmission medium. Electronic and paper formats are both specifically included.

3. The admitting clerk enters the patient into the hospital's health information system (HIS) and the emergency department tracking system, which displays his status on secured monitors.

- The HIS and tracking systems must have the security features required by HIPAA.
- The emergency department tracking system monitors cannot display information that can be viewed by other patients, family members, or employees and staff without proper authority or the need to know.

4. The physician, after examining the patient, orders laboratory testing from the emergency department terminal.

- The provider must have received privacy and security training developed by the hospital.
- The provider must be authenticated by the system and her authority to access the laboratory ordering function confirmed.
- The hospital or its designee must certify the security of systems and networks processing and communicating this request.
- The terminal on which the provider is requesting laboratory testing must be secured from view and use by unauthorized personnel.

5. Emergency department software identifies the patient as qualifying for a research study. The research coordinator is notified and arrives in the department to obtain the patient's informed consent.

- Clinical research studies can access patient information without patient authorization provided that the research protocol has been approved by the Institutional Review Board or privacy board.
- Research study design falls under specific waiver requirements that HIPAA delegates to the Institutional Review Board or privacy board.

6. While in the emergency department, hospital accounting contacts the patient's insurance company online. The insurance company requests additional information to confirm eligibility.

- The eligibility transaction must comply with the relevant transaction, coding, and identifier standards.
- A business associate agreement must exist between the hospital and the insurance company.
- The associate agreement must comply with the following minimum standards.
  - The insurance company must have policies and procedures in place to assure that it requests only the minimum relevant information.
  - Because the insurance company is a covered HIPAA entity, the hospital can presume that any request for information will be for the minimum necessary information.
  - Online transactions between the hospital and the insurance company must be encrypted.

7. After the patient has been treated and released, the hospital patient accounting office submits a bill to the patient's insurance company.

- The standard transaction must comply with the HIPAA transaction code set and identifier standard.
- The insurance company must accept the bill in this format and cannot delay payment because it is so submitted.

These multiple layers of authentication, privacy, security, and data standardization now permeate all aspects of healthcare in the post-HIPAA United States. Each of these specific regulations is discussed in greater detail in other sections of this book. They are briefly presented here for the benefit of the non-HIPAA professional.

INFORMATICS TECHNOLOGIES IN HEALTHCARE

As HIPAA regulations redefine the rules for health information management in modern day healthcare, new information technology applications are also revolutionizing the tools available for information capture and management. Currently, healthcare lags all other major industry sectors in the application of informatics technology. Although automated information systems have been widely used in healthcare for reporting and archiving laboratory information and for claims filling, the usage of these systems to record patient medical information has been limited. Briefly, these technologies require that patient-encounter data be digitized for processing, storage, and retrieval. Even today only a small but growing percentage of health providers captures patient-encounter information electronically. The vast majority of medical recordkeeping and prescription creation occurs by manually writing on a paper document as it has been done for generations.

The reasons for the slow adoption of these technologies by health providers are complex. In general, there has been little standardization of how individual providers manage their clinical workflows. Providers develop their own personal patterns of productivity. A process as ubiquitous as generating a clinical encounter note varies widely in style and content between providers. Some providers prefer to generate these notes during the patient encounter, others between encounters, and still others at the end of the clinic day. These patterns of workflow, once established, are very difficult to change. Practitioners routinize these flows not only for productivity, but also for safety reasons. This routinization is similar to a pilot's review of the preflight checklist as he prepares for take-off. By standardizing the approach to each patient encounter, a provider assures that no pertinent information or examination is omitted or overlooked. These issues create significant challenges in constructing a single informatics solution that permits different practitioners to function efficiently in multiple clinical settings and across multiple personal styles. Design difficulties have arisen in crafting an application user interface that does not reduce productivity if a provider is unable to use a keyboard. Writing on a paper document has long been a very efficient way to capture encounter information, but writing legibility has long been recognized to diminish as writing speed increases. Poor provider penmanship has always presented a daunting challenge for those health personnel tasked with interpreting these enigmatic clinic notes. However, the error rates associated with these illegible notes have only recently been quantified and are discussed in more detail below. Increasingly, written documentation is an inefficient technique for sharing information because a paper record can only be in one place at a time. With society's increasing mobility and the movement toward more distributed access to healthcare, transition from handwritten documents to electronic medical records is becoming an essential element for providing patient care.[8]

In addition to increasing the availability of patients' medical information for care purposes, digitalization also increases efficiencies for those who manage medical claims. Additionally, it allows medical researchers to more easily retrieve and analyze information from large clinical databases facilitating medical outcome studies. Electronic patient records also allow providers responsible for oversight of the medical management of large patient populations to actively track utilization patterns and other important practice parameters.

Finally, perhaps the most significant driver influencing the transition from handwritten notes and prescriptions to electronic capture is patient safety. In 1999 the Institute of Medicine stunned the country when it revealed that more people are killed annually by medication errors than die in motor vehicle accidents. By using information technology to provide decision support and order entry of medications and produce unequivocally legible orders, patient safety can be greatly improved.[9]

The benefits of moving from a paper-based system to an electronic system are numerous: new efficiencies in matching care needs and care resources, more comprehensive health management capabilities, and most important, improvement in patient safety. These benefits touch every member of society who will seek medical care in the future. However, for the transition from paper-based to electronic medical records to occur, patients must be assured that the information will be appropriately managed and protected. Usage of the medical information must create a trail of accountability. HIPAA provides a regulatory construct that assures the patient that the most personal of all information, their medical record, will be protected from misuse.

CONCLUSION

HIPAA represents a good faith attempt by the federal government to improve employees' access to health insurance and to define new health information management requirements. As healthcare costs continue to consume an increasing percentage of the GNP and the mean age of the U.S. population continues to rise, new strategies must be developed to improve the efficiencies with which U.S. healthcare resources are managed. The HIPAA legislation is an important first step in developing these strategies.

From the patient's point of view, he will face an increasing number of job changes as society moves into the new millennium. From the healthcare management perspective, public health experts have long recognized the importance of providing uninterrupted wellness surveillance and continual management of chronic diseases. HIPAA provides a health-care bridge for employees when job change becomes necessary.

HIPAA also lays the groundwork for new health information management strategies. Central to the country's need to better manage healthcare resources is the need for improved access to patient health information. This applies not only to health claims processing, but also to healthcare providers and managers allowing reduction in diagnostic redundancies and better coordination of patient routing through the healthcare continuum. For health information to be appropriately collected and distributed for these purposes, privacy and security policies defined by HIPPA are essential to assuage the public's concerns.

Although HIPAA has been criticized by many for its expense of implementation and its lack of specific guidance to organizations on how to comply, it is destined to become a cornerstone in this nation's necessary reengineering of its healthcare delivery system.

REFERENCES

1. Health Insurance Portability and Accountability Act of 1996 (HIPAA). 104P.L. 191;110 Stat.1936.
2. Price Water House. 2001. "Coopers health cast 2010," *E-Health Quarterly*, June.
3. Annas, George J. 2003. "HIPAA regulations — A new era of medical-record privacy?" *New England Journal of Medicine* 348: 1486–1490.
4. Ishe, Jonathan. "HIPAA: An overview." Paper undergoing review for journal publication.
5. Annas, George J. 2003. "HIPAA regulations — A new era of medical-record privacy?" *New England Journal of Medicine* 348: 1486–1490.
6. Price Water House. 2001. "Coopers health cast 2010." *E-Health Quarterly,* June.
7. Tan, Joseph K. 2001. *Health Management Information Systems.* 2nd ed., Aspen Publishers, New York.
8. Shortliffe, Edward, Ed. 2000. *Medical Informatics: Computer Applications in Health Care and Biomedicine.* 2d Ed., New York: Springer.
9. Richardson, William C. 2000. *To Err Is Human: Building a Safer Health System.* National Academy Press, Washington, D.C.

11

INTEROPERABILITY AND BUSINESS CONTINUITY INVOLVING HIPAA EDI TRANSACTIONS

Mark Lott

INTRODUCTION

The Common Conformance Assessment Program (CCAP) is a proactive business intelligence process for developing and maintaining interoperability of HIPAA transaction software. This process includes the strategy, planning, and execution deliverables that explain both the theory and practical application of a national configuration management process used to align compliance edits across the industry. This initiative will assist both covered entities and vendors in reducing trading partner compliance differences and maintaining compliance while promoting operational and fiscal stability across the healthcare industry.

The deadline for incorporating HIPAA transactions was October 16, 2003. Installing and using these new formats is just the first of many steps needed to enable successful EDI transactions for healthcare. Now that the new transactions are running in many production environments, there are several key factors to consider in developing coherent policies and procedures concerning the implementation and ongoing compliance with the HIPAA transactions regulations. This chapter addresses the requirement for creating and maintaining transaction interoperability among all healthcare trading partners.

The HIPAA implementation guides will continue to undergo changes in both definition and meaning during the course of their use. Due to all the subsequent changes, continual testing and software maintenance will be required. This will also lead to many variations of what will denote a compliant transaction based on each organization's configuration management plan. In order for the entire healthcare industry to be successful using these new transaction formats, all organizations must incorporate interoperability as a primary initiative and industrywide solution. This initiative provides the ability for all EDI translators, EDI validators, EDI vendors, and covered entities with key business intelligence decisions on the accuracy of their software systems in relation to the comprehensive set of HIPAA compliance edits. For HIPAA transactions to be interchanged easily among trading partners, compliance edits must be viewed by all trading partners the same way. Various and incongruent compliance edit coding will lead to transactions being rejected by trading partners based on differences in compliance understanding as opposed to data quality. The process for resolving compliance differences can be cumbersome and time consuming for organizations that cannot agree on a similar interpretation of the HIPAA implementation guides.

Implementation guides and their associated edits will change and improve over time. Once an edit is altered in definition or format, changes must occur in all healthcare technology software departments. The configuration management process involved in incorporating these changes must be accomplished in a manner that will continue to keep all trading partners in synch. When a HIPAA implementation guide edit is changed all affected organizations must have a process to have that change reflected in production environments simultaneously with that of their trading partners. The adverse effect of improper configuration management on a national scale will be incongruence of compliance edit definition. In other words, when one covered entity changes a compliance edit all other healthcare organizations must interpret the compliance edit the same way. This process of interoperability of HIPAA transactions must occur on a national level where software changes can be filtered down from the largest to the smallest in a process that continues to foster compliance interoperability among healthcare trading partners.

In addition to the prerequisites for creating a national interoperability program, the process must also clearly function for all types of organizations and be administered in a vendor-neutral environment. There is a multitude of differing software platforms in use throughout the healthcare industry and any solution must take this inherent market condition into consideration in the development of any interoperability program. The successful accomplishment of a national program must address the needs of all various types of healthcare organizations affected by the HIPAA transaction regulations. Inherent within the aspects of software testing is that no one vendor product can ever be determined to be unequivocally correct at all times, therefore a national interoperability program must be accomplished through the use of testing artifacts including predefined test conditions, HIPAA test files, easily understood expected results, and an associated software interoperability testing methodology. These artifacts can then be utilized by all types of healthcare organizations to align HIPAA compliance edits within their associated software testing and production environments.

STRATEGY

It is clear that a national configuration management plan is needed within the healthcare technology marketplace in relation to the ongoing maintenance of HIPAA implementation guide edits. There is an inherent difficulty in programming and testing of all the variations that exist within a healthcare transaction along with a multitude of different interpretations of what denotes a compliant transaction. This testing process must have an overall strategy to identify and uncover the compliance differences of each product and promote software testing best practices to ensure widespread adoption by all involved in the healthcare industry. It is this major aspect of HIPAA software testing and implementation that HCCO created and maintains as the Common Conformance Assessment Program, better known in the industry by its acronym CCAP.

The CCAP process is a national configuration management plan and testing methodology designed to keep all healthcare participants in the forefront of ensuring the highest quality HIPAA compliance edits. CCAP brings covered entities, vendors, and the standards community together in a collaborative, vendor-neutral environment to perform detailed testing and analysis of HIPAA compliance edits and deliver a proactive solution that will ease production support and maintenance challenges associated with HIPAA transactions and code sets. CCAP has garnered widespread support among industry participants including all HIPAA third-party EDI validators and over 90 percent of EDI translators. This allows for continuous testing and maintaining synchronization of compliance edits on a national level.

The healthcare industry is faced with many challenges under HIPAA and it is vitally important for business continuity that this process be in place to address the alignment of compliance edits across all vendors and covered entities for easier trading partner communication. HIPAA transactions and code sets will only work successfully when all trading partners have a common understanding of compliance within their technology solutions. It is also an important consideration that any rulings or determinations arising from the Centers for Medicare and Medicaid Services (CMS) enforcement complaint process are incorporated on a national scale for participants to maintain continual compliance with the established regulations and implementation guides.

The testing strategy encompassing CCAP entails using a two-layer methodology to create and maintain compliance synchronization. The first strategy uses a collaborative vendor-neutral testing environment where all participants are tested concurrently and compliance results are compared across the various technology solutions. This allows for all participants to debug their software against other industry participants on a national level. Through this interoperability testing process the testing artifacts undergo a rigorous testing process and upon completion of the initial testing phase the artifacts and especially the expected results have been verified in accordance with compliance edit definitions. For the most part, the pre-defined test conditions uncover compliance edit differences in vendor products without the need for X12 clarifications. There are times when test participants are equally divided on the interpretation of a compliance edit and the meaning in the implementation guide may be a little unclear. A small percentage of test conditions then requires the change control process to forward a request to X12 for compliance issue resolution. Once a resolution is determined by X12, the test conditions and expected results are adjusted accordingly and the vendors alter their programming to agree with this new definition. Upon completion of this initial phase of testing, the test conditions, test files, and expected results are bundled for dissemination by the healthcare industry as a whole.

This begins the second part of the testing strategy, which involves the dissemination of test results by the rest of the healthcare technology sector. The industry can utilize the CCAP testing artifacts against their own internal EDI compliance process through the use of the test files and expected results to ensure that their internal software analyzes the compliance test cases in accordance with the agreed-upon expected results from the national testing process.

Test conditions are created in one of four test input processes. The first process involves creating technical test cases based on the definitions present within the HIPAA implementation guides themselves. These types of test cases are finite in nature although very significant in the number of test conditions needed to prove overall conformance. These types of test conditions are tested quarterly for all HIPAA transaction sets and changes to compliance edits within vendor systems when identified are incorporated into their software maintenance release. The second input process involves creating healthcare business scenarios reflecting common transactions occurring within production environments. These test conditions are much more complicated to create and verify due to inherent data element and loop dependencies within an EDI transaction. This type of test case is very valuable to the industry because it reflects what is occurring in the industry's production systems. This process also identifies where many missing data elements arise due to certain information being required in a HIPAA transaction that is not required within the previous healthcare file formats such as NSF or UB92.

The third input process incorporates vital healthcare industry feedback into test-case creation through the use of a compliance edit resolution process. This important aspect of testing utilizes healthcare stakeholders who discover compliance edit differences among themselves and their trading partners, and specific test requests are created and tested on a national level attempting to determine the correct interpretation. If an interpretation is not easily determined by the national CCAP effort then the request is forwarded to X12 to follow the normal compliance edit issue resolution process.

The fourth input process incorporates any compliance rulings emanating from the national CMS HIPAA transaction enforcement process. Any CMS ruling that alters or changes a predefined compliance edit definition or understanding is incorporated back into a test condition and tested on a national level through the normal process and CCAP testing methodology.

COMPLIANCE EDIT TESTING

The process of a complex national healthcare interoperability program can be greatly understood and simplified through information sharing and illustrating the process through case studies. It is hoped that the presented examples will provide clear insight into the process, methodology, and purpose behind an interoperability testing model for HIPAA transactions. This section examines in detail several actual test cases and the alignment of compliance edits that have occurred during the CCAP process.

As explained previously, CCAP participants include most of the major vendors involved in determining HIPAA compliance of EDI transactions within many of largest healthcare application systems' front-end edit processes. This HIPAA compliance determination is accomplished through EDI validation rules incorporated with the EDI translator technology or through a third-party EDI validation module. It is within these front-end application systems where interoperability will have the greatest impact and benefit on the greatest number of covered entities and in the alignment on a national level of HIPAA compliance edits.

Let us first examine a set of compliance edits that caused some confusion within the industry in the beginning stages of HIPAA transaction implementation. This example concerns data elements within all of the

HIPAA transaction sets. These edits were (a) leading zeroes and (b) trailing spaces present within a data element. These two edits were inconsistently applied across most of the various vendors and covered entities. This was also very clearly evident within the first round of technical testing scenarios within CCAP back in 2002. There was initial confusion on the interpretation of key verbiage within the implementation guides concerning the words, "must and must not" and conversely "should and should not." The word "must" contains definitive logic as to a yes or no result whereas "should" is not as definitive and would be seen as an industry recommendation only. In regard to (b) trailing spaces, many otherwise valid transactions were being rejected for noncompliance within the CCAP testing effort for data elements containing trailing spaces. Many programmers incorrectly interpreted the implementation guide language that states "*trailing spaces should be suppressed unless to satisfy minimum length requirements*" and software code was designed to reject for compliance purposes the appearance of trailing spaces with HIPAA data elements. The correction that was made after subsequent testing and discussion with X12 was that trailing spaces should be suppressed was a recommendation but must not accompany a compliance rejection because "should" does not equate to the stricter language of "must."

The solution for all CCAP test participants was to change the programming code to either ignore the edit or to issue a warning level advisement only. Although it is true that elements containing trailing spaces are considered bad X12 form, it was determined through this collaborative interoperability testing effort that transactions must not be rejected for the presence of such data. Upon resolution of this particular test condition, all vendors changed their code and through upcoming software releases the configuration management occurred easily at a national level. A similar test case uncovered commonalities in the way (a) leading zeroes within data elements were being validated for HIPAA compliance and a similar change occurred for this compliance understanding across the healthcare industry as well.

The HIPAA implementation guides are very complex and X12 did an excellent job compiling them given the extraordinary human resource and volunteer effort required. As with any complex task there is the possibility that errors may still be present even if at a very low level as compared to the number of possible testable conditions. During the CCAP testing effort a clarification was needed concerning the 270 HIPAA Transaction. Through this interoperability testing an error in the implementation guide was discovered. Upon the execution of the 270 test files, participating vendors disagreed on the error reporting involving the INS segment in the 2100D Loop. This test condition and expected result was designed to test the mandated search field functionality. The INS segment was used in addition to the other search field options within the 270 transaction set.

The majority of vendors reported an error condition due to the fact that other search option fields were used and the INS segment must not be used for this functionality. Other vendors reported this test condition either as a warning or as a nonerror in relation to compliance edits. CCAP forwarded this request to the appropriate X12 workgroup that developed the 270/271 implementation guide for author clarification and resolution. The test condition and associated error was as follows:

> *The Segment INS in Loop 2100D should not be used because one or more of the mandated search option fields has been populated. Refer to section 1.3.8, page 22.*

Response from the X12 workgroup was that the overall goal was not to restrict additional information. This test condition uncovered an error in the implementation guide in relation to this edit. The new verbiage for the INS segment within the 2100D Loop, Note 1 in the 004050 version of the implementation guide is as follows:

> *Required when using a search option other than the mandated search option identified in Section 1.3.8 if that alternate search option requires either the relationship to the subscriber in 2100C or the dependent's birth sequence in the case of multiple births with the same birth date. If not required, this segment may be provided at the sender's discretion.*

> *Upon clarification from X12 on this compliance edit, the vendors agreed to alter the programming logic to account for a relaxation in the strictness of this edit and pay particular attention to the use of "should not" instead of "must not" within the current 4010A implementation guidelines.*

- 837P — Value of element LX01 is incorrect.
- 837I — Element NM103 is missing. This element's user option is "Must Use."
- 837D — Segment AMT (COB Patient Responsibility Amount) is missing. It's required if patient is responsible for payment according to another payer's adjudication (CAS01 with "PR" is used in loop 2320).
- 278RQ — 2000F DTP01="472" is not used when 2000F HI is present.

CASE STUDIES

There are clear and demonstrable methods for explaining the benefits of the CCAP interoperability testing process. These can be defined by examining the outcomes that occur from this type of testing effort on the organizations this program was designed to benefit. Test conditions are designed to serve a specific purpose and within this CCAP effort, one of the first goals that must be accomplished is the alignment of compliance edits across all the major national vendors that in turn represent well over 90 percent of all installed compliance technology in the nation. A secondary goal within this process is to provide the ability to respond quickly to impromptu test case requests for compliance differences uncovered between vendors within production environments in real time.

As with all software vendors, periodic software upgrades and maintenance releases are common. These occur throughout the software life cycle and contain new features and bug fixes. Within the CCAP testing methodology is a plan to incorporate all changes discovered during the testing effort to be released within each vendor's update schedules. It is not possible to have compliance edit updates released to the healthcare industry all at the same time given each vendor's own software development and release life cycle. It is possible though through this initiative to have releases occur at the earliest possible timeframe. When discrepancies are found through diligent testing across all vendors then defects can be corrected and released to the industry in a congruent manner. This is an important benefit to the end users of each software vendor in that compliance changes will have a configuration management process in place affording the best possible chance for all end users to remain in synch with their trading partners. This would otherwise not be possible without CCAP as vendors would not be aware of changes in other vendor systems until a file was rejected for compliance differences in their respective production environments and would add significant cost to each organization's production support budget and resource hours.

In relation to real-time compliance edit testing requests, this occurs when one vendor's and/or covered entity's production support department discovers that transactions are not flowing smoothly due to a difference in compliance edit definition between two separate software infrastructures. Two choices are possible upon an occurrence of this type. The first is for the two organizations to discuss and resolve the compliance difference and have one of the systems change the way the compliance edit is handled. This is fine for getting the transaction to process but leaves out the fact that software infrastructures across their other trading partners may not have the same compliance edit understanding, which will cause a ripple effect of changes needed throughout the entire healthcare transaction supply chain. This type of quick fix in production has the ability to have adverse effects on all types of trading partners and their associated vendors.

The second alternative to handling this type of production discrepancy is to forward the test condition causing the error to the CCAP testing process. It is here that the compliance edit change can be tested against all the major software vendors in the market, and upon a decision as to the correct compliance determination all vendors can change their systems simultaneously to prevent later adverse effects in production systems. This also allows for a static test case to be developed and stored in the CCAP regression test bed along with the verifiable expected result for use by downstream systems and smaller covered entities and vendors to ensure their software systems are also up to date with any compliance changes discovered through this interoperability testing process.

What should become fairly evident throughout this testing methodology is that no one entity or vendor can change compliance edits within a vacuum. When a change is made to one compliance system, at a minimum the change should be tested by other systems to ensure the same compliance edit interpretation exists across all application system infrastructures. The error in question might involve a compliance edit that on the surface appears simple in nature such as testing for an excluded segment or missing data within an NM1 data element. Through the experience of the CCAP interoperability testing process to date, it is incorrect to assume that although the compliance edit appears on the surface to be a simple coding fix, it still requires testing by all entities involved. As the widespread use of HIPAA transactions sets increases, the ability to maintain interoperability will become even more important as the industry moves into greater use of the transactions and especially true with the more complex edits and business functionality required for coordination of benefits within the 837 transactions and electronic payment and remittances using the 835 transaction.

CONCLUSION

The CCAP interoperability testing process provides many industry benefits that may not be obvious at first glance. The CCAP process allows all competing vendors to test against each other within a neutral environment for the benefit of their internal testing staff, their end users, and the healthcare industry as a whole. For HIPAA to work successfully within the transactions arena all organizations must have the same understanding of compliance. It does not benefit healthcare as a whole to have inconsistent application of compliance edits across vendors. Eventually all compliance edits must be coded the same way for all involved and the CCAP testing process facilitates this process to occur in a more organized and faster manner than if it were to happen naturally on its own. Within this process is the ability for all national software products to change compliance edit logic simultaneously and communicate these changes to their clients in a timely manner.

The CCAP process also allows for a national repository of test cases, expected results, and issue resolution to be assembled as this function does not occur within healthcare today. There is a clear need for a process that can perform this function at both the national and local levels of healthcare. When one major covered entity changes its coding of a compliance edit, there must be a process that informs all other industry organizations in order for that compliance edit to be tested against all compliance engines, not just one. When CMS or X12 changes an interpretation of a compliance edit, there also must be a specifically designed process in place to both inform the industry of the change and to create applicable test cases and expected results for all organizations to effectively test the new compliance interpretation.

Healthcare cannot afford to assume that everyone will be aware of where to look for changes to compliance guides, understand how to test for the new change, or understand how to inquire of a third-party vendor to ensure all industry changes have been applied to its software package. In addition, healthcare should not depend on a trickle-down effect to occur. This means that major covered entities and vendors that participate within X12 would be aware of changes more quickly and would alter their compliance programming logic sooner than the smaller entities and vendors. This has the unfortunate possibility of leading to compliance rejections in production for edits that were changed by the larger organizations, whereas the smaller ones would discover the changes through file rejections in productions. This would lead to increased production support costs across all healthcare organizations, in the larger covered entities and vendors by answering requests of why files that were accepted previously are now being rejected and in the smaller organizations by having to understand the new compliance edit changes and quickly recode them to ensure successful file processing. Through this example it is clear that a national and local level policy, procedure, and methodology must be in place to assist healthcare in going forward with the HIPAA compliance initiatives.

In conclusion, the industry as a whole needs to promote healthcare working together to establish a common baseline for understanding and programming compliance edits, keeping the industry up to date with any changes to or clarification of compliance interpretation, and providing useful and valuable test cases and expected results that can be reused throughout all future regression testing phases for all healthcare-related organizations. This interoperability testing process has the opportunity to save organizations hundreds of critical resource hours and thousands of dollars in testing and production costs over the lifespan of HIPAA transaction sets. It is in the best interest of every organization to ensure interoperable software solutions for their clients and their trading partners. Ultimately this collaborative approach will produce a consistent compliance solution that will enable successful implementation and maintenance of HIPAA Transaction and Code Sets initiatives, minimize compliance costs, and help promote continued healthcare business continuity.

12

THE ROLE OF DHHS, CMS, OCR, AND OHS

Todd Fitzgerald, CISSP, CISA

INTRODUCTION

It has finally happened, a cure has been found for Alzheimer's disease and cancer. Heart attacks are a thing of the past due to a new vitamin supplement that prevents blocked arteries before they occur. The spread of AIDS has been slowed to where the number of people afflicted with the terminal disease is negligible. People from all races, ethnic backgrounds, and income levels are all nourished with the proper diet and have access to the food they need to maintain a healthy active lifestyle. Automobiles are technologically advanced with built-in sensors that detect oncoming cars and prevent accidents. Due to healthy diets older Americans are no longer homebound. Infants no longer have health problems thanks to genetic advances and are free from child abuse, living in households without being subjected to domestic violence. When the few drugs that are still needed are required, the honor system is used for drug manufacturers because all companies have proved they are concerned about safety of food and drug products, thus making oversight of the clinical trials and manufacturing processes unnecessary. People taking illegal drugs and excessive amounts of alcohol are also a thing of the past as we all now know those are harmful for our health. Electronic health transactions and health insurers are a thing of the past, as they are no longer necessary due to the wonderful health to which we have evolved.

Yes, unfortunately, this was a dream or possibly a script for a Hollywood movie, and not our reality today or the foreseeable future. Every one of us has been touched by one of more of these illnesses or situations in our lives, be it a family member, relative, co-worker, or close friend. The reality is that our health is at the core of our existence and one day, we wake up and find our lives or the lives of someone close to us has irreversibly changed. Why is it that one only thinks about being healthy when one becomes sick? Should we not wake up every day and be thankful for the good health and the doctors, nurses, and specialists that have prepared for our medical emergency? Should we not be thankful for a healthcare system comprised of the infrastructure of available hospitals, physicians' offices, health insurers, and governmental oversight to ensure appropriate treatment and payment of our medical needs? Should we not be thankful that people are dedicating their lives to research in hopes of finding cures to these diseases? This may not be the first thought of the day when we wake up, but the system is in place, and although not perfect, people working in the system have a single goal in mind: to improve the quality of healthcare for all individuals.

DEPARTMENT OF HEALTH AND HUMAN SERVICES HAS A LARGE JOB

All of the situations above, with the exception of creating accident-prevention automobiles (Detroit car manufacturers *are* researching technological sensing methods to minimize serious accidents), fall under the purview of the Department of Health and Human Services (DHHS). DHHS has a critical role in protecting the health of all Americans by providing essential services such as medical and science research, immunization services to prevent the outbreak of infectious diseases, financial assistance to low-income families, improving maternal and infant health, prevention of child abuse and domestic violence, substance abuse and prevention, services for older Americans, Native-American services, ensuring food and drug safety, and providing health insurance for elderly and disabled Americans (Medicare) and for low-income people (Medicaid). With over 300 programs, a 2003 fiscal year budget of $502 billion and over 65,000 employees, DHHS plays a significant role in advancing the healthcare of the United States.

The Department of Health and Human Services is made up of twelve operating divisions, also known as agencies, and nine staff divisions. The agencies, number of employees, and latest budget numbers are provided in Table 12.1. Leadership for the department is provided by the Office of the Secretary. As part of the administrative simplification legislation enacted by Congress, the secretary of DHHS was required to adopt security standards to reasonably protect health information. Administrative simplification also required the secretary to adopt a suite of national uniform standards for transactions, unique health identifiers, and code sets in support of processing electronic transactions to improve the effectiveness and efficiency of the healthcare system. The secretary was also required

Table 12.1   Operating Divisions/Agencies within the Department of Health and Human Services

Operating Division/Agency	Employees	2003 Fiscal Year Budget (Billons $)
National Institutes of Health (NIH)	17,693	27.2
Food & Drug Administration (FDA)	10,479	1.7
Centers for Disease Control and Prevention (CDC)	8,668	6.8
Agency for Toxic Substances and Disease Registry	*	*
Indian Health Service (IHS)	14,961	3.5
Health Resources & Services Administration	1,937	7.1
Substance Abuse & Mental Services Administration	588	3.2
Agency for Healthcare Research & Quality	294	.309
Centers for Medicare & Medicaid Services (CMMS)	4,661	413
Administration for Children & Families	1,512	47.5
Administration on Aging	124	1.4
Program Support Center	*	*
Other Offices with DHHS		
Office of Public Health & Science (PHS)	*	*
Office of the DHHS Inspector General (OIG)	*	*
DHHS Office for Civil Rights (OCR)	*	*
Office of the Secretary	*	*

* Unknown.

Source: Department of Health and Human Services Web site.

to provide recommendations for protecting the confidentiality of information. It was then up to the secretary to determine the appropriate operating divisions within DHHS that would be most suited for the development of the standards, communication of the standards and associated outreach activities, and the compliance enforcement.

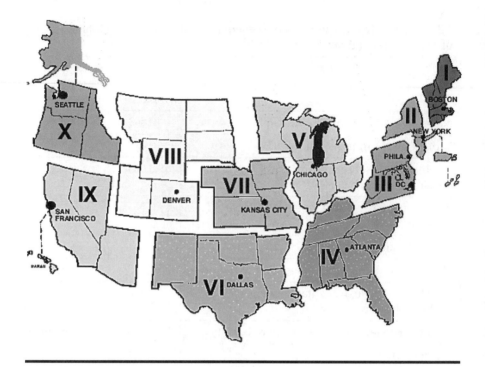

Figure 12.1 Department of Health and Human Services Regions (Source: Department of Health & Human Services Web site)

DHHS is divided into ten geographic regions, as shown in Figure 12.1. Each region has employees that are part of the different operating divisions within DHHS, such as the Office of the Secretary, Office of Civil Rights, Centers for Medicare and Medicaid Services, and so forth. This structure permits regional-focused support and understanding of issues affecting the local areas.

DHHS HIPAA RESPONSIBILITIES

The secretary of DHHS has designated several agencies to be responsible for the Health Insurance Portability & Accountability Act of 1996 (HIPAA). Although there are agencies within the department that provide support and influence for HIPAA in an indirect manner (such as the Office of Inspector General, which provides audit controls oversight for Medicare and state health programs), the following departments have been designated specific roles with respect to the provisions of the Administrative Simplification Act by the secretary of DHHS:

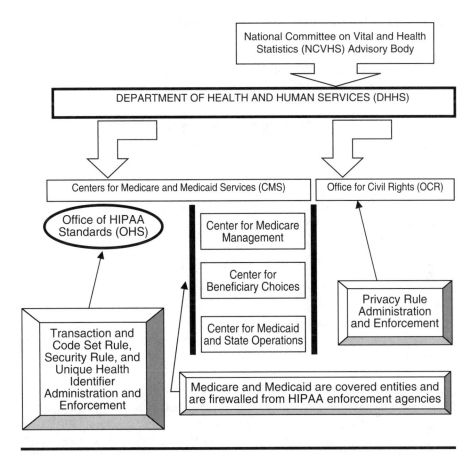

Figure 12.2   DHHS HIPAA Agencies

- *Department of Health and Human Services (DHHS)* — Responsible for promulgating standards
- *Office of Civil Rights (OCR)* — Administration and enforcement of the HIPAA privacy rule
- *Centers for Medicare and Medicaid Services (CMS)* — Administration and enforcement of transaction and code set standards, security rule, and insurance portability provisions
- *Office of HIPAA Standards (OHS)* — Located within CMS to provide oversight for all HIPAA standards except privacy

The various organizations and how they relate to HIPAA are shown in Figure 12.2.

Table 12.2   Administrative Rule-Making Process

Administrative Simplification Rule-Making Process
DHHS implementation team drafts Notice of Proposed Rule-Making (NPRM) for review
DHHS Data Council Committee on Health Data Standards reviews
Advisors to DHHS Secretary (division agency heads) agree
Office of Management and Budget (OMB) reviews
Proposed NPRM published in *Federal Register*
Public comments are solicited for 60-day period
Comments open for public view
Comments are analyzed and content summarized by implementation team
Final rule is published; standards become effective 24 months after adoption, 36 months for small health plans

Administrative Simplification Rule-Making Process

Before delving into the specific departments that have a role within HIPAA, their objectives, and their processes for ensuring compliance with the adopted rules, it would be beneficial to understand the rule-making process that is utilized in the creation of the various rules and their subsequent modification.

Each provision of the Administrative Simplification must follow a rule-making process intended to achieve consensus within the Department of Health and Human Services and other federal departments. When the rule is approved within the government, the public has the opportunity to comment on the proposal, and then these comments are evaluated in the determination of the final rule. Once the rules have gone through this process, they have the force of federal law. The Department of Health and Human Services implementation teams draft Notices of Proposed Rule Making (NPRMs), which are subsequently published in the *Federal Register* after review within the federal government according to the process shown in Table 12.2. Once the NPRMs are published, they are available for a 60-day public comment period that provides for input and for interested parties to influence the outcome of the final regulation. After the publication of the final rule, most large health plans, clearinghouses, and providers have 24 months to be in compliance, and smaller parties have 36 months to be in compliance.

The proposed security and electronic signature standards were originally published in the *Federal Register* on August 12, 1998. The security rule was delayed on several occasions, as resources were committed to and focused on the proposed transaction and code set and privacy rules, both of which generated a large number of public comments. These public comments must be reviewed, and the numbers can be large. Over 17,000 public comments were received on the transaction and code sets NPRM and several thousand on the privacy and security rules. The transaction and code set compliance date was also delayed by one year, to October 16, 2003 as long as the covered entity filed an extension request by October 15, 2002. In addition, the security rule was initiated during the Clinton administration and was carried over into the Bush administration, which created political challenges for expedient passage of the rule. As a result, the language was rewritten during 2002 to coincide with the privacy rule (compliance date of April 14, 2003), which needed to go through the DHHS clearance process prior to final rule publication. The Centers for Medicare and Medicaid Services provided their best estimates several times during 2002 of publication of the final security rule, and the rule was subsequently published on February 20, 2003.

Office of Civil Rights

The Office of Civil Rights (OCR) ensures that people have equal access and opportunity to participate in and receive the services of all DHHS programs without facing unlawful discrimination. With their past experience in voluntary dispute resolution, investigations, enforcement, policy management, and technical capabilities, OCR was positioned as the logical choice for the enforcement of the HIPAA privacy rule. Although their staffing levels started out very small with a handful of people, DHHS has indicated that staffing would be increased to handle the complaints as the volume increased, subject to budgetary constraints.

In their role of providing administration and enforcement of the privacy rule, OCR provides guidance to provide clarification of the rules provisions and answer common questions related to the rule. Searchable Frequently Asked Questions (FAQs) are posted to the OCR Web site at http://hhs.gov/ocr/hipaa/assist.html. The database of searchable questions is very extensive and is updated as more questions are presented to OCR. OCR participates in hundreds of conferences among trade groups, professional associations, and regional conferences hosted by DHHS. Through these conferences, OCR shares information related to some of the misunderstandings or misinterpretation of the privacy rule within the industry. Due to the size, complexity, company functions, and interrelationships of the rule, these variances in interpretation can be expected. The best way to ensure that the intended interpretation of the privacy rule is achieved is to utilize the resources provided by OCR. Chances are that some other organization has encountered a similar situation, where the FAQ may answer the concern. OCR and CMS work together to provide support for the privacy, security, and transaction and code sets of HIPAA and as such have implemented a toll-free hotline for information.

As the OCR deems necessary, they will also issue guidance, such as that issued on December 4, 2002 to clarify the expectations around the interpretations of the privacy rule. Guidance has covered topic areas such as incidental uses and disclosures, minimum necessary, personal representatives, business associates, uses and disclosures for the treatment, payment and healthcare operations, marketing, public health, research, worker's compensation laws, notice, and government access.

The Privacy Rule Complaint Process

Enforcement is complaint-driven and OCR will investigate all complaints to determine if an individual's privacy rights have been violated under the HIPAA regulations. When OCR has determined that violations have occurred, they can impose monetary penalties of up to $100 per violation, up to $25,000/year for each requirement that is violated. Potential criminal penalties would be handled by the Department of Justice (DOJ) for consideration and determination of further action. These penalties include up to $50,000 and one year in jail for certain offenses, up to $100,000 and five years in prison if the offenses are committed under false pretenses, and up to $250,000 and ten years in prison if the offenses are committed with the intent to sell, transfer, or use protected health information (PHI) for commercial advantage, malicious harm, or personal gain. The covered entity has a right to notice and a hearing before the civil money penalty is final.

Each complaint made to the Office of Civil Rights concerning a violation from a covered entity (health plan, healthcare clearinghouse, or any healthcare provider who creates certain healthcare transactions electronically) must be made in writing within 180 days of when the person filing the complaint had knowledge of the act that occurred. Exceptions may be made to the 180-day period if "good cause" can be shown. OCR has developed a complaint form and has made it available on their Web site and through their regional offices. OCR requests that the complaints be addressed to the appropriate OCR regional manager of the local office.

The philosophy of the OCR is to promote voluntary compliance, investigate and resolve those complaints that are received, and determine those cases where exceptions may be valid. OCR seeks to resolve matters by informal means prior to issuing any findings of noncompliance under the existing authority to investigate and resolve complaints and to engage in compliance reviews. OCR may begin an investigation, however, voluntary resolution of the issues is still possible. OCR issued an interim enforcement rule with request for comments in April 2003 outlining rules of procedure for the imposition of Civil Monetary Penalties (CMP) on covered entities that violate the standards of the HIPAA rule.

OCR makes a form available to file complaints with information requested such as the requestor's contact information, individual whose rights have been potentially violated (if not the person filing the complaint), dates of the occurrences, and a description of what happened. The request does not need to use a form if the appropriate information is provided in a letter to OCR. Once OCR receives the information, they will investigate it and maintain the confidentiality of the protected information. Because they are a government agency and this is considered a government record, they must protect the information according to the Privacy Act of 1974. They may release identifying information about individuals when it is necessary for the investigation of the health privacy violation allegations.

No civil money penalties are provided if the person did not know and by exercising reasonable diligence would not have known of the violation. If the covered entity can show that the failure to comply was due to reasonable cause versus willful neglect and corrects the situation within 30 days, then no civil money penalties will be awarded. In addition, if the offense is punishable by a criminal sanction, then no civil monetary penalties will be awarded. OCR has the capability to grant exceptions as they determine are warranted, grant extensions of the 30-day period, and reduce the CMP if the amount appears excessive related to the violation or the infraction was due to a reasonable cause versus willful neglect.

Centers for Medicare and Medicaid Services (CMS) Organization

The Centers for Medicare and Medicaid Services administer the Medicare and Medicaid programs. Approximately 44 million elderly and disabled Americans are served through these programs, constituting one in every four Americans. These numbers are expected to increase to 77 million by 2030 as the baby boomer generation and some of their children will be supported by the system. Medicaid is a joint federal–state program serving low-income persons. The agency was established in 1977 as the Health Care Financing Administration (HCFA) and was renamed CMS on July 1, 2001 to position the agency to place increased attention on the responsiveness to beneficiaries, providers, and quality improvement. CMS accounts for approximately one third of the nation's healthcare spending and is responsible for the administration of health insurance for the largest number of lives.

When the name change occurred in 2001, three offices were created to support the reforms including the Center for Beneficiary Choices, which promotes beneficiary informed choices for their healthcare decisions; the Center for Medicare Management, which manages the traditional fee-for-service Medicare program and the development and implementation of payment policies/management of the Medicare carriers and fiscal intermediaries; and the Center for Medicaid and State Operations to support the programs that are administered by the states, such as Medicaid for low-income groups, the State Children's Health Insurance Program, private insurance, survey and certification, and the Clinical Laboratory Improvement Amendments. As part of introducing legislation for Medicare reform, CMS developed a proposal for Congress permitting the competitive bidding of claim processing services. Over 22,000 people are involved in processing 900 million Medicare claims each year through private health insurance companies contracted by CMS.

CMS is made up of ten regional offices with the central office in Baltimore, Maryland. CMS enters into agreements with fiscal intermediaries (Part A) and carriers (Part B) to facilitate the processing of claims. The intermediaries make the payments to the providers to reimburse for the services provided based upon the reasonable cost of the covered services and items and the customary charges associated with the services. The contracted intermediaries provide safeguards for the fiscal information, communicate with providers, conduct audits of provider records, assist in the beneficiary appeals process, and provide information for institutions that wish to qualify as healthcare providers.

As with the Office of Civil Rights, CMS is focused on providing increased levels of outreach through the establishment of more information through decision-making tools on the Web sites, 24-hour support of the 1-800-Medicare hotline, national advertising campaigns, assigning individuals within the department as key contacts, and being responsive to healthcare groups such as beneficiaries, health plans, providers, and physicians.

CMS and HIPAA

On October 15, 2002, the secretary of Health and Human Services named CMS as the agency to enforce the HIPAA transaction and code set standards. In this role, CMS was made responsible for the establishment and operation of enforcement processes and the development of regulations for transaction and code sets, security, and identifiers for providers, insurers, and employers for use in the electronic transactions. CMS was the agency within DHHS that issued the final security standards (February 20, 2003) and the transaction and code set standards. As modifications to these standards become necessary, CMS is the agency which ensures that the process is followed to ensure appropriate input is received.

The administrative simplification part of the Social Security Act requires the Health and Human Services secretary to adopt standards for electronic transactions to improve the effectiveness and efficiency of the healthcare administrative system. By implementing standard formats to be used between trading partners, the costs and time associated with transmitting, storing, and processing can be substantially reduced. Electronic Data Interchange (EDI) has been around for many years, however, different payers, clearinghouses, and vendor software have implemented their own unique coding systems, which limits the ability to achieve the total cost benefit of EDI.

To facilitate the adoption of standard transactions, administrative simplification (under Section 1172, Part C of Title XI of the Social Security Act) requires that any standard adopted by the secretary must have been developed, adopted, or modified by a Standard Setting Organization (SSO). The standard-setting organizations for transactions and code sets are the Accredited Standards Committee ASC X12N and the National Council for Prescription Drug Programs (NCPDP). The SSO must consult with one of the Data Content Committees (DCCs) while developing, modifying, or adopting the standard. There are also organizations and a process for updating the standards, known as Designated Standard Maintenance Organizations (DSMOs), which manage and process the changes to the adopted standards (see Table 12.3). In the case of any other standard (not adopted, modified, or developed by an SSO), the secretary is required to consult with the DCCs and also must consult with the National Committee on Vital and Health Statistics (NCVHS), which is designated by HIPAA as the advisor to the secretary of DHHS. The secretary may adopt a different standard if the standard will substantially reduce administrative costs to healthcare plans and providers, provided that the required rule-making procedures are followed.

Because the responsibility for the privacy rule administration and enforcement rests with the Office of Civil Rights, coordination between CMS and OCR must take place for outreach, enforcement, and issues that overlap each other. Privacy and security are so related, wherein true privacy cannot be obtained without adequate application of security controls, that the agencies understand the importance of working together. Many of the outreach programs that have been initiated by CMS have combined privacy and security into one educational track, and have kept the transaction and code sets or EDI discussions in another track. A representative from the Office of Civil Rights is typically on the agenda to address privacy concerns. The basis for the security rule from the beginning was to ensure the privacy of the aggregated protected health information versus incorporating security for the sake of security, so this collaboration between departments is expected. During roundtable conference calls sponsored by the Department of Health and Human Services, questions related to transactions and code sets and security standards are typically directed to CMS representatives and questions related to privacy

Table 12.3   Transaction and Code Set Standards Committees

Organization	Web Site
Standards Setting Organization (SSO)	
Accredited Standards Committee X12N (ASC X12N)	www.x12.org
National Council for Prescription Drug Programs (NCPDP)	www.ncpdp.org
Designated Standard Maintenance Organization (DSMO)	
Health Level Seven, Inc. (HL 7)	www.hl7.org
National Uniform Billing Committee (NUBC)	www.nubc.org
National Uniform Claim Committee (NUCC)	www.nucc.org
Dental Content Committee of the American Dental Association	www.ada.org
ASC X12N	(see above)
NCPDP	(see above)
Data Content Committees (DCCs)	
NUBC	(see above)
NUCC	(see above)
Workgroup for Electronic Data Interchange (WEDI)	www.wedi.org
American Dental Association (ADA)	(see above)
Advisor to Secretary of DHHS	
National Committee on Vital and Health Statistics (NCVHS)	http://ncvhs.hhs.org

are directed to the OCR, leveraging the specific knowledge within the respective organization.

CMS Transaction and Code Set Enforcement Approach

With CMS's role in managing the Medicare and Medicaid programs, they have been able to influence the adoption of national standards. For providers that were utilizing electronic transactions, failure to submit the claim transaction in the correct "HIPAA Compliant" standard format would mean that the claim would not be accepted by Medicare and could negatively affect cash flow for the provider. The original date for this compliance was October 16, 2002, however, through the Administrative Simplification Compliance Act (ASCA), Public law 107-105, healthcare providers, clearinghouses, and large health plans were granted an extension to October 16, 2003 provided they submitted a plan to the secretary of DHHS of how they would attain compliance by that date. The plans needed to include the budget, schedule, work plan, and implementation strategy for becoming compliant, specification of the use of contractors or vendors to complete the testing, and assessments of any compliance problems and the timeframe for testing, which could start no later than April 16, 2003. The summary of the testing plan and a form were provided for filing to obtain the extension. Small plans were not granted a further extension, so the date for all plans (provided the compliance extension was requested) was October 16, 2003. By requiring extension plans and a start date for testing of no later than April 16, 2003 versus granting a blanket extension to all plans, ASCA was advocating that steps needed to be taken to achieve the October 16, 2003 compliance date sooner rather than later.

As the October 16, 2003 date was approaching, it became clear that many of the covered entities would not be compliant by the date, so on July 24, 2003 CMS issued a guidance document with respect to compliance expectations for the transaction and code set provisions of HIPAA. The goals of the guidance were twofold: (1) to move covered entities towards compliance, and (2) to avoid disruption of cash flow. There was some concern by CMS and within the industry that organizations would "drop to paper" as a mechanism to maintain their cash flow (because paper-submitters would not be subject to the HIPAA regulations). CMS did not want this to happen, as this would produce the exact opposite objectives of HIPAA, which are to improve the effectiveness and efficiency of the healthcare system. By reverting to paper submissions, increased handling costs would be incurred, and data entry of claims and the successes of the EDI transactions would be undone. By the same token, disrupting the cash flow to providers by not paying their claim submissions based upon the legacy formats would cause financial problems for the providers, especially those that have very thin operating margins.

CMS did not have the authority to change the date of the compliance, as the date was established by an act of law (HIPAA) and the subsequent Administrative Simplification Compliance Act, which required covered entities to comply with the electronic and code set provisions adopted by the secretary by October 16, 2003. However, CMS does have the discretion as to how they will enforce the standards, due to the flexibility granted in Section 1176(b) of the Social Security Act. Similar to the approach utilized by the OCR for the privacy rule, CMS decided to utilize the following approach to their enforcement after the October 16, 2003 date:

■ *Complaint-Driven.* Complaints would be submitted to CMS before an action would be taken. CMS is not "looking for" covered entities whom they believe to be out of compliance. Again, the mission of CMS with respect to transactions and code sets is to move the industry towards voluntary compliance to reap the benefits of the implementation and position the industry towards lower administrative costs.

■ *Good Faith Efforts.* Under Section 1176(b) of the Social Security Act, DHHS may not impose a civil money penalty if the failure to comply "was due to reasonable cause and not to willful neglect; and . . . is corrected during the 30-day period beginning on the first date the person liable for the penalty knew, or by exercising reasonable diligence would have known, that the failure to comply occurred." The secretary has the authority to extend the period to fix the noncompliance based upon the nature and the extent of the failure to comply. To achieve this, CMS was looking for evidence that plans made sustained and demonstrable progress towards compliance *before and after* the deadline. Some examples that CMS would regard as "good faith efforts" for a health plan included:

  – Demonstrated outreach efforts such as letters, conferences, phone calls, mailings, and Web site information
  – Encouraging providers or those who submit claims on their behalf (i.e., billing services, clearinghouses) to begin testing
  – Maintaining testing schedules and statistics of testers

■ *Contingency Plan.* As long as the organization could demonstrate the outreach and testing efforts were occurring, they could implement a contingency plan to ensure that payments would continue to be made to providers. As a result of this, many health plans decided to continue accepting the legacy format EDI transactions at the same time as accepting the HIPAA compliant, 4010A transactions as their contingency plans. This action served the purpose of minimizing disruption to the cash flow, while increasing efforts were underway to move the noncompliant providers to full HIPAA compliance.

■ *Documentation.* Covered entities were expected to document their good faith efforts in the event a complaint was filed with them. Documentation of the outreach activities, testing schedules, statistics, communications with other trading partners, and any other activities taken to move towards compliance would be helpful in determining whether the noncompliance was reasonable under the circumstances.

It should be clearly understood at this point that although CMS does not have the authority to change the dates implemented by law, they do have the authority to develop mechanisms for enforcement. CMS has stated at numerous outreach conferences that they will not be tolerant of the noncompliance issue indefinitely. CMS will issue guidance and requirements to the industry to achieve the appropriate goals. CMS's desire is that the healthcare industry work together to resolve the issues and where this is not possible, the resources provided by CMS are utilized to attain the compliance among health plans, clearinghouses, and providers that communicate through electronic transactions.

CMS Office of HIPAA Standards (OHS)

The agency within CMS that has been designated the responsibility for the enforcement of the transaction and code sets and security is the Office of HIPAA Standards (OHS). Because OHS is the enforcement mechanism for all covered entities, and Medicare (a covered entity) is also within CMS, the divisions operate independently and are completely detached from the Medicare program. OHS will handle complaints against Medicare, as a covered entity, and process them according to the protocols established for any other covered entity.

OHS does not want to become involved in every dispute and desires that trading partners work collaboratively to resolve the issues. Filing complaints with CMS should be regarded as a "last resort" to get an issue resolved. When complaints are filed, OHS will look at the complaint and make an assessment as to whether the noncompliance was the result of willful neglect or it was reasonable, were there mitigating factors, and when does the covered entity expect to become fully compliant. OHS will look at the severity of the complaint and address each one as resources permit, utilizing tools such as Corrective Action Plans (CAP) and imposition of CMP as noted in the preceding section.

To facilitate the compliant process, OHS has implemented the Administrative Simplification Enforcement Tool (ASET), which is a Web-based, Internet-accessible tool where complaints can be filed. When a valid complaint is received, OHS notifies the covered entity that a complaint has been filed against it. OHS will then facilitate the resolution of the dispute, whereby the covered entity will have the opportunity to demonstrate compliance, its good faith efforts to comply, or submit a corrective action plan. Complaints need to be specific and be directed towards noncompliance. OHS has received complaints regarding a covered entity that are general in nature, such as the organization not liking the way the covered entity does business or not liking portions of the HIPAA rule!

Table 12.4   Upcoming Standard/Rule Expected Dates

Standard/Rule	Date
National provider ID	Expected December 26, 2003
National plan ID	Expected 2004
Enforcement rule	Expected 2004
Claims and attachment standard proposed rule	Expected Spring 2004
Modification II	Expected Summer 2004

Source: Office of HIPAA Standards (OHS).

There is not much that OHS can do with these complaints, as they are not related to issues of noncompliance. It warrants restating, that filing a complaint should be viewed as a last resort.

To further OHS's goals of voluntary compliance and providing technical assistance, they are engaged in other initiatives such as developing the FAQs for transactions and code sets and FAQs for security by working with various industry groups to facilitate compliance, provide clarification on confusing issues, and develop enforcement strategies. New code sets, rules, and modifications will continue to emerge to address issues. OHS will continue to work towards these goals and achieve the approval of new standards given the resource limitations, and compete with other priority focuses within CMS, such as Medicare Contractor Reform. Target dates (give or take a few months), as of this writing, have been established by OHS for some future deliverables, which are subject to change with the priorities, as shown in Table 12.4.

CMS Security Standard Approach

The final security rule was published in the *Federal Register* on February 20, 2003 and became effective April 21, 2003, meaning a compliance date of April 21, 2005 for all covered entities except small health plans and April 21, 2006 for all small health plans that are subject to HIPAA (according to the requirements specified in the regulation). Therefore, compliance with the final security rule does not begin until these dates. However, there exists the often-referred-to "mini-security rule" within the privacy rule, whereby the covered entity "must have in place the appropriate administrative, technical and physical safeguards to protect the privacy of health information," which still provides an avenue for a noncompliance condition to be filed with respect to security.

As previously noted, the privacy rule complaints are handled by the Office of Civil Rights and the security rule complaints by the Office of HIPAA Standards. OCR and OHS work closely together, as security and privacy are interdependent.

The goals of OHS with respect to the final security rule are consistent with the approach taken for the privacy rule and transaction and code set compliance: move entities towards voluntary compliance and enforcement will be complaint-based. Complaints will not be taken by OHS on the final security rule until after the compliance dates of April 21, 2005 and April 21, 2006. Again, the focus is on compliance, not complaints or fines. There is a significant amount of work that is necessary to address the 18 security standards and OHS expects that organizations are working towards the compliance dates. OHS is continually working on additional guidance and technical assistance and openly solicits input from industry on critical issues in meeting the requirements of the rule.

In determining whether an organization has not complied with the final security rule, OHS will look at the following areas:

- *Willful versus recalcitrant entities* — Was the intent to completely ignore the standard or was there some other explanation for not achieving compliance?
- *Administrative versus substantive noncompliance* — If the standard was not followed and the condition that resulted did not constitute a serious security threat, then the noncompliance may be of a more administrative nature. For example, there may be a data backup procedure that is executed every day religiously by the network engineer and the tapes are taken off-site on a periodic basis. The network engineer records every tape that is created and ensures successful completion of the tape backup process. However, no policies or documented procedures were created, because this had been operated as a one-person task in that office. At the time, no real security problem was created (i.e., inability to recover electronic protected health information if lost), but has the potential to create a problem if the network engineer is sick, on vacation, or leaves the company. The knowledge of the backup operation would be lost and could present a higher risk to the organization protecting the information assets. This may be viewed as an administrative issue versus substantive. If, on the other hand, there are two or three network engineers and there is no consistent method of backing up the tapes, and a server is lost and the backup required to restore the electronic health information is not available, this may be viewed as a substantive issue.

- *Entity decision versus entity ignoring* — Covered entities need to make deliberate decisions based upon a risk analysis to determine which security measures are appropriate for their particular environment. Ignoring the security standards is making a decision, but not a decision that involves conscious rational thought to come up with alternatives and decide the most appropriate control. The decision may end up being the same decision (not to do anything and accepting the associated risk), however, many times this will not be the choice as there are usually some controls that can be put in place to improve the security.

- *Number of standards/implementation specifications violated* — The greater the number of standards and implementation specifications that are violated, the less likely that security is really being taken seriously within the covered entity. Many of the standards are derived from security industry practices that are "good business" to practice. In addition, the greater the number of standards violated, the more risks there are to the covered entity and those that do business with it.

- *Time elapsed* — Consider the case whereby an organization has performed a vulnerability assessment as part of the risk analysis to see where vulnerabilities are present that could be exploited on the network servers, workstations, and networking devices (i.e., routers, firewalls, switches, hubs). If the organization finds a few hundred vulnerabilities and still has those same vulnerabilities a year later, without any attention paid to addressing them or development of a plan to address the high-risk items immediately, then it would be difficult to indicate that the organization is paying the proper attention to security. There may be mitigating factors; however, these would need to be analyzed to determine if they were reasonable and appropriate under the circumstances.

- *Reasonableness of the entity's plan* — Security is an ongoing process to reduce the residual risk. How has the covered entity planned to mitigate the threats and implement security safeguards? Has the covered entity made this into a ten-year project due to the complexity? Or does the plan for an insurance company paying out millions of claims and having revenues in the billions show a $100,000 a year security budget? Or does the plan purchase an insurance policy to avoid implementing any security controls? Reasonableness is a subjective measure and it would be in the covered entities' best interests to understand what other organizations of their size, type, system complexity, and resources available (technical and financial) are committing to their security programs and their approaches in moving towards compliance with the final security rule.

The OHS expects organizations to move towards compliance by the established regulatory dates. At this time, there are no plans for contingency planning and OHS has stated that there will not be one as there was with the transaction and code sets standard. The rationale is that many of the security standards are largely a function that a covered entity must perform within its organization and are not as dependent upon two parties to complete the effort. Granted, there is communication between parties, such as through e-mail and data transmission, where interoperability issues need to be worked through; however, many requirements can be addressed within the organization. Agreements with business associates also need to ensure that the appropriate controls are being specified. OHS will issue additional guidance as necessary to support the move towards compliance.

National Health Information Infrastructure

In today's world, organizations are very focused on compliance, meeting the regulations or the standards that have been agreed upon as necessary by governmental agencies and industry standards committees. To some organizations that are very bottom-line focused and think of "today's environment," this may represent the "minimum necessary" to meet the standard. Those organizations that see the value of the information may already be thinking of a different tomorrow; one where the information can reduce medical costs and increase the care levels of the beneficiaries. However, the prevailing mood seems to be one of "How compliant are we" versus "What benefits can moving in this direction provide me?" A common analogy applied to the healthcare industry is that of the banking industry with their use of ATM cards. People think nothing of having an ATM card and getting information and primarily cash out of their accounts and expect to have this availability within walking distance. However, attainment of the same level of access to our healthcare information is not available today. It does beg the question of whether knowledge and access to our financial assets is more important than knowledge and access to our personal health information. It does provide cause for pause.

That National Health Information Infrastructure is an initiative initiated in the Department of Health and Human Services to improve the effectiveness, efficiency, and overall quality of health within the United States through promoting a set of interoperable technologies, standards, systems, values, and laws to enable decision making when the information is available and needed. The initiative is voluntary and is not intended to form a centralized database of health information, but rather enable access to the information at the point of care. Errors can be reduced, patient safety increased, quality of treatment improved, and early detection of bioterrorism through the detection of patterns can be accomplished. Consumers would have more information available to evaluate their health-care options and healthcare costs would be better understood.

According to the proponents of the National Health Information Infra-structure, healthcare error rates are too high, quality is inconsistent, research results are not rapidly used, costs are escalating, new technologies continue to drive up costs, baby boomers will greatly increase demand, and our capacity for early detection of bioterrorism is minimal. Addition-ally, it is estimated that 20 percent of the labs and x-rays that are completed are done because the prior results are unavailable, one in seven hospi-talizations is performed because prior patient information is unavailable, community health information exchange could save $84 billion/year, pub-lic health could be immediately notified of infectious diseases and potential outbreaks, and efficiency gains in information technology could exceed $120 billion/year.

Has "compliance" been mentioned yet? No, the vision of the Depart-ment of Health and Human Services is much larger than advocating merely compliance and imposing civil monetary penalties on those that do not comply. Although these controls are important, sight of the larger vision should not be lost. Healthcare can be improved with the establishment of standardized electronic medical records that can be accessed when needed, securely, and with privacy intact. The physicians can make increased informed choices about the appropriate treatment, information can be processed at a lower cost, and unnecessary procedures can be avoided. The standards that are being put into place today as well as those that are under development are moving healthcare towards an environment where these ideas may be possible. The average baby boomers think nothing of checking their bank balances online, privately and securely. Why is that? The answer lies in the long-standing trust that consumers have had with the banking industry, coupled with the assurances of safety (through limits to personal liability on credit cards of $50 or less), and assurances of secure transmission and protection of the financial infor-mation. Someday we will move to the same point, with the adoption of standards that permit the interoperability of the health information — stored in a distributed fashion, but accessed at the point of care. The National Health Information Infrastructure can move us towards that goal.

CONCLUSION: DHHS AND THE REST OF US

Will Alzheimer's be cured someday? Will cancer be a distant memory for many Americans like polio became? Will the spread of AIDS cease to become a major health risk? Will everyone have access to the necessary healthcare, regardless of income level? We can hope for these ideals, and can move closer to them. The Department of Health and Human Services invests much in the way of resources in the areas of research, public health support, and efforts to reduce the administrative costs and increase the efficiency of the healthcare system. By reducing the administrative costs, more of the healthcare dollar is available for initiatives that could provide healthcare where needed, such as providing necessary healthcare to the uninsured or enabling access of information to improve the quality of care to individuals who are homebound.

For future leveraging of the health information to be possible, the standards adoption must occur today. The Department of Health and Human Services is "driving the bus" and it is up to each health plan, clearinghouse, and provider to get on board to move the healthcare system to the next level. Yes, information does need to be electronic. Yes, it does need to be private and disclosed only to those who have a legitimate need to know the information. Yes, it does need to be secured appropriately so that the confidentiality is maintained, the information is kept accurate, and it is available to the physician and healthcare practitioner at the point of service, as well as to the processing systems necessary to reduce the administrative costs.

The DHHS, through its various departments, will continue to be in the driver's seat. They will come out with more standards, more rules, more guidance, more enforcement communications, and more modifications to the existing standards and rules. As children, most of us remember getting on a school bus. As children, our parents would wait for the bus to come and would make sure that we were safely on the bus. All we knew is that we were going to school, and did not really understand the path to get there. That was OK, because we trusted our parents, and trusted that the bus driver knew the way. As we gained more experience with riding the bus, we too began to learn the path and what would come next. We were given minimal standard instructions as to how to behave and to "just sit down" and enjoy the ride according to the rules. There was disruption within the bus along the way, as not all the other kids would behave, and some thought gum in the hair was appropriate. Some kids were even thinking about their future after the bus ride, and others were just "in the moment." When there were different requirements to do more than the normal ride to school, such as field trips or traveling to a band or choral concert, there was more money added to purchase a more comfortable coach bus for the long trip. Without the expenditures, safety was at question as well as the comfort (health) of the students on the longer trips.

The bus ride has started the journey. Some will be short trips; some will be longer, requiring more planning and more interaction between the passengers and the bus driver. The department is driving the bus and has a vision of all the places where it would like to go. We should expect the bus to change, the drivers to be different from time to time, but we need to maintain our trust in the vision of the department to get us to our destination, which is more efficient and effective healthcare.

REFERENCES

1. Health Insurance Reform: Security Standards; Final Rule, February 20, 2003, *Federal Register* 45 CFR Parts 160, 162 and 164, Department of Health and Human Services.
2. Health Insurance Reform: Standards for Electronic Transactions; Announcement of Designated Standard Maintenance Organizations; Final Rule and Notice, August 17, 2000, *Federal Register* 45 CFR Parts 160 and 162, Department of Health and Human Services.
3. Health Insurance Reform: Modifications to Electronic Data Transaction Standards and Code Sets; Final Rule February 20, 2003, *Federal Register* 45 CFR Part 162, Office of the Secretary, DHHS.
4. Health Insurance Portability and Accountability Act of 1996, August 21, 1996, Public Law 104–191.
5. The Health Insurance Portability and Accountability Act of 1996 (HIPAA), Centers for Medicare and Medicaid Services, http://cms.hhs.gov/hipaa.
6. HIPAA Administrative Simplification, Centers for Medicare and Medicaid Services, http://cms.hhs.gov/hipaa/hipaa2.
7. Standards for Privacy of Individually Identifiable Health Information; Final Rule August 14, 2002, *Federal Register* 45 CFR Parts 160 and 164, Department of Health and Human Services.
8. "Enforcing HIPAA: Who, When and How" presented by Stanley Nachimson, Office of HIPAA Standards, Centers for Medicare and Medicaid Services at 2003 Healthsec, September 23, 2003, Chicago.
9. "Compliance with HIPAA Regulations: Where are we now, how are things going? What's coming up next?" presented by Dianne Faup, J.D., Senior Policy Advisor, Office of HIPAA Standards, Department of Health and Human Services at 2003 CMS Great Lakes HIPAA Implementation Summit, December 4, 2003, Schaumburg, IL.
10. Administrative Simplification Enforcement Tool Web site (htct.hhs.gov).
11. Department of Health and Human Services Web site (www.hhs.gov).
12. "Federal Update: HIPAA Rule Schedule, Enforcement, and CHI" presented by Jared Adair, Director Office of HIPAA Standards, BCBSA HIPAA Implementation Team Conference, August 20, 2003, San Francisco.
13. "The National Health Information Infrastructure and Future of E-Health" presented by William Yasnoff, M.D., Ph.D., Senior Advisor, National Health Information Infrastructure, Department of Health and Human Services, December 5, 2003, 2003 Great Lakes HIPAA Implementation Summit, December 5, 2003, Schaumburg, IL.

V

SECURITY, PRIVACY, AND CONTINUITY

13

THE HIPAA SECURITY RISK ANALYSIS

Caroline Ramsey Hamilton

INTRODUCTION

Risk analysis (also known as risk assessment) is the cornerstone of any information security program, and it is the fastest way to gain a complete understanding of a healthcare organization's security profile — its strengths and weaknesses, its vulnerabilities and exposures. A risk analysis is a key requirement of the HIPAA final security rule. The security rule requires covered entities (CEs) to "conduct an accurate and thorough assessment of the potential risks and vulnerabilities to the confidentiality, integrity, and availability of electronic protected health information held by the covered entity." The rule further states that "[t]he required risk analysis is also a tool to allow flexibility for entities in meeting the requirements of this final rule. . . . "

In the CFR 164.308, under Administrative safeguards, the rule states that

(a) A covered entity must, in accordance with § 164.306:
  (1) (i) Standard: Security management process. Implement policies and procedures to prevent, detect, contain, and correct security violations.
  (ii) Implementation specifications:
    (A) Risk analysis *(Required)*. Conduct an accurate and thorough assessment of the potential risks and vulnerabilities to the confidentiality, integrity, and availability of electronic protected health information held by the covered entity.
    (B) Risk management *(Required)*. Implement security measures sufficient to reduce risks and vulnerabilities to a reasonable and appropriate level to comply with § 164.306(a).
    (C) Sanction policy *(Required)*. Apply appropriate sanctions against workforce members who fail to comply with the security policies and procedures of the covered entity.

Healthcare organizations are justifiably nervous about embarking on such a complicated project because risk analyses have not been widely used outside of government agencies but the risk analysis process will benefit the organization in many ways, not just in meeting a requirement. Properly done, risk analysis also measures overall HIPAA compliance, as well as standing up in a court of law to confirm that the organization has properly addressed relevant security risks. In addition, the risk analysis will put a management component into the security program, which will justify and validate the security program.

If you've been selected to manage the security risk analysis project, your first task is to determine the scope of the effort. Should it include the entire organization's data processing components, only the networks, or just the key databases? Do you have to include every single PC and network connection? How do you calculate the value of patient information? Should you use an automated package? Which one? Should you hire an outside consulting company to help or should you let them do the whole thing?

Most important, what results should you expect, and how can you convey these results to management in a meaningful way? This last question is a key consideration. A short concise report is much more valuable than a lengthy report that contains a jumble of confusing numbers and no specific recommendations. To gain the support of senior management, you'll need to give them a clear picture of your critical and sensitive assets, with detailed information on which ones are most in need of protection and how they should be protected.

WHAT IS RISK ANALYSIS?

A formal, quantitative risk analysis is the foundation and starting point of a good risk management program. A risk analysis can be called by many names: risk assessment, management review, gap analysis, risk management, vulnerability assessment, loss prevention, review of a sensitive application, or information security audit. Each name refers to the same function — analyzing an information system, an organization, a physical facility, or a business process in order to assess its existing security profile, and to identify the safeguards needed to bring the system's security up to the desired level. A risk analysis also provides a means of analyzing all potential threats to an organization, as well as their likelihood of occurrence. Risk analysis gives you a clear picture of your loss potential if certain threats materialize. It establishes expected losses from defined threats based on asset exposures, vulnerabilities, and estimated probabilities of occurrence. It identifies the problems you could expect to encounter with your information systems or facilities, whether that includes managing sensitive patient databases, making sure that physical controls are in place, or limiting access to information to individuals who need that access to do their jobs.

A simple definition is: risk analysis is a method of determining what kinds of controls are needed to protect an organization's information systems and other assets and resources not just adequately, but cost-effectively.

The risk analysis process analyzes a set of five variables, and comes up with recommended actions based on the relationships of these variables to each other.

You need to ask these questions:

- What are you trying to protect, how much is it worth, and how much depends on it?
- What could potentially threaten the asset?
- What weakness exists that would allow the threat to materialize?
- What kind of loss could you have should the threat materialize?
- What controls could you put into place that would reduce the loss if a threat occurred, or eliminate the threat altogether?

A risk analysis analyzes the relationship between five critical components:

1. *Assets* — The resources the organization wants to protect, including computers, networks, applications, databases, hardware, software, facilities, and protected health information (e-PHI).
2. *Threats* — The events that could occur, and cannot ever be completely eliminated, although you can reduce the likelihood of occurrence, or mitigate their impact. Even stringent security cannot eliminate every threat. Threats include events such as hurricanes, earthquakes, viruses, hackers, data destruction, data modification, theft of protected health information, fire, false alarms, bomb threats, sabotage, fraud, or embezzlement.
3. *Vulnerabilities* — Weaknesses or "windows of opportunity" that could allow a threat to materialize. For example, not having a current and up-to-date security plan could cause employees to allow unauthorized access to systems by leaving systems logged on when they are not in use.
4. *Losses* — Anything that can be taken away from the organization. This includes loss of data integrity of protected health information by modification, destruction, theft of equipment, delays or denials of service, or even loss of life. For example, a list of Alzheimer's patients was stolen from a local hospital, and was used to present false invoices to the individuals who then sued the hospital for releasing personal information.

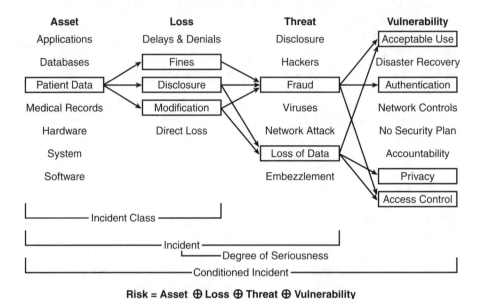

Linking Relationships

Asset	Loss	Threat	Vulnerability
Applications	Delays & Denials	Disclosure	Acceptable Use
Databases	Fines	Hackers	Disaster Recovery
Patient Data	Disclosure	Fraud	Authentication
Medical Records	Modification	Viruses	Network Controls
Hardware	Direct Loss	Network Attack	No Security Plan
System		Loss of Data	Accountability
Software		Embezzlement	Privacy
			Access Control

Incident Class

Incident

Degree of Seriousness

Conditioned Incident

Risk = Asset ⊕ Loss ⊕ Threat ⊕ Vulnerability

Figure 13.1   Relationship among the Different Elements

5. *Safeguards* — Administrative, physical, or technical controls designed to provide protection against threats and reduce identified vulner-abilities. Examples of safeguards could include cipher locks and terminals that log off automatically, biometric devices for user authentication, such as biometric mice, doing background checks on key personnel, and having an emergency mode operation plan.

Figure 13.1 illustrates the relationship between the different elements of a security risk analysis.

THE "CLASSIC" METHOD OF RISK ANALYSIS

In the traditional method of risk analysis, created by the U.S. National Institute of Standards and Technology (NIST) and influenced by audit standards, a questionnaire is used to survey users and determine whether the existing controls and standards are actually in use. Ask a security manager whether a password program is in place and whether all users are complying, and you will usually get an affirmative answer. However, if you ask 60 system users individually if they are using their passwords, you will generally find something quite different. You may also find that one group of users doesn't turn their computers off when they go to lunch because they don't want to have to log on again. A new employee's background check hasn't been finished, so the supervisor lends him a password until the check is complete. Many users have their "secret" passwords (yes — their pet's name) stuck on a Post-it™ note above their terminals.

RISK ASSESSMENT METHODOLOGY

The risk assessment process includes gathering information about the assets of the organization, including all information assets, such as networks, data centers, computers, hardware, software, and data/information; as well as physical assets, such as the personnel who staff the organization, the network users, the physical facility, and dozens of other organizational resources. In addition, the risk assessment process includes finding sources for comprehensive threat data, which may be gathered from internal sources such as incident report data, intrusion detection software, or threat data such as crime statistics, industry standards, and benchmarking data, and historical data about what has happened in the organization previously.

Vulnerability assessment is a key component of the risk assessment. Vulnerability data can come from two sources, however, a combination of both is recommended. The first source is a survey to find the weaknesses in the organization, asking the organization's personnel a controlled set of questions that validate compliance with the HIPAA final security rule or HIPAA privacy rule. The second source is technical vulnerability scanning reports and penetration tests that give very microlevel details about the weaknesses in the configuration of a network. Vulnerability data is then matched to see what combination of asset/threat/vulnerability could trigger a loss, and then it is decided what safeguards might be put in place to reduce or eliminate the potential loss.

STEPS IN A RISK ASSESSMENT

There are six basic steps in a risk assessment:

1. Set parameters for risk analysis
2. Define system assets
3. Determine relevant threat profiles
4. Survey all system users to discover vulnerabilities
5. Analyze all data
6. Write the report

THE VULNERABILITY ASSESSMENT

Risk assessment is composed of two parts: the vulnerability assessment and the countermeasure (safeguard) assessment. The vulnerability assessment looks at an existing system or facility and evaluates its existing security, including how personnel are complying with existing policies and guidelines. The result of the vulnerability assessment will present a detailed road map of all the existing weaknesses in the present system, including information on how widespread the problem is, and which individuals identified the weakness (vulnerability).

Surveying people who use the system under review is a critical part of the vulnerability assessment. Although paper surveys are laborious and difficult to aggregate, automated questionnaires now exist that allow risk analysts to interview users electronically. Survey questions start with a control standard that outlines the official policy of the organization. Questions should be set up to validate compliance against published policies, guidelines, and directives. There is little point in asking questions unrelated to requirements, because the organization would find it difficult to enforce compliance if it were not a requirement.

The risk analysis manager is the analyst in charge. However, there may be other individuals in the organization who can make major contributions. According to the audit guidelines for risk assessment, the more people you interview, the more likely you are to find vulnerabilities. Individuals should not be asked to answer more than 50 to 100 questions that are directly related to their jobs. For example, network users might answer questions related to whether they use their passwords, whether they log off their terminals when they leave their station, or whether they have attended basic data security training. The human resources manager or admissions clerk will answer a few general questions, but also more specific questions related to their job.

SURVEY QUESTIONS

Asking good questions is the very heart of the risk assessment and also forms the core of the vulnerability assessment. Questions should always be compliance-based and directly linked to the control standards that make up the final security rule or the privacy rule. If you ask questions that are not linked directly to the standard, and discover major problems, the path will not exist to force compliance. Limiting the number of questions to ask is one of the most difficult aspects of the analysis.

Employees may be nervous when they are asked to answer questions related to how they perform their jobs. It is important to make sure that these individuals understand that the risk analysis is a legal requirement for the organization and that any data gathered in the risk assessment will be seen by only one individual (the risk analysis manager), and that their comments will not be reviewed by their supervisor, nor will they end up in their personnel files.

Random surveys are often used to predict election results, from local precincts in a particular city, to federal elections, where the network news teams are able to predict the final results from a profile of only a few key states. In these examples, random samples are usually less than one percent. In a risk analysis, a random sample is not desirable. Instead, the objective should be to question as many people as possible. The more individuals you question, the better the chances that you will discover vulnerabilities. It is unrealistic to think that people will answer more than 50 to 100 questions.

To avoid individuals having to answer questions that do not relate to their area, in a risk assessment, questions are divided into job categories, or what are called "functional areas." Functional areas are pieces of a job. By dividing up questions into these categories, for example, Michael Smith may answer 20 questions for network users, 20 questions for personnel management (which is his area), and 15 general administration questions. More specialized personnel, such as facilities managers, the physical security officer, or legal counsel, will answer questions that relate only to their particular area.

Questions start as control standards. The standard might be: "CFR 164.308(a) (7) (Required Element) — Establish and implement procedures to create and maintain retrievable exact copies of electronic protected health information." The question statement asks the users how well they comply with this standard on a percentage scale from 0 to 10. The zero answer means the user never complies with the standard. An answer of 10 means the user complies with the standard 100 percent of the time, and the user is encouraged to answer with any percentage in between. In addition, users should be allowed two additional options in answering. The first is the opportunity to answer "not applicable," if the question doesn't apply to them; and second, to answer "I don't know," if they don't know the answer. This question process also serves as a training exercise, and a security awareness process.

THE TECHNICAL VULNERABILITY ASSESSMENT

Technical vulnerability assessments use scanning tools to survey the actual network and report the technical weaknesses that are discovered. Products can use passive analysis or active probing methods to identify security vulnerabilities, which may increase the efficiency of vulnerability identification and reduce false positive results. These technical assessments can

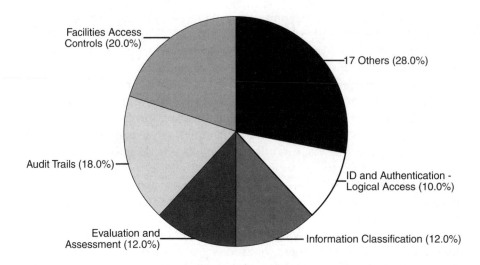

Figure 13.2   Weaknesses Discovered

differentiate between infrastructure devices (such as routers, switches, and firewalls) and host devices (user workstations or servers (such as e-mail servers or Web servers). Technical vulnerability tools can find vulnerabilities in Network TCP/IP hosts, UNIX hosts, Windows NT hosts, Web servers, mail servers, FTP servers, firewalls, routers, and switches.

VULNERABILITY ASSESSMENT RESULTS

At a very high level, the vulnerability assessment will analyze and summarize the results of the all the weaknesses that were discovered in the systems under review, as illustrated in Figure 13.2.

ENROLLING THE ORGANIZATION IN RISK MANAGEMENT

Risk assessment is a management process and, by its nature, should involve the whole organization. Because the vulnerability discovery process will include questioning many different parts of the organization, it is vitally important to the eventual acceptance of the risk assessment findings that different departments be involved in the initial setting up of the analysis. Midlevel managers may feel threatened that another group is asking questions of "their" employees. They may worry that the findings could reflect negatively on their performance as supervisors. In addition, if the survey questions are not approved prior to their use by the various supervisors and department heads, the results they generate might be discounted and not taken seriously.

For these reasons, it is important to set up a risk analysis team within the organization. The team members will include representatives from each department included in the analysis process. Team members will review questions, identify the correct standards for their areas, assist the risk analyst in arriving at current asset replacement values, and serve as administrative support for the surveys in their respective areas of responsibility.

THE COST BENEFIT — ESTABLISHING RETURN-ON-INVESTMENT (ROI)

The cost benefit analysis combines information from the vulnerability assessment along with relevant threat data and asset information such as present day replacement values, criticality, integrity, and availability of the information contained in the system under review, as well as how completely safeguards are currently being implemented. In reviewing the existing security controls, it's important to indicate percentages of current implementation. For example, maybe the visitor-badging policy is only 70 percent implemented, meaning that it is implemented on weekdays, but not on weekends. In actual risk assessments, completing implementation of an existing control to 100 percent is often the most cost-effective solution.

The result of the cost benefit analysis will be to create a Return-On-Investment ratio (ROI), balancing the value of the information against the cost of controls to protect it. By establishing return-on-investment data, managers and directors at healthcare organizations can make more informed decisions regarding which controls to implement, based not only on initial cost to implement, but also on the current threat exposure of the organization and their contribution to meeting the requirements of the final security rule.

The accountability that is a built-in component of risk assessment is increasingly attractive to top-level management, both in the federal sector as well as in private industry, where board members and shareholders want quantitative numbers to use in assessing the security level of an organization and making the resultant management recommendations.

A typical cost benefit analysis graph is shown in Figure 13.3.

AUTOMATING THE PROCESS

Automating the risk assessment process is a major improvement over doing it manually. Just ask Daniel W. Sedano, CISSP and manager, Information Security at Community Medical Centers in Fresno, California and someone who's on the front lines of the HIPAA risk analysis:

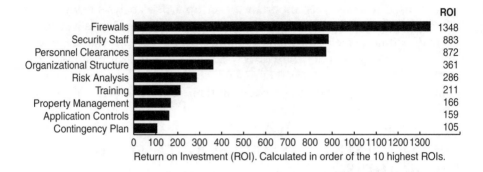

Figure 13.3   Cost Benefit Analysis

Without the help of software, it's a very cumbersome task. It's not impossible, but it would take months just to complete the risk assessment, not to mention the volumes of paper involved. I often tell people that using tools like HIPAA-Watch, allows a covered entity to make scalable and reasonable business decisions. With a fully automated program, you can do it three times faster, and the results are much more accurate.

■ Automating the security risk assessment required for HIPAA has some key advantages over the manual process.
■ The level of effort is greatly reduced, often by 50 percent or more.
■ Major cost savings can be realized on subsequent analyses when systems have to be recertified, as the HIPAA final security rule requires.
■ Automation makes it easier to consider the effects of different safeguards. It allows you to play "What if?" to help develop the best level of protection for the least cost.
■ Automated packages are adaptable to many environments, even new systems or new facilities being developed.
■ Many automated packages can produce both quantitative and qualitative results.
■ Updated data can be easily added at any point of the assessment.

SELECTING AN AUTOMATED RISK ASSESSMENT PACKAGE TO MEET THE RISK ANALYSIS REQUIREMENT OF THE HIPAA FINAL SECURITY RULE

Ten years ago, few security risk assessment packages were available, and they were generally cumbersome, based on spreadsheets, and difficult to use. In recent years, however, several PC-based risk assessment packages have been developed and marketed. These packages automate many of the labor-intensive tasks involved in a security risk assessment. Automated methodologies generally provide either quantitative or qualitative results; a few can do both. Very few risk assessment programs are suited to doing the gap analysis and risk assessments required for HIPAA. The newness of the content and the difficulty some programs have in updating have limited the availability of these programs.

In evaluating automated tools, consider the guidelines provided in the National Institute of Standards and Technology (NIST) Special Publication 500-174, *Guide for Selecting Automated Risk Assessment Tools*. It recommends that packages include three fundamental components:

1. *Data Collection.* The method used to compile asset information, data on the operational environment of the system under review, as well as collection of questionnaire data from assessment participants.
2. *Data Assessment.* Techniques can include statistical methods, sampling techniques, the Delphi process, Monte Carlo modeling, regression analysis, and use of expert systems.
3. *Report Generation.* The form taken by the output data from the risk assessment, how the report is configured, whether it can be tailored to individual needs, and whether the report includes graphics.

In addition, you will probably want to consider the following factors.

1. *Program Operation.* Does the methodology meet existing risk assessment guidelines? Has it been tested in a regulatory environment so you can be sure it meets federal requirements? Does it comply with a methodology that has already been endorsed by your agency or organization?
2. *Compliance with Requirements.* Does the program include the exact regulatory requirements? Does it include gap analysis to measure compliance with privacy regulations and the administrative, technical, and physical requirements of HIPAA?
3. *Ease of Use.* Is the program easily installed and implemented without needing a consultant?
4. *Tailoring.* Can the program be easily tailored so that its screens reflect your organizational environment?
5. *Question Development.* Does the program allow you to create your own questions, and to modify existing questions and standards?
6. *Questionnaire Distribution.* Can questionnaires be distributed to survey recipients by e-mail, diskette, or over a network, to both end users and administrative and medical personnel? Can questions

be answered, and returned on disk or via network, and automatically uploaded?

7. *Report Generation.* Does the program write the report automatically? Can it be easily changed and adjusted by the user?

8. *Usefulness to Management.* Are graphics easy to understand? Is the report written in nontechnical, easy-to-understand language?

9. *Vendor Support.* What support does the vendor provide in training in the use of the package? Is there a mechanism to keep users informed of product enhancements? Is telephone support provided at no additional charge?

10. *Updates and Enhancements.* Is the product upgraded by a major release at least annually, or whenever the regulations change?

11. *Cost.* Is the cost reasonable when balanced against the performance and output of the product?

RISK ASSESSMENT IS GOOD MANAGEMENT

Many healthcare managers face gap analysis and risk analysis with a groan, seeing only a complicated project without any redeeming attributes. Risk assessment as a management tool is actually a vital element in the overall management of patient records, medical records, or any information system. Because of the different interpretations of the term "risk management," there has been a great deal of confusion about risk assessment/risk management. This accounts for the reluctance of many healthcare managers to incorporate risk analysis and assessment into their HIPAA toolbox.

The U.S. General Accounting Office (GAO) recently reported on using risk assessment to deal with biological terrorism, and said, "We have previously reported on the value of a new approach of using sound threat and risk assessments for focusing programs and investments to combat terrorism. Without such assessments, there is little or no assurance that programs and spending are focused in the right areas in the right amounts."

THE FUTURE OF RISK ASSESSMENT

Commenting on the future of risk assessment in the HIPAA environment, Gary Swindon, former Chief Security and Privacy Officer for WebMD and Security Officer for Orlando Regional Health Care, said:

> Any program that seeks to achieve HIPAA compliance must have an enduring quality since, by its very definition, HIPAA is forever. Nowhere is a solid risk management program more important — just as HIPAA will endure, risks will change with time and efforts to contain them, forcing the risk management

effort to take on similar "enduring" qualities in order to be of value to the company.

With requirements increasing as fast as the losses, the final question remaining for HIPAA managers to think about security risk assessment is not whether they have to do it, or can afford to do it, but whether they can afford *not* to do it.

14

HIPAA SECURITY COMPLIANCE: WHAT IT MEANS FOR DEVELOPERS, VENDORS, AND PURCHASERS

Keith Pasley, CISSP

INTRODUCTION

For market efficiencies to be gained, sellers must understand the needs of their buyers. Creators of products must develop with the needs of the customer in mind. Purchasers need to feel comfortable that they are getting what they paid for. How do the dynamics of the HIPAA final security rule regulatory environment affect the market participants?

Good communication and a common interpretation of the HIPAA security rules between vendor and potential customers is essential when working with vendors of products that are targeting the Health Information Portability and Accountability (HIPAA) security compliancy market, which includes "covered entities."[1]

Most vendors base their product road maps on feedback from customers and selected groups of users and industry subject matter experts. In the case of HIPAA compliancy products, whether a billing system, computerized patient records products, e-mail software, or any other related products, the security rule helps promote a common understanding of security intent based on the high-level goals set by the U.S. federal government regarding the security of electronically transmitted or received Protected Health Information (PHI).

One of the determining factors that leads to vendors developing products that accurately provide the product characteristics desired by the target audience is to truly understand the environment of the customer.

0-8493-2211-1/05/$0.00+$1.50
© 2005 by CRC Press LLC

Part of the regulatory environment of the healthcare industry is the HIPAA security rule. This chapter deals primarily with the technical standards section of the final HIPAA security rule.

What do vendors need to know about creating products that truly embody the needs of the HIPAA security rule compliance market? Is there a methodology that purchasers can use to evaluate whether a product meets the relevant HIPAA standards for their organization?

What questions should be asked of vendors to determine whether their product will fit in with the HIPAA security compliance goals of covered entities?

The following discussion is not intended to be exhaustive on all aspects of implementing the technical standards section of the HIPAA security rule, but rather to serve as a basis for discussion among software developers, vendors, and potential customers in the HIPAA security compliance market when determining systems requirements. The HIPAA security compliance market is defined as the group of buyers and sellers of products/services that claim to help, in some way, covered entities to comply with one or more aspects of the HIPAA security rule.

HIPAA SECURITY RULE: WHAT SOFTWARE DEVELOPERS SHOULD KNOW

Do you develop software that has even the remote possibility of being used by a HIPAA covered entity? If so, what should you know about the HIPAA security rule when developing software? Most of the security rule standards are increasingly becoming "good programming" and may already be incorporated in the systems development cycle of software vendors. However, there are some HIPAA security concepts that need to be emphasized to software developers, should their software be used by businesses that are considered "covered entities" under HIPAA security regulations.

PHI-Related Software Development

HIPAA defines protected health information as "any information, whether oral or recorded in any form or medium" that

- "[i]s created or received by a health care provider, health plan, public health authority, employer, life insurer, school or university, or health care clearinghouse"; and
- "[r]elates to the past, present, or future physical or mental health or condition of an individual; the provision of health care to an individual; or the past, present, or future payment for the provision of health care to an individual."

In short, PHI is information that is identifiable to a certain person that includes health information. PHI data is the target of protection, as covered by the security rule. The security rule for PHI only applies if the PHI data is electronically transmitted or received by a covered entity. If the data is covered by the HIPAA security rule then the law requires the customer (covered entity) to: "Implement technical policies and procedures for electronic information systems that maintain electronic PHI to allow access only to those persons or software programs that have been granted access rights as specified." Thus the covered entity is mandated to protect the PHI while allowing only authorized access, as needed.

Covered entities have been advised by the HIPAA regulators to work with their software vendors in producing software that will help their security rule compliance efforts. Therefore, when performing the requirements analysis phase of systems design, you may be prompted by customers, who are covered entities, to provide an explanation of how your system design features map to various HIPAA security rule standards. In other cases, software applications will have to be redesigned or modified to fit specific security compliance objectives of individual covered entities. In many cases, HIPAA security rule technical standards compliance will be gained by small adjustments to the existing security posture of the covered entity. In such cases, the ability to integrate into existing security architectures will be a key to effecting compliance.

If you are developing PHI-related software applications one person on the client side who will probably have input into the design requirements is the Information Security Officer (ISO). Covered entities are mandated by HIPAA to designate someone as the ISO, the person responsible for implementing HIPAA security rules. The ISO can be someone with a security background or can literally be anyone designated as such, regardless of experience. ISO responsibilities include setting up user accounts, controlling authorization and access controls, and emergency access contingency plans. These will be major discussion points in developing requirements for software systems that must comply with the HIPAA security rule.

Reasonably Anticipated Threat Protection

It is impossible to build a system that is completely secure. The stated objective of the security rule is to establish standards to "protect against reasonably anticipated threats or hazards and improper use or disclosure." Viruses, malicious code, password cracking, social engineering, and other threats that are common to most business networks must be considered in designing PHI-related software systems. The HIPAA security rule provides criminal and civil liability in cases where covered entities experience security breaches due to not implementing required standards as proscribed by the security rule. Healthcare-informed software developers will understand that this reason, along with the anticipated savings opportunity, will be a major reason for the covered entities to seek compliance. Keep in mind that the security rule sets the minimum standard of securing data. Good security practice generally provides for much more protection than is simply covered by the security rule. It is likely that HIPAA security rule compliance, in some cases, will be a subset of an already existing organizational security policy and architecture.

Software developers should be aware of the goals of the HIPAA security and privacy rules: providing confidentiality, integrity, and availability of protected health information. PHI data must be accessible to authorized entities and persons, kept private from unauthorized viewing, and protected from unauthorized modification or deletion.

Also, note that there are 18 technical security standards and 36 implementation specifications of which developers should be aware. Security rule implementation specifications contain more detailed instructions on either required implementation steps or optional choices in implementing HIPAA security standards. When working with PHI-related customer applications be aware that some implementation specifications are required and some are addressable. Addressable means that implementation of an implementation specification is an option. Covered entities are given flexibility in implementation depending on such factors as the security risk involved, size of the organization, cost of the procedures to comply, technical infrastructure, and capabilities. What does this mean to software developers? It is because of this flexibility that covered entities in the same line of business may have different implementations of the same standard. The important point is that during the early phase of software design, think in terms of risks associated with the application, reasonably anticipated threats to the security of the application, and flexibility of implementation specifications based on unique requirements of covered entities.

HIPAA SECURITY RULE: HOW VENDORS CAN HELP

One interesting statement in the regulatory impact analysis section of the security rule sheds light on the implications of the HIPAA security rule to vendors:

Impact on System Vendors

> Systems vendors that provide computer software applications to health care providers and other billers [companies that provide billing services] of health care services would likely be

affected. These vendors would have to develop software solutions that would allow health plans, providers, and other users of electronic transactions to protect these transactions and the information in their databases from unauthorized access to their systems. Their costs would also probably be passed along to their customer bases.

The intent of the security rule is to encourage vendors to work with the healthcare industry to create solutions and standards that are presently absent. To this end software vendors play an important role in enabling the HIPAA security rule. Vendors will need to create easy to implement/manage, cost-effective, and easy to integrate solutions. Integration is important due to the business goal of extending the value of systems in which covered entities have invested. For example, standards-based solutions tend to work better together due to common agreement on the definition of protocols and certain APIs. The information security marketplace is starting to reach consensus on more security standards than ever before.

Successful vendors serving this market will be aware of the healthcare industry environment. The healthcare industry is looking for solutions that include improving business operating efficiency and streamlining access to information. Other common goals of healthcare include balancing the need for security and the ability for clinicians to easily access the information they require to provide superior patient care. Healthcare is faced with a rapidly changing business environment with the challenge of industrywide government regulation. Vendors will need to be more adept at responding to change more quickly in order to effectively serve this market. For example, it is no longer acceptable in healthcare to produce any financial system or patient care applications that do not include basic security, such as unique user accounts or policy-based access controls.

Scalable Solutions

The security rules are designed to scale from small doctors to the large university medical campus. Because both organizations transmit and receive the covered transactions electronically to some degree, both need to comply with the security rule. However, the extent of compliance can be different depending on such factors as the security risk involved. What does this mean to software developers? It means that no vendor will really have a product that will, for example, "solve all your HIPAA compliance issues." What will be applicable to one healthcare covered entity may not be in another, even though they are in the same HIPAA compliance market segment.

Vendors will need to take the HIPAA scalability intent in as a factor when designing and marketing products for the HIPAA compliance market. As an over-simplified example, a vendor might create a product that provides e-mail encryption. The informed vendor will know that not every covered entity will need or want the vendor's e-mail encryption product due to how the covered entity designates itself within the HIPAA framework.

With this knowledge, the vendor may develop the product to embody the security rule scalability concept "designed into" it. In this example, the product feature that addresses the scalability aspect of the encryption specification in the security rule could be that the product allows encryption enforcement based on business policy. In such a product, perhaps when the device detects an e-mail receiver address and document type that matches a "Use encryption when sending this type of document to this destination" policy, the device would enforce encryption. In another case, however, if the device detects an e-mail receiver address and document type that matches a "Do *not* use encryption when sending this type of document to this destination," the device would merely perform a data integrity check only with the document being sent in cleartext. If the mechanics of making the policy enforcement decisions can be configured so that end users do not need to be aware of the enforcement action (user intervention), so much the better. In such a case, there is no need for an end user to determine policy enforcement because the end user is not the security expert. The end user just wants to send an e-mail and business management wants to ensure the e-mail is sent appropriately. This is a simple example of the requirements gathering thought process that a vendor could use to demonstrate an understanding of the real needs of the HIPAA compliance market. This is, of course, a grossly simplified example that establishes a process that vendors can use when creating product requirements based on a real understanding of the HIPAA security rule as it applies to various businesses that are covered entities. It is not just a matter of assuming that all healthcare organizations will want to use a product in the same way. Rather, vendors should expect that covered entities will want specific flexibility in products due, again, to how the covered entity designates itself with respect to the provisions in the HIPAA security rule and the covered entity's unique operating environment.

Security solutions that will most successfully adapt to the HIPAA compliance market will embody the intent of the security rule in whatever respect is appropriate based on the common understanding, between the HIPAA compliance market and the vendor community, of the security rule requirements of individual covered entities.

The general requirements of the HIPAA security rule are that covered entities must protect against reasonably anticipated threats or hazards to the security or integrity of information. Covered entities must also protect against reasonably anticipated uses and disclosures not permitted by privacy rules. What does this mean to vendors? It means that "reasonable" can mean low-tech. Also, "protect" can mean not just highly sophisticated next-generation technology but it also can mean the use of fairly mainstream security technology such as firewalls, virtual private networks, antivirus, and some detect/response capabilities. Services such as risk assessments, security architecture and design, policy life-cycle management, and security outsourcing will be important areas of need for covered entities. Depending on the risk, based on the content and business impact if lost or exposed, it could also mean no change from what the covered entity is already doing. This highlights another point that bears repetition — the HIPAA security rule sets a baseline, a minimum standard for the industry, and is based on security best practices, other preexisting security standards work, and industry consensus. Therefore, the HIPAA security rule is a subset of the broader, plain old "good security" practices. This means that any organization that has a well thought out and executed security plan will need minimum adjustments to comply with the rule.

A couple of approaches that software vendors can take come to mind. One approach is to study the needs of the broader healthcare market in order to offer solutions that can cost-effectively benefit organizations based on economies of scale. For example, outsourced services, so-called managed service providers, are based on this approach. Another strategy is to divide the market into segments, and then provide solutions based on healthcare market segments that are underserved. An example of this is the so-called "boutique" vendors who serve a highly focused, narrowly defined target submarket.

Due to the mandatory nature and time-based urgency of the security rule, many vendors are suddenly proclaiming their products' "HIPAA-compliance" in an effort to extend their products to a captured audience. This is helpful to the HIPAA compliance market inasmuch as the vendors can demonstrate that their preexisting products' features can provide value by addressing one or more of the 18 standards in the security rule technical safeguards section in a clear, concise, and compelling manner.

Vendors will keep in mind that the security rule is risk-based as compared to vulnerability-based. What does this mean for vendors? Informed vendors will demonstrate that their product is a tool used to reduce risk as this is the general intent of the security rule and the specific objective of the standards

HIPAA SECURITY RULE: MAKING PRODUCT SELECTIONS

Before making product selections it is important that the decision to purchase security controls be based on the risk analysis as mandated by HIPAA security rule sec 164.308(a) (1). An output from the analysis will be a business impact analysis.

After performing a risk assessment, a covered entity will have some idea of the amount of risk exposure it has in relation to the security rule standards. Based on the business impact analysis included in the risk assessment, a covered entity will have some quantitative or qualitative measurement based on the consequences of an exploited vulnerability that reasonably should have been mitigated. Using that metric, for example, a covered entity can then make a business decision as to what procedure or technology will be purchased or applied to lower the risk of exposure to a relevant threat. Purchasers should budget enough to manage a risk to an acceptable level and not a penny more (despite what a vendor tells you). So, instead of relying on a vendor to provide an arbitrary statement of risk, as part of a marketing campaign, for example, covered entities will have a risk assessment performed in advance of purchasing security technology, if at all possible or practical. In the case of risk that can be measured in dollars, this risk management-based approach will help covered entities understand the monetary value of specific risks to specific assets. This approach will help entities from overspending in areas that present low risk with respect to HIPAA security rule compliance. Covered entities are certainly encouraged to go beyond the minimum standards outlined in the security rule as they see fit. Vendors are certainly willing to go beyond the security compliance agenda as well.

NOTE

1. Covered entities include the following business classifications: health plans, healthcare providers, and health care clearinghouses.

BIBLIOGRAPHY

1. 45 CFR Parts 160, 162, and 164 Health Insurance Reform: Security Standards; Final Rule.
2. Fodor, Joseph. HIPAA and the EHR: Making technical safeguard changes. *Journal of AHIMA* 75, 1 (January 2004): 54–55.
3. Kaelin, Mark. Ignore the HIPAA security rules at your own considerable risk. | Builders.Com, November 7, 2003.
4. Amatayakul, Margret. Rethinking initial HIPAA Efforts, *RHIA, CHPS, FHIMSS AHIMA Journal*, November 2, 2003.
5. http://www.hipaadvisory.com/regs/PenaltiesbyZon.htm.
6. http://www.wedi.org/snip/public/articles/hipaa_glossary.pdf.
7. http://www.wedi.org/snip/public/articles/dis_viewArticle.cfm?ID=202.
8. HIPAA Security Standards-Final Rule presentation Stanley Nachimson, Office of HIPAA Standards CMS, June 2003.
9. http://www.sanctuminc.com/pdf/HIPAA_Advisory.pdf.
10. http://www.cms.hhs.gov/hipaa/hipaa2/education/Feb2003RoundTrans.pdf.
11. http://www.cms.hhs.gov/hipaa/hipaa2/education/Aug22trans-ed.pdf.
12. http://www.eventstreams.com/cms/tm_001/Questionstoaskvendors.pdf.

15

ISSUES AND CONSIDERATIONS FOR BUSINESS CONTINUITY PLANNING UNDER HIPAA

Kevin C. Miller

INTRODUCTION

The Health Insurance and Portability Act (HIPAA) of 1996 requires organizations that, "maintain or transmit health information shall maintain reasonable and appropriate administrative, technical, and physical safeguards." Among the safeguards mentioned include protecting against any "reasonably anticipated threats or hazards to the security or integrity of the information. . . . "

The final security rule as published by the Department of Health and Human Services (DHHS) requires organizations to implement a contingency plan to protect Private Health Information (PHI). The requirements regarding a contingency plan (also called a Business Continuity Plan (BCP)) are deliberately left vague due to the fact that organizations differ. As the final security rule states, "A contingency plan may involve highly complex processes in one processing site, or simple manual processes in another. The contents of any given contingency plan will depend upon the nature and configuration of the entity devising it."

This chapter provides a road map for building a continuity plan and discusses the BCP requirements and recommendations of the final security rule.

Business continuity planning as a discipline evolved from the information technology field. Computers became the norm in the workplace in the 1970s, and companies increasingly began to rely on technology.

As data began to take on new importance, disaster recovery planning, the recovery of information, became commonplace at large organizations. Over the years it has evolved from being strictly IT focused to being a comprehensive discipline that covers technology, people, facilities, and procedures, thus the new term "business continuity planning."

During a disaster, many privacy and security initiatives may become ineffective or disabled. This is true no matter the nature of a disaster, whether it is natural (tornado, hurricane, earthquakes, etc.), intentionally manmade (war, act of terrorism, hacking, etc.), or an accidental disaster (power outage, equipment failures, software errors, etc.). For this reason, the Department of Health and Human Services (DHHS) requires organizations that handle private health information to implement a business continuity plan.

BCP BEST PRACTICES

Aside from being regulated by HIPAA, a solid business continuity plan ensures an organization's survivability in the event of an unforeseen business disruption. In addition, it illustrates to customers, investors, and other stakeholders the organization's commitment to longevity and fiscal responsibility.

Some experts liken BCP to insurance. Others prefer to think of it as complementary to insurance. If a major disaster wipes out your entire corporate headquarters, an insurance policy may compensate you for the loss of property, but how do you recover the lost business, the damage to your reputation, and the lost patients? Your customers won't wait until you rebuild your business. They will simply find a competitor to supply the same or similar product or service. Business continuity planning when done properly will help an organization get back to business in the most cost-effective and efficient manner.

The first and often most difficult step for most organizations is to gather senior executive support. It can be a daunting task to convince bottom-line people to spend money on a program that does not produce any revenue. Fortunately for healthcare professionals, this process is streamlined. Because HIPAA requires companies that handle private health information to have written contingency plans, the senior executives have no choice but to support the program or risk the regulatory penalties.

A mistake often made by first-time planners is to rush in and begin making preparations. They feel that they, or the organization's managers, intuitively know what the most important processes, applications, or business functions are within their organization. This is not always the case.

In a sense, you must start your plan — with a plan. The following five steps are a recommended course of action when starting a new business continuity program.

- *Step One:* Initiation
- *Step Two:* Business impact analysis
- *Step Three:* Business continuity strategies
- *Step Four:* Plan construction
- *Step Five:* Plan exercise and maintenance

STEP ONE: INITIATION

During the initiation phase, the business continuity planner will gather information. Items to be reviewed and collected include: pertinent laws or regulations, any existing BCP plans or policies, and statistics on local events such as floods, tornados, or power outages.

Also during the initiation phase, the decision needs to be made as to where the BCP function should reside within an organization. Traditionally, many organizations place BCP under the IT department. A survey of BCP professionals found that as of May 2003, 51 percent of the respondents reported that the IT department had the ultimate responsibility for BCP. (See Figure 15.1 for complete results of the survey.)

To many this would seem the logical place to place BCP, especially because the majority of other requirements of HIPAA will be placed under the purveyance of the IT department as well. Although placing BCP under the IT department may be the most popular choice, it may not be the

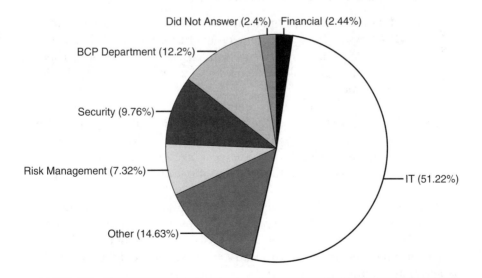

Figure 15.1   Which department in your organization is ultimately responsible for business continuity planning? (Strohl Systems/Contingency Planning & Management, October 2002.)

best choice. Having the BCP program report to the IT department may lead an organization to see BCP issues only as technological problems rather than business challenges.

But this is not to say that the IT department is always the wrong place to put a BCP program. As with many issues in BCP, decisions are based on a variety of unique characteristics within an organization and a thorough evaluation of the issues should be conducted before a decision is to be made.

After the decision has been made about which department will have authority over the BCP program, the budget needs to be addressed. Keep in mind that BCP is not a one-time project, but a program that needs annual funding. When budgeting, the organization needs to decide how the program will be run. Will there be a central BCP office that develops plans for each department, or will each department be responsible for writing its own plans with guidance from those responsible for the planning program? If the first option is chosen, the budget process should be straightforward. If the latter is chosen, then it may be best to divide the budget among departments.

Other considerations during the initiation phase include choosing the BCP team members, delineating the roles of the team members, and defining the scope of the BCP program.

STEP TWO: BUSINESS IMPACT ANALYSIS

Any comprehensive BCP program must begin with a Business Impact Analysis (BIA). A BIA is a management-level assessment of financial and operational impacts that would result from a business disruption. The BIA highlights costs and possible losses associated with recovering business functions over time.

A sound BIA should identify extraordinary expenses that could be incurred from a disaster, the organization's current state of preparedness, any single points of failure, technology requirements for recovery, special recovery resources needed, and the organization's critical information systems. The results of the BIA are used as the foundation of the continuity plan.

Organizations new to planning seriously should consider getting outside help in the form of an experienced consultant to help conduct the BIA. Because the BIA is serving as the basis for any continuity decisions, any overlooked questions at the start can result in a continuity plan that is less than sound.

An important point to remember with BIAs: Once is not enough. Because of the ever-changing aspects of technology and business, BIAs should be conducted and reviewed on a regular basis. As indicated in

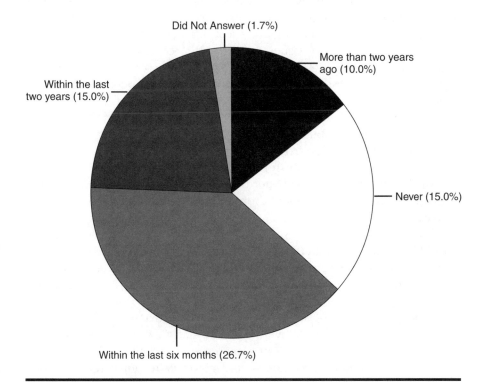

Figure 15.2 When was the last time that you conducted a business impact analysis? (Strohl Systems/Contingency Planning & Management, October 2002.)

Figure 15.2, the majority of healthcare organizations conducted a BIA within a year of the January 2003 survey.

The first step in the BIA process is to prepare a survey. The survey should include queries that will help determine the following:

- Financial impacts on the organization resulting from each business operation's inability to conduct operations for a prolonged period of time
- Operational impacts relating to each business operation
- Extraordinary expenses involved in continuity operations after a disruption
- Current state of preparedness to resume business operations
- Seasonal impacts relating to each business operation
- Technology requirements for resumption and recovery
- Other special resumption and recovery resources
- Information systems support for resumption of time-sensitive operations

Survey questions should run the gamut of the BCP process: from identification of workaround procedures, to software required to accomplish tasks, to the amount of money lost if a department were down for a given time period. Key issues that are often overlooked include regulatory fines and penalties incurred (a significant issue with HIPAA), the possibility of lost customers, service level agreement penalties, potential drop-off in product or service quality, and the impact a disaster would have on union contracts and employee turnover.

The survey is distributed to department heads and other critical personnel for input and is an extremely important step in gaining awareness, ownership, and participation from department managers. The more comprehensive the survey is, the better the information received. But a survey that is too long will receive less thorough answers. In addition, surveyors will waste a lot of time tracking down delinquent recipients, too overwhelmed by the enormity of the document to provide answers. A balance should be struck between the need for accurate and complete information and the need to be concise and efficient. Before sending the survey to all recipients, it is a good idea to try it out on a few test recipients. Speak to them and gauge their general impressions of the document. Fine tune and improve the survey before going live to the masses.

The end result of the BIA will be charts, statistics, and costs associated with any business disruption. You should discover time-sensitive business operations, resumption timeframes, and recovery resource requirements. In addition, the BIA will show the organization's current level of preparedness. The survey answers are combined and analyzed in order to build the organization's planning strategy.

STEP THREE: BUSINESS CONTINUITY STRATEGIES

Business continuity planning is not a one-size-fits-all proposition. Many factors are considered when determining the best strategy for a particular organization. HIPAA addresses this fact and is deliberately left flexible.

The final security rule states that organizations that handle private health information must "establish (and implement as needed) policies and procedures for responding to an emergency or other occurrence (for example, fire, vandalism, system failure, and natural disaster) that damages systems that contain electronic protected health information."

It requires organizations to develop a data backup plan, a disaster recovery plan, and an emergency mode operation plan. It does not provide specifics on what needs to be incorporated into any of these plans. Because each organization is different, and the HIPAA regulations are vague on the subject, it is impossible to say how all organizations should strategize to meet their business continuity needs. It is best to use the

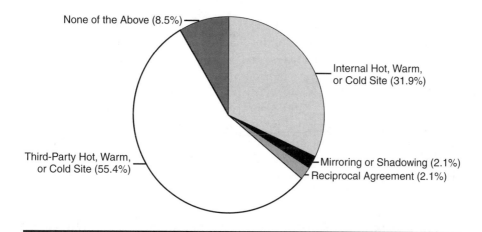

Figure 15.3   What is your primary alternate site strategy in your business continuity program? (Strohl Systems/Contingency Planning & Management, October 2002.)

results of the BIA to build a plan that provides senior management with an adequate risk comfort level.

Most large organizations choose to outsource their data recovery and disaster recovery plans (see Figure 15.3). But over the last few years that trend has been changing and many companies (particularly in the heavily regulated financial industry) are choosing to bring their alternate sites in-house.

STEP FOUR: PLAN CONSTRUCTION

In general, the plan should document procedures and resources necessary to recover critical business functions. It also should include information about who can declare a disaster and under what circumstances. It should identify recovery teams, team members, and each team's responsibilities. The plan should contain contact lists of critical personnel, vendors, regulatory agencies, and partners. In addition, a plan should describe the responsibilities and procedures to be followed by each continuity team and contain contact lists of critical personnel.

Plans should also identify any interdependencies within the business and with critical vendors. For example, if a particular business function absolutely needs e-mail to perform its mission, the e-mail system becomes a critical function for the organization.

STEP FIVE: PLAN EXERCISE AND MAINTENANCE

HIPAA states that contingency plan testing and revision procedures are addressable. It does not indicate how often tests and revisions should be conducted, but BCP best practices indicate that plans should be tested on at least an annual basis. In addition, changes should be made to the plan any time key personnel change; new products, services, or procedures are introduced; or after reorganizations.

Through testing, companies can establish realistic recovery time objectives, needed resources, and appropriate personnel. An untested plan, sitting on a shelf gathering dust, will fail more often than not. There are four types of tests. Choosing which test works for a financial institution depends on the objective of the planners. Using automated BCP software and experienced consultants can help with plan testing and maintenance. Types of tests include:

- *Structured Walkthrough* — The most basic type of test. A structured walkthrough takes place in a group-meeting type of setting, where the main goal is to confirm that critical personnel from all areas are familiar with the BCP. These types of tests take the least amount of time (typically about two to three hours) to conduct. A scenario is given by the team leaders (e.g., a power outage), and subsequent questions are asked such as, "What will you do in the first two hours?" or, "What should you have accomplished by now?" After each hourly increment, teams are polled again to gauge their progress. The only downsides to this type of test are that it usually doesn't involve the entire organization, nor does it test the team's ability to execute it.

- *Tactical Exercise* — Also known as a tabletop exercise, a tactical exercise is the most popular type of test used by consultants. The main goals here are to practice team interaction, as well as decision-making and problem-solving skills during a full-blown simulation that typically lasts between six to eight hours. During a tactical exercise, the first three to five days of the recovery effort are simulated (not in real-time, of course), with a few twists and turns included. The given scenario typically will unfold slowly, because in real life, that's how a situation develops. There are usually four to seven timed segments, each providing a little more information about the scenario. After each of these segments, teams participating in the test exchange report to one another, which serves as the only form of communication among them. A complete audit trail of the exercise is kept that will help determine the test's strengths and weaknesses.

- *Technical Test* — Also known as a hot site test, a technical test deals exclusively with the IT side of a recovery, and will take place at an alternate site, which will most likely be your organization's hot site. The main goal of a technical test is to see if your company's

IT team can get some portion of the production processes up and running at the alternate site. Although quite disruptive, it's still very necessary to prove that your company can do business in the event of a disaster. This is a very specialized test, and will utilize only a small portion of your recovery team.

■ *Full-Scale Exercise* — By far, the most comprehensive test is the full-scale exercise, also known as the operational exercise. During this test, all or most of the BCP is put into action. The main goal here is simple — to simulate an actual recovery situation as closely as possible. The exercises in this case usually are longer, and will evolve and develop just as they would in an actual crisis. Full-scale exercises are similar to tactical exercises in that they re-create an actual scenario, but have a much broader scope both in terms of teams involved and the number of business and technical functions required.

CONCLUSION

In order to be compliant with the April 2005 deadline, healthcare companies should begin the BCP process immediately by conducting a business impact analysis. Not only is having a business continuity plan now mandated by HIPAA, it is prudent business. A healthcare organization does not want to discover that it is out of business at a time when patients need it most.

VI

APPENDICES

Appendix

A

PART I: A HIPAA GLOSSARY

AAHomecare See the American Association for Homecare.

Accredited Standards Committee (ASC) An organization that has been accredited by ANSI for the development of American National Standards.

ACG Ambulatory Care Group.

ACH See Automated Clearinghouse.

ADA See the American Dental Association.

ADG Ambulatory Diagnostic Group.

Administrative Code Sets Code sets that characterize a general business situation, rather than a medical condition or service. Under HIPAA, these are sometimes referred to as nonclinical or nonmedical code sets. Compare to medical code sets.

Administrative Services Only (ASO) An arrangement whereby a self-insured entity contracts with a Third-Party Administrator (TPA) to administer a health plan.

Administrative Simplification (A/S) Title II, Subtitle F of HIPAA, which gives HHS the authority to mandate the use of standards for the electronic exchange of healthcare data; to specify what medical and administrative code sets should be used within those standards; to require the use of national identification systems for healthcare patients, providers, payers (or plans), and employers (or sponsors); and to specify the types of measures required to protect the security and privacy of personally identifiable healthcare information. This is also the name of Title II, Subtitle F, Part C of HIPAA.

AFEHCT See the Association for Electronic Health Care Transactions.

AHA See the American Hospital Association.

AHIMA See the American Health Information Management Association.

AMA See the American Medical Association.

Ambulatory Payment Class (APC) A payment type for outpatient PPS claims.

Amendment See Amendments and Corrections.

Amendments and Corrections In the final privacy rule, an amendment to a record would indicate that the data is in dispute while retaining the original information, whereas a correction to a record would alter or replace the original record.

American Association for Homecare (AAHomecare) An industry association for the home care industry, including home IV therapy, home medical services and manufacturers, and home health providers. AAHomecare was created through the merger of the Health Industry Distributors Association's Home Care Division (HIDA Home Care), the Home Health Services and Staffing Association (HHSSA), and the National Association for Medical Equipment Services (NAMES).

American Dental Association (ADA) A professional organization for dentists. The ADA maintains a hardcopy dental claim form and the associated claim submission specifications, and also maintains the Current Dental Terminology (CDT) medical code set. The ADA and the Dental Content Committee (DeCC), which it hosts, have formal consultative roles under HIPAA.

American Health Information Management Association (AHIMA) An association of health information management professionals. AHIMA sponsors some HIPAA educational seminars.

American Hospital Association (AHA) A healthcare industry association that represents the concerns of institutional providers. The AHA hosts the NUBC, which has a formal consultative role under HIPAA.

American Medical Association (AMA) A professional organization for physicians. The AMA is the secretariat of the NUCC, which has a formal consultative role under HIPAA. The AMA also maintains the Current Procedural Terminology (CPT) medical code set.

American Medical Informatics Association (AMIA) A professional organization that promotes the development and use of medical informatics for patient care, teaching, research, and healthcare administration.

American National Standards (ANS) Standards developed and approved by organizations accredited by ANSI.

American National Standards Institute (ANSI) An organization that accredits various standards-setting committees, and monitors their compliance with the open rule-making process that they must follow to qualify for ANSI accreditation. HIPAA prescribes that the standards mandated under it be developed by ANSI-accredited bodies whenever practical.

American Society for Testing and Materials (ASTM) A standards group that has published general guidelines for the development of standards, including those for healthcare identifiers. ASTM Committee E31 on Healthcare Informatics develops standards on information used within healthcare.

AMIA See the American Medical Informatics Association.

ANS See American National Standards.

ANSI See the American National Standards Institute. Also see Part II, 45 CFR 160.103.

APC See Ambulatory Payment Class.

A/S, A.S., or AS See Administrative Simplification.

ASC See Accredited Standards Committee.

ASO See Administrative Services Only.

ASPIRE AFEHCT's Administrative Simplification Print Image Research Effort work group.

Association for Electronic Health Care Transactions (AFEHCT) An organization that promotes the use of EDI in the healthcare industry.

ASTM See the American Society for Testing and Materials.

Automated Clearinghouse (ACH) See Health Care Clearinghouse.

BA See Business Associate.

BBA The Balanced Budget Act of 1997.

BBRA The Balanced Budget Refinement Act of 1999.

BCBSA See Blue Cross and Blue Shield Association.

Biometric Identifier An identifier based on some physical characteristic, such as a fingerprint.

Blue Cross and Blue Shield Association (BCBSA) An association that represents the common interests of Blue Cross and Blue Shield health plans. The BCBSA serves as the administrator for the Health Care Code Maintenance Committee and also helps maintain the HCPCS Level II codes.

BP See Business Partner.

Business Associate (BA) A person or organization that performs a function or activity on behalf of a covered entity, but is not part of the covered entity's workforce. A business associate can also be a covered entity in its own right. Also see Part II, 45 CFR 160.103.

Business Model A model of a business organization or process.

Business Partner (BP) See Business Associate.

Business Relationships

(a) The term agent is often used to describe a person or organization that assumes some of the responsibilities of another one. This term has been avoided in the final rules so that a more HIPAA-specific meaning could be used for business associate. The term business partner (BP) was originally used for business associate.

(b) A Third-Party Administrator (TPA) is a business associate that performs claims administration and related business functions for a self-insured entity.

(c) Under HIPAA, a healthcare clearinghouse is a business associate that translates data to or from a standard format on behalf of a covered entity.

(d) The HIPAA Security NPRM used the term Chain of Trust Agreement to describe the type of contract that would be needed to extend the responsibility to protect healthcare data across a series of sub-contractual relationships.

(e) A business associate is an entity that performs certain business functions for you, and a trading partner is an external entity, such as a customer, with whom you do business. This relationship can be formalized via a trading partner agreement. It is quite possible to be a trading partner of an entity for some purposes, and a business associate of that entity for other purposes.

Cabulance A taxi cab that also functions as an ambulance.

CBO Congressional Budget Office or Cost Budget Office.

CDC See the Centers for Disease Control and Prevention.

CDT See Current Dental Terminology.

CE See Covered Entity.

CEFACT See United Nations Centre for Facilitation of Procedures and Practices for Administration, Commerce, and Transport (UN/CEFACT).

CEN European Center for Standardization, or Comité Européen de Normalisation.

Centers for Disease Control and Prevention (CDC) An organization that maintains several code sets included in the HIPAA standards, including the ICD-9-CM codes.

Center for Healthcare Information Management (CHIM) A health information technology industry association.

CFR or C.F.R. Code of Federal Regulations.

Chain of Trust (COT) A term used in the HIPAA Security NPRM for a pattern of agreements that extend protection of healthcare data by requiring that each covered entity that shares healthcare data with another entity require that that entity provide protections comparable to those provided by the covered entity, and that that entity, in turn, require that any other entities with which it shares the data satisfy the same requirements.

CHAMPUS Civilian Health and Medical Program of the Uniformed Services.

CHIM See the Center for Healthcare Information Management.

CHIME See the College of Healthcare Information Management Executives.

CHIP Child Health Insurance Program.

Claim Adjustment Reason Codes A national administrative code set that identifies the reasons for any differences, or adjustments, between the original provider charge for a claim or service and the payer's payment for it. This code set is used in the X12 835 Claim Payment & Remittance Advice and the X12 837 Claim transactions, and is maintained by the Health Care Code Maintenance Committee.

Claim Attachment Any of a variety of hardcopy forms or electronic records needed to process a claim in addition to the claim itself.

Claim Medicare Remark Codes See Medicare Remittance Advice Remark Codes.

Claim Status Codes A national administrative code set that identifies the status of healthcare claims. This code set is used in the X12 277 Claim Status Notification transaction, and is maintained by the Health Care Code Maintenance Committee.

Claim Status Category Codes A national administrative code set that indicates the general category of the status of healthcare claims. This code set is used in the X12 277 Claim Status Notification transaction, and is maintained by the Health Care Code Maintenance Committee.

Clearinghouse See Health Care Clearinghouse.

CLIA Clinical Laboratory Improvement Amendments.

Clinical Code Sets See Medical Code Sets.

CM See ICD.

COB See Coordination of Benefits.

Code Set Under HIPAA, this is any set of codes used to encode data elements, such as tables of terms, medical concepts, medical diagnostic codes, or medical procedure codes. This includes both the codes and their descriptions. Also see Part II, 45 CFR 162.103.

Code Set Maintaining Organization Under HIPAA, this is an organization that creates and maintains the code sets adopted by the secretary for use in the transactions for which standards are adopted. Also see Part II, 45 CFR 162.103.

College of Healthcare Information Management Executives (CHIME) A professional organization for healthcare Chief Information Officers (CIOs).

Comment Public commentary on the merits or appropriateness of proposed or potential regulations provided in response to an NPRM, an NOI, or other federal regulatory notice.

Common Control See Part II, 45 CFR 164.504.

Common Ownership See Part II, 45 CFR 164.504.

Compliance Date Under HIPAA, this is the date by which a covered entity must comply with a standard, an implementation specification, or a modification. This is usually 24 months after the effective data of the associated final rule for most entities, but 36 months after the effective data for small health plans. For future changes in the standards, the compliance date would be at least 180 days after the effective data, but can be longer for small health plans and for complex changes. Also see Part II, 45 CFR 160.103.

Computer-Based Patient Record Institute (CPRI)—Healthcare Open Systems and Trials (HOST) An industry organization that promotes the use of healthcare information systems, including electronic healthcare records.

Contrary See Part II, 45 CFR 160.202.

Coordination of Benefits (COB) A process for determining the respective responsibilities of two or more health plans that have some financial responsibility for a medical claim. Also called cross-over.

CORF Comprehensive Outpatient Rehabilitation Facility.

Correction See Amendments and Corrections.

Correctional Institution See Part II, 45 CFR 162.103.

COT See Chain of Trust.

Covered Entity (CE) Under HIPAA, this is a health plan, a healthcare clearinghouse, or a healthcare provider who transmits any health information in electronic form in connection with a HIPAA transaction. Also see Part II, 45 CFR 160.103.

Covered Function Functions that make an entity a health plan, a healthcare provider, or a healthcare clearinghouse. Also see Part II, 45 CFR 164.501.

CPRI-HOST See the Computer-Based Patient Record Institute—Healthcare Open Systems and Trials.

CPT See Current Procedural Terminology.

Cross-Over See Coordination of Benefits.

Cross-Walk See Data Mapping.

Current Dental Terminology (CDT) A medical code set, maintained and copyrighted by the ADA, that has been selected for use in the HIPAA transactions.

Current Procedural Terminology (CPT) A medical code set, maintained and copyrighted by the AMA, that has been selected for use under HIPAA for noninstitutional and nondental professional transactions.

Data Aggregation See Part II, 45 CFR 164.501.

Data Condition A description of the circumstances in which certain data is required. Also see Part II, 45 CFR 162.103.

Data Content Under HIPAA, this is all the data elements and code sets inherent in a transaction, and not related to the format of the transaction. Also see Part II, 45 CFR 162.103.

Data Content Committee (DCC) See Designated Data Content Committee.

Data Council A coordinating body within HHS that has high-level responsibility for overseeing the implementation of the A/S provisions of HIPAA.

Data Dictionary (DD) A document or system that characterizes the data content of a system.

Data Element Under HIPAA, this is the smallest named unit of information in a transaction. Also see Part II, 45 CFR 162.103.

Data Interchange Standards Association (DISA) A body that provides administrative services to X12 and several other standards-related groups.

Data Mapping The process of matching one set of data elements or individual code values to their closest equivalents in another set of them. This is sometimes called a cross-walk.

Data Model A conceptual model of the information needed to support a business function or process.

Data-Related Concepts

(a) Clinical or medical code sets identify medical conditions and the procedures, services, equipment, and supplies used to deal with them. Nonclinical, nonmedical, or administrative code sets identify or characterize entities and events in a manner that facilitates an administrative process. HIPAA defines a data element as the smallest unit of named information. In X12 language, that would be a simple data element. But X12 also has composite data elements, which aren't really data elements, but are groups of closely related data elements that can repeat as a group. X12 also has segments, which are also groups of related data elements that tend to occur together, such as street address, city, and state. These segments can sometimes repeat, or one or more segments may be part of a loop that can repeat. For example, you might have a claim loop that occurs once for each claim, and a claim service loop that occurs once for each service included in a claim. An X12 transaction is a collection of such loops, segments, etc. that supports a specific business process, whereas an X12 transmission is a communication session during which one or more X12 transactions is transmitted.

(b) Data elements and groups may also be combined into records that make up conventional files, or into the tables or segments used by database management systems, or DBMS. A designated code set is a code set that has been specified within the body of a rule. These are usually medical code sets. Many other code sets are incorporated into the rules by reference to a separate document, such as an implementation guide, that identifies one or more such code sets.

These are usually administrative code sets.

(c) Electronic data is data that is recorded or transmitted electronically, whereas nonelectronic data would be everything else. Special cases would be data transmitted by fax and audio systems, which is, in principle, transmitted electronically, but which lacks the underlying structure usually needed to support automated interpretation of its contents.

(d) Encoded data is data represented by some identification or classification scheme, such as a provider identifier or a procedure code. Nonencoded data would be more nearly freeform, such as a name, a street address, or a description. Theoretically, of course, all data, including grunts and smiles, is encoded.

(e) For HIPAA purposes, internal data, or internal code sets, are data elements that are fully specified within the HIPAA implementation guides. For X12 transactions, changes to the associated code values and descriptions must be approved via the normal standards development process, and can only be used in the revised version of the standards affected. X12 transactions also use many coding and identification schemes that are maintained by external organizations. For these external code sets, the associated values and descriptions can change at any time and still be usable in any version of the X12 transactions that uses the associated code set.

(f) Individually identifiable data is data that can be readily associated with a specific individual. Examples would be a name, a personal identifier, or a full street address. If life were simple, everything else would be nonidentifiable data. But even if you remove the obviously identifiable data from a record, other data elements present can also be used to re-identify it. For example, a birth date and a zip code might be sufficient to re-identify half the records in a file. The re-identifiability of data can be limited by omitting, aggregating, or altering such data to the extent that the risk of it being re-identified is acceptable.

(g) A specific form of data representation, such as an X12 transaction, will generally include some structural data that is needed to identify and interpret the transaction itself, as well as the business data content that the transaction is designed to transmit. Under HIPAA, when an alternate form of data collection such as a browser is used, such structural or format-related data elements can be ignored as long as the appropriate business data content is used.

(h) Structured data is data the meaning of which can be inferred to at least some extent based on its absolute or relative location in a separately defined data structure. This structure could be the blocks on a form, the fields in a record, the relative positions of data elements in an X12 segment, etc. Unstructured data, such as a memo or an image, would lack such clues.

Data Set See Part II, 45 CFR 162.103.

DCC See Data Content Committee.

D-Codes A subset of the HCPCS Level II medical code set with a high-order value of "D" that has been used to identify certain dental procedures. The final HIPAA transactions and code sets rule states that these D-codes will be dropped from the HCPCS, and that CDT codes will be used to identify all dental procedures.

DD See Data Dictionary.

DDE See Direct Data Entry.

DeCC See Dental Content Committee.

Dental Content Committee (DeCC) An organization hosted by the American Dental Association that maintains the data content specifications for dental billing. The Dental Content Committee has a formal consultative role under HIPAA for all transactions affecting dental healthcare services.

Descriptor The text defining a code in a code set. Also see Part II, 45 CFR 162.103.

Designated Code Set A medical code set or an administrative code set that HHS has designated for use in one or more of the HIPAA standards.

Designated Data Content Committee or Designated DCC An organization that HHS has designated for oversight of the business data content of one or more of the HIPAA-mandated transaction standards.

Designated Record Set See Part II, 45 CFR 164.501.

Designated Standard A standard that HHS has designated for use under the authority provided by HIPAA.

Designated Standard Maintenance Organization (DSMO) See Part II, 45 CFR 162.103.

DHHS See HHS.

DICOM See Digital Imaging and Communications in Medicine.

Digital Imaging and Communications in Medicine (DICOM) A standard for communicating images, such as x-rays, in a digitized form. This standard could become part of the HIPAA claim attachments standards.

Direct Data Entry (DDE) Under HIPAA, this is the direct entry of data that is immediately transmitted into a health plan's computer. Also see Part II, 45 CFR 162.103.

Direct Treatment Relationship See Part II, 45 CFR 164.501.

DISA See the Data Interchange Standards Association.

Disclosure Release or divulgence of information by an entity to persons or organizations outside of that entity. Also see Part II, 45 CFR 164.501.

Disclosure History Under HIPAA this is a list of any entities that have received personally identifiable healthcare information for uses unrelated to treatment and payment.

DME Durable Medical Equipment.

DMEPOS Durable Medical Equipment, Prosthetics, Orthotics, and Supplies.

DMERC See Medicare Durable Medical Equipment Regional Carrier.

Draft Standard for Trial Use (DSTU) An archaic term for any X12 standard that has been approved since the most recent release of X12 American National Standards. The current equivalent term is "X12 standard."

DRG Diagnosis Related Group.

DSMO See Designated Standard Maintenance Organization.

DSTU See Draft Standard for Trial Use.

EC See Electronic Commerce.

EDI See Electronic Data Interchange.

EDIFACT See United Nations Rules for Electronic Data Interchange for Administration, Commerce, and Transport (UN/EDIFACT).

EDI Translator A software tool for accepting an EDI transmission and converting the data into another format, or for converting a non-EDI data file into an EDI format for transmission.

Effective Date Under HIPAA, this is the date that a final rule is effective, which is usually 60 days after it is published in the *Federal Register*.

EFT See Electronic Funds Transfer.

EHNAC See the Electronic Healthcare Network Accreditation Commission.

EIN Employer Identification Number.

Electronic Commerce (EC) The exchange of business information by electronic means.

Electronic Data Interchange (EDI) This usually means X12 and similar variable-length formats for the electronic exchange of structured data. It is sometimes used more broadly to mean any electronic exchange of formatted data.

Electronic Healthcare Network Accreditation Commission (EHNAC) An organization that tests transactions for consistency with the HIPAA requirements, and that accredits healthcare clearinghouses.

Electronic Media See Part II, 45 CFR 162.103.

Electronic Media Claims (EMC) This term usually refers to a flat file format used to transmit or transport claims, such as the 192-byte UB-92 Institutional EMC format and the 320-byte Professional EMC NSF.

Electronic Remittance Advice (ERA) Any of several electronic formats for explaining the payments of healthcare claims.

EMC See Electronic Media Claims.

EMR Electronic Medical Record.

EOB Explanation of Benefits.

EOMB Explanation of Medicare Benefits, Explanation of Medicaid Benefits, or Explanation of Member Benefits.

EPSDT Early and Periodic Screening, Diagnosis, and Treatment.

ERA See Electronic Remittance Advice.

ERISA The Employee Retirement Income Security Act of 1974.

ESRD End-Stage Renal Disease.

FAQ(s) Frequently Asked Question(s).

FDA Food and Drug Administration.

FERPA Family Educational Rights and Privacy Act.

FFS Fee-for-Service.

FI See Medicare Part A Fiscal Intermediary.

Flat File This term usually refers to a file that consists of a series of fixed-length records that include some sort of record type code.

Format Under HIPAA, these are those data elements that provide or control the enveloping or hierarchical structure, or assist in identifying data content, of a transaction. Also see Part II, 45 CFR 162.103. Also see Data-Related Concepts.

FR or F.R. Federal Register.

GAO General Accounting Office.

GLBA The Gramm–Leach–Bliley Act.

Group Health Plan Under HIPAA this is an employee welfare benefit plan that provides for medical care and that either has 50 or more participants or is administered by another business entity. Also see Part II, 45 CFR 160.103.

HCFA See the Health Care Financing Administration. Also see Part II, 45 CFR 160.103.

HCFA-1450 HCFA's name for the institutional uniform claim form, or UB-92.

HCFA-1500 HCFA's name for the professional uniform claim form. Also known as the UCF-1500.

HCFA Common Procedural Coding System (HCPCS) A medical code set that identifies healthcare procedures, equipment, and supplies for claim submission purposes. It has been selected for use in the HIPAA transactions. HCPCS Level I contains numeric CPT codes that are maintained by the AMA. HCPCS Level II contains alphanumeric codes used to identify various items and services that are not included in the CPT medical code set. These are maintained by HCFA, the BCBSA, and the HIAA. HCPCS Level III contains alphanumeric codes that are assigned by Medicaid state agencies to identify additional items and services not included in levels I or II. These are usually called "local" codes, and must have "W," "X," "Y," or "Z" in the first position. HCPCS Procedure Modifier Codes can be used with all three levels, with the WA–ZY range used for locally assigned procedure modifiers.

HCPCS See HCFA Common Procedural Coding System. Also see Part II, 45 CFR 162.103.

Health and Human Services (HHS) The federal government department that has overall responsibility for implementing HIPAA.

Health Care See Part II, 45 CFR 160.103.

Health Care Clearinghouse Under HIPAA, this is an entity that processes or facilitates the processing of information received from another entity in a nonstandard format or containing nonstandard data content into standard data elements or a standard transaction, or that receives a standard transaction from another entity and processes or facilitates the processing of that information into nonstandard format or nonstandard data content for a receiving entity. Also see Part II, 45 CFR 160.103.

Health Care Code Maintenance Committee An organization administered by the BCBSA that is responsible for maintaining certain coding schemes used in the X12 transactions and elsewhere. These include the Claim Adjustment Reason Codes, the Claim Status Category Codes, and the Claim Status Codes.

Health Care Component See Part II, 45 CFR 164.504.

Healthcare Financial Management Association (HFMA) An organization for the improvement of the financial management of healthcare-related organizations. The HFMA sponsors some HIPAA educational seminars.

Health Care Financing Administration (HCFA) The HHS agency responsible for Medicare and parts of Medicaid. HCFA has historically maintained the UB-92 institutional EMC format specifications, the professional EMC NSF specifications, and specifications for various certifications and authorizations used by the Medicare and Medicaid programs. HCFA also maintains the HCPCS medical code set and the Medicare Remittance Advice Remark Codes administrative code set.

Healthcare Information Management Systems Society (HIMSS) A professional organization for healthcare information and management systems professionals.

Health Care Operations See Part II, 45 CFR 164.501.

Health Care Provider See Part II, 45 CFR 160.103.

Health Care Provider Taxonomy Committee An organization administered by the NUCC that is responsible for maintaining the Provider Taxonomy coding scheme used in the X12 transactions. The detailed code maintenance is done in coordination with X12N/TG2/WG15.

Health Industry Business Communications Council (HIBCC) A council of healthcare industry associations that has developed a number of technical standards used within the healthcare industry.

Health Informatics Standards Board (HISB) An ANSI-accredited standards group that has developed an inventory of candidate standards for consideration as possible HIPAA standards.

Health Information See Part II, 45 CFR 160.103.

Health Insurance Association of America (HIAA) An industry association that represents the interests of commercial healthcare insurers. The HIAA participates in the maintenance of some code sets, including the HCPCS Level II codes.

Health Insurance Issuer See Part II, 45 CFR 160.103.

Health Insurance Portability and Accountability Act of 1996 (HIPAA) A federal law that allows persons to qualify immediately for comparable health insurance coverage when they change their employment relationships. Title II, Subtitle F, of HIPAA gives HHS the authority to mandate the use of standards for the electronic exchange of healthcare data; to specify what medical and administrative code sets should be used within those standards; to require the use of national identification systems for healthcare patients, providers, payers (or plans), and employers (or sponsors); and to specify the types of measures required to protect the security and privacy of personally identifiable healthcare information. Also known as the Kennedy–Kassebaum Bill, the Kassebaum–Kennedy Bill, K2, or Public Law 104-191.

Health Level Seven (HL7) An ANSI-accredited group that defines standards for the cross-platform exchange of information within a healthcare organization. HL7 is responsible for specifying the Level Seven OSI standards for the health industry. The X12 275 transaction will probably incorporate the HL7 CRU message to transmit claim attachments as part of a future HIPAA claim attachments standard. The HL7 Attachment SIG is responsible for the HL7 portion of this standard.

Health Maintenance Organization (HMO) See Part II, 45 CFR 160.103.

Health Oversight Agency See Part II, 45 CFR 164.501.

Health Plan See Part II, 45 CFR 160.103.

Health Plan ID See National Payer ID.

HEDIC The Healthcare EDI Coalition.

HEDIS Health Employer Data and Information Set.

HFMA See the Healthcare Financial Management Association.

HHA Home Health Agency.

HHIC The Hawaii Health Information Corporation.

HHS See Health and Human Services. Also see Part II, 45 CFR 160.103.

HIAA See the Health Insurance Association of America.

HIBCC See the Health Industry Business Communications Council.

HIMSS See the Healthcare Information Management Systems Society.

HIPAA See the Health Insurance Portability and Accountability Act of 1996.

HIPAA Data Dictionary or HIPAA DD A data dictionary that defines and cross-references the contents of all X12 transactions included in the HIPAA mandate. It is maintained by X12N/TG3.

HISB See the Health Informatics Standards Board.

HL7 See Health Level Seven.

HMO See Health Maintenance Organization.

HPAG The HIPAA Policy Advisory Group, a BCBSA subgroup.

HPSA Health Professional Shortage Area.

Hybrid Entity A covered entity whose covered functions are not its primary functions. Also see Part II, 45 CFR 164.504.

IAIABC See the International Association of Industrial Accident Boards and Commissions.

ICD & ICD-n-CM & ICD-n-PCS International Classification of Diseases, with "n" = "9" for Revision 9 or "10" for Revision 10, with "CM" = "Clinical Modification," and with "PCS" = "Procedure Coding System."

ICF Intermediate Care Facility.

IDN Integrated Delivery Network.

IG See Implementation Guide.

IHC Internet Healthcare Coalition.

IIHI See Individually Identifiable Health Information

Implementation Guide (IG) A document that explains the proper use of a standard for a specific business purpose. The X12N HIPAA IGs are the primary reference documents used by those implementing the associated transactions, and are incorporated into the HIPAA regulations by reference.

Implementation Specification Under HIPAA, this is the specific instruction for implementing a standard. Also see Part II, 45 CFR 160.103. See also Implementation Guide.

Indirect Treatment Relationship See Part II, 45 CFR 164.501.

Individual See Part II, 45 CFR 164.501.

Individually Identifiable Health Information (IIHI) See Part II, 45 CFR 164.501.

Information Model A conceptual model of the information needed to support a business function or process.

Inmate See Part II, 45 CFR 164.501.

International Association of Industrial Accident Boards and Commissions (IAIABC) One of their standards is under consideration for use for the First Report of Injury standard under HIPAA.

International Classification of Diseases (ICD) A medical code set maintained by the World Health Organization (WHO). The primary purpose of this code set was to classify causes of death. A U.S.

extension, maintained by the NCHS within the CDC, identifies morbidity factors, or diagnoses. The ICD-9-CM codes have been selected for use in the HIPAA transactions.

International Organization for Standardization (ISO) An organization that coordinates the development and adoption of numerous international standards. "ISO" is not an acronym, but the Greek word for "equal."

International Standards Organization See International Organization for Standardization (ISO).

IOM The Institute of Medicine.

IPA Independent Providers Association.

IRB Institutional Review Board.

ISO See the International Organization for Standardization.

JCAHO See the Joint Commission on Accreditation of Healthcare Organizations.

J-Codes A subset of the HCPCS Level II code set with a high-order value of "J" that has been used to identify certain drugs and other items. The final HIPAA transactions and code sets rule states that these J-codes will be dropped from the HCPCS, and that NDC codes will be used to identify the associated pharmaceuticals and supplies.

JHITA See the Joint Healthcare Information Technology Alliance.

Joint Commission on Accreditation of Healthcare Organizations (JCAHO) An organization that accredits healthcare organizations. In the future, the JCAHO may play a role in certifying these organizations' compliance with the HIPAA A/S requirements.

Joint Healthcare Information Technology Alliance (JHITA) A healthcare industry association that represents AHIMA, AMIA, CHIM, CHIME, and HIMSS on legislative and regulatory issues affecting the use of health information technology.

Law Enforcement Official See Part II, 45 CFR 164.501.

Local Code(s) A generic term for code values that are defined for a state or other political subdivision, or for a specific payer. This term is most commonly used to describe HCPCS Level III Codes, but also applies to state-assigned Institutional Revenue Codes, Condition Codes, Occurrence Codes, Value Codes, etc.

Logical Observation Identifiers, Names and Codes (LOINC) A set of universal names and ID codes that identify laboratory and clinical observations. These codes, which are maintained by the Regenstrief Institute, are expected to be used in the HIPAA claim attachments standard.

LOINC See Logical Observation Identifiers, Names and Codes.

Loop A repeating structure or process.

LTC Long-Term Care.

Maintain or Maintenance See Part II, 45 CFR 162.103.

Marketing See Part II, 45 CFR 164.501.

Massachusetts Health Data Consortium (MHDC) An organization that seeks to improve healthcare in New England through improved policy development, better technology planning and implementation, and more informed financial decision making.

Maximum Defined Data Set Under HIPAA, this is all of the required data elements for a particular standard based on a specific implementation specification. An entity creating a transaction is free to include whatever data any receiver might want or need. The recipient is free to ignore any portion of the data that is not needed to conduct their part of the associated business transaction, unless the inessential data is needed for coordination of benefits. Also see Part II, 45 CFR 162.103.

MCO Managed Care Organization.

M+CO Medicare Plus Choice Organization.

Medicaid Fiscal Agent (FA) The organization responsible for administering claims for a state Medicaid program.

Medicaid State Agency The state agency responsible for overseeing the state's Medicaid program.

Medical Code Sets Codes that characterize a medical condition or treatment. These code sets are usually maintained by professional societies and public health organizations. Compare to administrative code sets.

Medical Records Institute (MRI) An organization that promotes the development and acceptance of electronic healthcare record systems.

Medicare Contractor A Medicare Part A Fiscal Intermediary, a Medicare Part B Carrier, or a Medicare Durable Medical Equipment Regional Carrier (DMERC).

Medicare Durable Medical Equipment Regional Carrier (DMERC) A Medicare contractor responsible for administering Durable Medical Equipment (DME) benefits for a region.

Medicare Part A Fiscal Intermediary (FI) A Medicare contractor that administers the Medicare Part A (institutional) benefits for a given region.

Medicare Part B Carrier A Medicare contractor that administers the Medicare Part B (Professional) benefits for a given region.

Medicare Remittance Advice Remark Codes A national administrative code set for providing either claim-level or service-level Medicare-related messages that cannot be expressed with a Claim Adjustment Reason Code. This code set is used in the X12 835 Claim Payment & Remittance Advice transaction, and is maintained by the HCFA.

Memorandum of Understanding (MOU) A document that provides a general description of the responsibilities that are to be assumed by two or more parties in their pursuit of some goal(s). More specific information may be provided in an associated SOW.

MGMA Medical Group Management Association.

MHDC See the Massachusetts Health Data Consortium.

MHDI See the Minnesota Health Data Institute.

Minimum Scope of Disclosure The principle that, to the extent practical, individually identifiable health information should only be disclosed to the extent needed to support the purpose of the disclosure.

Minnesota Health Data Institute (MHDI) A public–private partnership for improving the quality and efficiency of healthcare in Minnesota. MHDI includes the Minnesota Center for Healthcare Electronic Commerce (MCHEC), which supports the adoption of standards for electronic commerce and also supports the Minnesota EDI Healthcare Users Group (MEHUG).

Modify or Modification Under HIPAA, this is a change adopted by the secretary, through regulation, to a standard or an implementation specification. Also see Part II, 45 CFR 160.103.

More Stringent See Part II, 45 CFR 160.202.

MOU See Memorandum of Understanding.

MR Medical Review.

MRI See the Medical Records Institute.

MSP Medicare Secondary Payer.

NAHDO See the National Association of Health Data Organizations.

NAIC See the National Association of Insurance Commissioners.

NANDA North American Nursing Diagnoses Association.

NASMD See the National Association of State Medicaid Directors.

National Association of Health Data Organizations (NAHDO) A group that promotes the development and improvement of state and national health information systems.

National Association of Insurance Commissioners (NAIC) An association of the insurance commissioners of the states and territories.

National Association of State Medicaid Directors (NASMD) An association of state Medicaid directors. NASMD is affiliated with the American Public Health Human Services Association (APHSA).

National Center for Health Statistics (NCHS) A federal organization within the CDC that collects, analyzes, and distributes healthcare statistics. The NCHS maintains the ICD-n-CM codes.

National Committee for Quality Assurance (NCQA) An organization that accredits managed care plans, or Health Maintenance Organizations (HMOs). In the future, the NCQA may play a role in certifying these organizations' compliance with the HIPAA A/S requirements. The NCQA also maintains the Health Employer Data and Information Set (HEDIS).

National Committee on Vital and Health Statistics (NCVHS) A federal advisory body within HHS that advises the secretary regarding potential changes to the HIPAA standards.

National Council for Prescription Drug Programs (NCPDP) An ANSI-accredited group that maintains a number of standard formats for use by the retail pharmacy industry, some of which are included in the HIPAA mandates. Also see NCPDP . . . Standard.

National Drug Code (NDC) A medical code set that identifies prescription drugs and some over-the-counter products, and that has been selected for use in the HIPAA transactions.

National Employer ID A system for uniquely identifying all sponsors of healthcare benefits.

National Health Information Infrastructure (NHII) This is a health-care-specific lane on the information superhighway, as described in the National Information Infrastructure (NII) initiative. Conceptually, this includes the HIPAA A/S initiatives.

National Patient ID A system for uniquely identifying all recipients of healthcare services. This is sometimes referred to as the National Individual Identifier (NII), or as the Healthcare ID.

National Payer ID A system for uniquely identifying all organizations that pay for healthcare services. Also known as Health Plan ID or Plan ID.

National Provider ID (NPI) A system for uniquely identifying all providers of healthcare services, supplies, and equipment.

National Provider File (NPF) The database envisioned for use in maintaining a national provider registry.

National Provider Registry The organization envisioned for assigning National Provider IDs.

National Provider System (NPS) The administrative system envisioned for supporting a national provider registry.

National Standard Format (NSF) Generically, this applies to any nationally standardized data format, but it is often used in a more limited way to designate the Professional EMC NSF, a 320-byte flat file record format used to submit professional claims.

National Uniform Billing Committee (NUBC) An organization, chaired and hosted by the American Hospital Association, that maintains the UB-92 hardcopy institutional billing form and the data element specifications for both the hardcopy form and the 192-byte UB-92 flat file EMC format. The NUBC has a formal consultative role under HIPAA for all transactions affecting institutional healthcare services.

National Uniform Claim Committee (NUCC) An organization, chaired and hosted by the American Medical Association, that maintains the HCFA-1500 claim form and a set of data element specifications for professional claims submission via the HCFA-1500 claim form, the Professional EMC NSF, and the X12 837. The NUCC also maintains the Provider Taxonomy Codes and has a formal consultative role under HIPAA for all transactions affecting nondental noninstitutional professional healthcare services.

NCHICA See the North Carolina Healthcare Information and Communications Alliance.

NCHS See the National Center for Health Statistics.

NCPDP See the National Council for Prescription Drug Programs.

NCPDP Batch Standard An NCPDP standard designed for use by low-volume dispensers of pharmaceuticals, such as nursing homes. Use of Version 1.0 of this standard has been mandated under HIPAA.

NCPDP Telecommunication Standard An NCPDP standard designed for use by high-volume dispensers of pharmaceuticals, such as retail pharmacies. Use of Version 5.1 of this standard has been mandated under HIPAA.

NCQA See the National Committee for Quality Assurance.

NCVHS See the National Committee on Vital and Health Statistics.

NDC See National Drug Code.

NHII See National Health Information Infrastructure.

NOC Not Otherwise Classified or Nursing Outcomes Classification.

NOI See Notice of Intent.

Nonclinical or Nonmedical Code Sets See Administrative Code Sets.

North Carolina Healthcare Information and Communications Alliance (NCHICA) An organization that promotes the advancement and integration of information technology into the healthcare industry.

Notice of Intent (NOI) A document that describes a subject area for which the federal government is considering developing regulations. It may describe the presumably relevant considerations and invite comments from interested parties. These comments can then be used in developing an NPRM or a final regulation.

Notice of Proposed Rulemaking (NPRM) A document that describes and explains regulations that the federal government proposes to adopt at some future date, and invites interested parties to submit comments related to them. These comments can then be used in developing a final regulation.

NPF See National Provider File.

NPI See National Provider ID.

NPRM See Notice of Proposed Rulemaking.

NPS See National Provider System.

NSF See National Standard Format.

NUBC See the National Uniform Billing Committee.

NUBC EDI TAG The NUBC EDI Technical Advisory Group, which coordinates issues affecting both the NUBC and the X12 standards.

NUCC See the National Uniform Claim Committee.

OCR See the Office for Civil Rights.

Office for Civil Rights The HHS entity responsible for enforcing the HIPAA privacy rules.

Office of Management and Budget (OMB) A federal government agency that has a major role in reviewing proposed federal regulations.

OIG Office of the Inspector General.

OMB See the Office of Management and Budget.

Open System Interconnection (OSI) A multilayer ISO data communications standard. Level Seven of this standard is industry-specific, and HL7 is responsible for specifying the level seven OSI standards for the health industry.

Organized Health Care Arrangement See Part II, 45 CFR 164.501.

OSI See Open System Interconnection.

PAG See Policy Advisory Group.

Payer In healthcare, an entity that assumes the risk of paying for medical treatments. This can be an uninsured patient, a self-insured employer, a health plan, or an HMO.

PAYERID HCFA's term for their pre-HIPAA National Payer ID initiative.

Payment See Part II, 45 CFR 164.501.

PCS See ICD.

PHB Pharmacy Benefits Manager.

PHI See Protected Health Information.

PHS Public Health Service.

PL or P. L. Public Law, as in PL 104-191 (HIPAA).

Plan Administration Functions See Part II, 45 CFR 164.504.

Plan ID See National Payer ID.

Plan Sponsor An entity that sponsors a health plan. This can be an employer, a union, or some other entity. Also see Part II, 45 CFR 164.501.

Policy Advisory Group (PAG) A generic name for many work groups at WEDI and elsewhere.

POS Place of Service or Point of Service.

PPO Preferred Provider Organization

PPS Prospective Payment System.

PRA The Paperwork Reduction Act.

PRG Procedure-Related Group.

Pricer or Repricer A person, an organization, or a software package that reviews procedures, diagnoses, fee schedules, and other data and determines the eligible amount for a given healthcare service or supply. Additional criteria can then be applied to determine the actual allowance, or payment, amount.

PRO Professional Review Organization or Peer Review Organization.

Protected Health Information (PHI) See Part II, 45 CFR 164.501.

Provider Taxonomy Codes An administrative code set for identifying the provider type and area of specialization for all healthcare providers. A given provider can have several Provider Taxonomy Codes. This code set is used in the X12 278 Referral Certification and Authorization and the X12 837 Claim transactions, and is maintained by the NUCC.

Psychotherapy Notes See Part II, 45 CFR 164.501.

Public Health Authority See Part II, 45 CFR 164.501.

RA Remittance Advice.

Regenstrief Institute A research foundation for improving healthcare by optimizing the capture, analysis, content, and delivery of healthcare information. Regenstrief maintains the LOINC coding system that is being considered for use as part of the HIPAA claim attachments standard.

Relates to the Privacy of Individually Identifiable Health Information See Part II, 45 CFR 160.202.

Required by Law See Part II, 45 CFR 164.501.

Research See Part II, 45 CFR 164.501.

RFA The Regulatory Flexibility Act.

RVS Relative Value Scale.

SC Subcommittee.

SCHIP The State Children's Health Insurance Program.

SDO Standards Development Organization.

Secretary Under HIPAA, this refers to the secretary of HHS or his or her designated representatives. Also see Part II, 45 CFR 160.103.

Segment Under HIPAA, this is a group of related data elements in a transaction. Also see Part II, 45 CFR162.103.

Self-Insured An individual or organization that assumes the financial risk of paying for healthcare.

Small Health Plan Under HIPAA, this is a health plan with annual receipts of $5 million or less. Also see Part II, 45 CFR 160.103.

SNF Skilled Nursing Facility.

SNOMED Systematized Nomenclature of Medicine.

SNIP See Strategic National Implementation Process.

Sponsor See Plan Sponsor.

SOW See Statement of Work.

SSN Social Security Number.

SSO See Standard-Setting Organization.

Standard See Part II, 45 CFR 160.103.

Standard-Setting Organization (SSO) See Part II, 45 CFR 160.103.

Standard Transaction Under HIPAA, this is a transaction that complies with the applicable HIPAA standard. Also see Part II, 45 CFR 162.103.

Standard Transaction Format Compliance System (STFCS) An EHNAC-sponsored WPC-hosted HIPAA compliance certification service.

State See Part II, 45 CFR 160.103.

State Law A constitution, statue, regulation, rule, common law, or any other state action having the force and effect of law. Also see Part II, 45 CFR 160.202.

State Uniform Billing Committee (SUBC) A state-specific affiliate of the NUBC.

Statement of Work (SOW) A document describing the specific tasks and methodologies that will be followed to satisfy the requirements of an associated contract or MOU.

STFCS See the Standard Transaction Format Compliance System.

Strategic National Implementation Process (SNIP) A WEDI program for helping the healthcare industry identify and resolve HIPAA implementation issues.

Structured Data See Data-Related Concepts.

SUBC See State Uniform Billing Committee.

Summary Health Information See Part II, 45 CFR 164.504.

SWG Sub-workgroup.

Syntax The rules and conventions that one needs to know or follow in order to validly record information, or interpret previously recorded information, for a specific purpose. Thus, a syntax is a grammar. Such rules and conventions may be either explicit or implicit. In X12 transactions, the data-element separators, the sub-element separators, the segment terminators, the segment identifiers, the loops, the loop identifiers (when present), the repetition factors, and so on, are all aspects of the X12 syntax. When explicit, such syntactical elements tend to be the structural, or format-related, data elements that are not required when a direct data entry architecture is used. Ultimately, however, there is not a perfectly clear division between the syntactical elements and the business data content.

TAG Technical Advisory Group.

TG Task Group.

Third-Party Administrator (TPA) An entity that processes healthcare claims and performs related business functions for a health plan.

TPA See Third-Party Administrator or Trading Partner Agreement.

Trading Partner Agreement (TPA) See Part II, 45 CFR 160.103.

Transaction Under HIPAA, this is the exchange of information between two parties to carry out financial or administrative activities related to healthcare. Also see Part II, 45 CFR 160.103.

Transaction Change Request System A system established under HIPAA for accepting and tracking change requests for any of the HIPAA mandated transactions standards via a single Web site. See www.hipaa-dsmo.org.

Translator See EDI Translator.

Treatment See Part II, 45 CFR 164.501.

UB Uniform Bill, as in UB-82 or UB-92.

UB-82 A uniform institutional claim form developed by the NUBC that was in general use from 1983 to 1993.

UB-92 A uniform institutional claim form developed by the NUBC that has been in general use since 1993.

UCF Uniform Claim Form, as in UCF-1500.

UCTF See the Uniform Claim Task Force.

UHIN See the Utah Health Information Network.

UN/CEFACT See the United Nations Centre for Facilitation of Procedures and Practices for Administration, Commerce, and Transport.

UN/EDIFACT See the United Nations Rules for Electronic Data Interchange for Administration, Commerce, and Transport.

Uniform Claim Task Force (UCTF) An organization that developed the initial HCFA-1500 Professional Claim Form. The maintenance responsibilities were later assumed by the NUCC.

United Nations Centre for Facilitation of Procedures and Practices for Administration, Commerce, and Transport (UN/CEFACT) An international organization dedicated to the elimination or simplification of procedural barriers to international commerce.

United Nations Rules for Electronic Data Interchange for Administration, Commerce, and Transport (UN/EDIFACT) An international EDI format. Interactive X12 transactions use the EDIFACT message syntax.

UNSM United Nations Standard Messages.

Unstructured Data See Data-Related Concepts.

UPIN Unique Physician Identification Number.

UR Utilization Review.

USC or U.S.C United States Code.

Use See Part II, 45 CFR 164.501.

Utah Health Information Network (UHIN) A public-private coalition for reducing healthcare administrative costs through the standardization and electronic exchange of healthcare data.

Value-Added Network (VAN) A vendor of EDI data communications and translation services.

Virtual Private Network (VPN) A technical strategy for creating secure connections, or tunnels, over the Internet.

VPN See Virtual Private Network.

Washington Publishing Company (WPC) The company that publishes the X12N HIPAA Implementation guides and the X12N HIPAA Data Dictionary, developed the X12 Data Dictionary, and hosts the EHNAC STFCS testing program.

WEDI See the Workgroup for Electronic Data Interchange.

WG Work Group.

WHO See the World Health Organization.

Workforce Under HIPAA, this means employees, volunteers, trainees, and other persons under the direct control of a covered entity, whether or not they are paid by the covered entity. Also see Part II, 45 CFR 160.103.

Workgroup for Electronic Data Interchange (WEDI) A healthcare industry group that lobbied for HIPAA A/S, and that has a formal consultative role under the HIPAA legislation. WEDI also sponsors SNIP.

World Health Organization (WHO) An organization that maintains the International Classification of Diseases (ICD) medical code set.

WPC See the Washington Publishing Company.

X12 An ANSI-accredited group that defines EDI standards for many American industries, including healthcare insurance. Most of the electronic transaction standards mandated or proposed under HIPAA are X12 standards.

X12/PRB The X12 Procedures Review Board.

X12 Standard The term currently used for any X12 standard that has been approved since the most recent release of X12 American National Standards. Because a full set of X12 American National Standards is only released about once every five years, it is the X12 standards that are most likely to be in active use. These standards were previously called Draft Standards for Trial Use.

XML Extensible Markup Language.

PART II: CONSOLIDATED HIPAA ADMINISTRATIVE SIMPLIFICATION FINAL RULE DEFINITIONS

45 CFR 160.103 Definitions [from the Final Privacy Rule]

Except as otherwise provided, the following definitions apply to this subchapter:

- *Act* means the Social Security Act.
- *ANSI* stands for the American National Standards Institute.

Business associate:

(1) Except as provided in paragraph (2) of this definition, *business associate* means, with respect to a covered entity, a person who: (i) On behalf of such covered entity or of an organized healthcare arrangement (as defined in § 164.501 of this subchapter) in which the covered entity participates, but other than in the capacity of a member of the workforce of such covered entity or arrangement, performs, or assists in the performance of:

    (A)   A function or activity involving the use or disclosure of individually identifiable health information, including claims processing or administration, data analysis, processing or administration, utilization review, quality assurance, billing, benefit management, practice management, and repricing; or

    (B)   Any other function or activity regulated by this subchapter; or (ii) Provides, other than in the capacity of a member of the workforce of such covered entity, legal, actuarial, accounting, consulting, data aggregation (as defined in § 164.501 of this subchapter), management, administrative, accreditation, or financial services to or for such covered entity, or to or for an organized healthcare arrangement in which the covered entity participates, where the provision of the service involves the disclosure of individually identifiable health information from such covered entity or arrangement, or from another business associate of such covered entity or arrangement, to the person.

(2) A covered entity participating in an organized healthcare arrangement that performs a function or activity as described by paragraph (1)(i) of this definition for or on behalf of such organized healthcare arrangement, or that provides a service as described in paragraph (1)(ii) of this definition to or for such organized healthcare arrangement, does not, simply through the performance of such function

or activity or the provision of such service, become a business associate of other covered entities participating in such organized healthcare arrangement.

(3) A covered entity may be a business associate of another covered entity.

Compliance date means the date by which a covered entity must comply with a standard, *implementation specification*, requirement, or *modification* adopted under this subchapter.

Covered entity means:

(1) A health plan.
(2) A health care clearinghouse.
(3) A health care provider who transmits any health information in electronic form n connection with a transaction covered by this subchapter.

Group health plan (also see definition of *health plan* in this section) means an employee welfare benefit plan (as defined in section 3(1) of the Employee Retirement Income and Security Act of 1974 (ERISA), 29 U.S.C. 1002(1)), including insured and self-insured plans, to the extent that the plan provides medical care (as defined in section 2791(a)(2) of the Public Health Service Act (PHS Act), 42 U.S.C. 300gg-91(a)(2)), including items and services paid for as medical care, to employees or their dependents directly or through insurance, reimbursement, or otherwise, that:

(1) Has 50 or more participants (as defined in section 3(7) of ERISA, 29 U.S.C. 1002(7)); or
(2) Is administered by an entity other than the employer that established and maintains the plan.

HCFA stands for Health Care Financing Administration within the Department of Health and Human Services.

HHS stands for the Department of Health and Human Services. *Health care* means care, services, or supplies related to the health of an individual. *Health care* includes, but is not limited to, the following:

(1) Preventive, diagnostic, therapeutic, rehabilitative, maintenance, or palliative care, and counseling, service, assessment, or procedure with respect to the physical or mental condition, or functional status, of an individual or that affects the structure or function of the body; and

(2) Sale or dispensing of a drug, device, equipment, or other item in accordance with a prescription.

Health care clearinghouse means a public or private entity, including a billing service, repricing company, community health management information system or community health information system, and "value-added" networks and switches, that does either of the following functions:

(1) Processes or facilitates the processing of health information received from another entity in a nonstandard format or containing nonstandard data content into standard data elements or a standard transaction.

(2) Receives a standard transaction from another entity and processes or facilitates the processing of health information into nonstandard format or nonstandard data content for the receiving entity.

Health care provider means a provider of services (as defined in section 1861(u) of the Act, 42 U.S.C. 1395x(u)), a provider of medical or health services (as defined in section 1861(s) of the Act, 42 U.S.C. 1395x(s)), and any other person or organization who furnishes, bills, or is paid for health care in the normal course of business.

Health information means any information, whether oral or recorded in any form or medium, that:

(1) Is created or received by a health care provider, health plan, public health authority, employer, life insurer, school or university, or health care clearinghouse; and

(2) Relates to the past, present, or future physical or mental health or condition of an individual; the provision of health care to an individual; or the past, present, or future payment for the provision of health care to an individual.

Health insurance issuer (as defined in section 2791(b)(2) of the PHS Act, 42 U.S.C. 300gg-91(b)(2) and used in the definition of health plan in this section) means an insurance company, insurance service, or insurance organization (including an HMO) that is licensed to engage in the business of insurance in a State and is subject to State law that regulates insurance. Such term does not include a group health plan.

Health maintenance organization (HMO) (as defined in section 2791(b)(3) of the PHS Act, 42 U.S.C. 300gg-91(b)(3) and used in the definition of *health plan* in this section) means a federally qualified HMO, an organization recognized as an HMO under State law, or a similar organization regulated for solvency under State law in the same manner and to the same extent as such an HMO.

Health plan means an individual or group plan that provides, or pays the cost of, medical care (as defined in section 2791(a)(2) of the PHS Act, 42 U.S.C. 300gg-91(a)(2)).

(1) *Health plan* includes the following, singly or in combination:
  (i) A group health plan, as defined in this section.
  (ii) A health insurance issuer, as defined in this section.
  (iii) An HMO, as defined in this section.
  (iv) Part A or Part B of the Medicare program under title XVIII of the Act.
  (v) The Medicaid program under title XIX of the Act, 42 U.S.C. 1396, et seq.
  (vi) An issuer of a Medicare supplemental policy (as defined in section 1882(g)(1) of the Act, 42 U.S.C. 1395ss(g)(1)).
  (vii) An issuer of a long-term care policy, excluding a nursing home fixed-indemnity policy.
  (viii) An employee welfare benefit plan or any other arrangement that is established or maintained for the purpose of offering or providing health benefits to the employees of two or more employers.
  (ix) The health care program for active military personnel under title 10 of the United States Code.
  (x) The veterans health care program under 38 U.S.C. chapter 17.
  (xi) The Civilian Health and Medical Program of the Uniformed Services (CHAMPUS) (as defined in 10 U.S.C. 1072(4)).
  (xii) The Indian Health Service program under the Indian Health Care Improvement Act, 25 U.S.C. 1601, et seq.
  (xiii) The Federal Employees Health Benefits Program under 5 U.S.C. 8902, et seq.
  (xiv) An approved State child health plan under title XXI of the Act, providing benefits for child health assistance that meet the requirements of section 2103 of the Act, 42 U.S.C. 1397, et seq.
  (xv) The Medicare+Choice program under Part C of title XVIII of the Act, 42 U.S.C. 1395w-21 through 1395w-28.
  (xvi) A high risk pool that is a mechanism established under State law to provide health insurance coverage or comparable coverage to eligible individuals.
  (xvii) Any other individual or group plan, or combination of individual or group plans, that provides or pays for the cost of medical care (as defined in section 2791(a)(2) of the PHS Act, 42 U.S.C. 300gg-91(a)(2)).

(2) *Health plan* excludes:
  (i) Any policy, plan, or program to the extent that it provides, or pays for the cost of, excepted benefits that are listed in section 2791(c)(1) of the PHS Act, 42 U.S.C. 300gg-91(c)(1); and
  (ii) A government-funded program (other than one listed in paragraph (1)(i)-(xvi) of this definition):
    (A) Whose principal purpose is other than providing, or paying the cost of, health care; or
    (B) Whose principal activity is:
      (1) The direct provision of health care to persons; or
      (2) The making of grants to fund the direct provision of health care to persons.

Implementation specification means specific requirements or instructions for implementing a standard.

Modify or *modification* refers to a change adopted by the Secretary, through regulation, to a standard or an implementation specification.

Secretary means the Secretary of Health and Human Services or any other officer or employee of HHS to whom the authority involved has been delegated.

Small health plan means a health plan with annual receipts of $5 million or less.

Standard means a rule, condition, or requirement:

(1) Describing the following information for products, systems, services or practices:
  (i) Classification of components.
  (ii) Specification of materials, performance, or operations; or
  (iii) Delineation of procedures; or
(2) With respect to the privacy of individually identifiable health information.

Standard setting organization (SSO) means an organization accredited by the American National Standards Institute that develops and maintains standards for information transactions or data elements, or any other standard that is necessary for, or will facilitate the implementation of, this part.

State refers to one of the following:

(1) For a health plan established or regulated by Federal law, State has the meaning set forth in the applicable section of the United States Code for such health plan.

(2) For all other purposes, State means any of the several States, the District of Columbia, the Commonwealth of Puerto Rico, the Virgin Islands, and Guam.

Trading partner agreement means an agreement related to the exchange of information in electronic transactions, whether the agreement is distinct or part of a larger agreement, between each party to the agreement. (For example, a trading partner agreement may specify, among other things, the duties and responsibilities of each party to the agreement in conducting a standard transaction.)

Transaction means the transmission of information between two parties to carry out financial or administrative activities related to health care. It includes the following types of information transmissions:

(1) Health care claims or equivalent encounter information.
(2) Health care payment and remittance advice.
(3) Coordination of benefits.
(4) Health care claim status.
(5) Enrollment and dis-enrollment in a health plan.
(6) Eligibility for a health plan.
(7) Health plan premium payments.
(8) Referral certification and authorization.
(9) First report of injury.
(10) Health claims attachments.
(11) Other transactions that the Secretary may prescribe by regulation.

Workforce means employees, volunteers, trainees, and other persons whose conduct, in the performance of work for a covered entity, is under the direct control of such entity, whether or not they are paid by the covered entity.

45 CFR 160.202 Definitions [from the Final Privacy Rule]

For purposes of this subpart, the following terms have the following meanings:

Contrary, when used to compare a provision of State law to a standard, requirement, or implementation specification adopted under this subchapter, means:

(1) A covered entity would find it impossible to comply with both the State and federal requirements; or
(2) The provision of State law stands as an obstacle to the accomplishment and execution of the full purposes and objectives of part C of title XI of the Act or section 264 of Pub. L. 104-191, as applicable.

More stringent means, in the context of a comparison of a provision of State law and a standard, requirement, or implementation specification adopted under subpart E of part 164 of this subchapter, a State law that meets one or more of the following criteria:

(1) With respect to a use or disclosure, the law prohibits or restricts a use or disclosure in circumstances under which such use or disclosure otherwise would be permitted under this subchapter, except if the disclosure is:
   (i) Required by the Secretary in connection with determining whether a covered entity is in compliance with this subchapter; or
   (ii) To the individual who is the subject of the individually identifiable health information.

(2) With respect to the rights of an individual who is the subject of the individually identifiable health information of access to or amendment of individually identifiable health information, permits greater rights of access or amendment, as applicable; provided that, nothing in this subchapter may be construed to preempt any State law to the extent that it authorizes or prohibits disclosure of protected health information about a minor to a parent, guardian, or person acting in *loco parentis* of such minor.

(3) With respect to information to be provided to an individual who is the subject of the individually identifiable health information about a use, a disclosure, rights, and remedies, provides the greater amount of information.

(4) With respect to the form or substance of an authorization or consent for use or disclosure of individually identifiable health information, provides requirements that narrow the scope or duration, increase the privacy protections afforded (such as by expanding the criteria for), or reduce the coercive effect of the circumstances surrounding the authorization or consent, as applicable.

(5) With respect to recordkeeping or requirements relating to accounting of disclosures, provides for the retention or reporting of more detailed information or for a longer duration.

(6) With respect to any other matter, provides greater privacy protection for the individual who is the subject of the individually identifiable health information.

Relates to the privacy of individually identifiable health information means, with respect to a State law, that the State law has the specific purpose of protecting the privacy of health information or affects the privacy of health information in a direct, clear, and substantial way.

State law means a constitution, statute, regulation, rule, common law, or other State action having the force and effect of law.

45 CFR 162.103 Definitions
[from the Final Transactions & Code Sets Rule]

For purposes of this part, the following definitions apply:

Code set means any set of codes used to encode data elements, such as tables of terms, medical concepts, medical diagnostic codes, or medical procedure codes. A code set includes the codes and the descriptors of the codes.

Code set maintaining organization means an organization that creates and maintains the code sets adopted by the Secretary for use in the transactions for which standards are adopted in this part.

Data condition means the rule that describes the circumstances under which a covered entity must use a particular data element or segment.

Data content means all the data elements and code sets inherent to a transaction, and not related to the format of the transaction. Data elements that are related to the format are not data content.

Data element means the smallest named unit of information in a transaction.

Data set means a semantically meaningful unit of information exchanged between two parties to a transaction.

Descriptor means the text defining a code.

Designated standard maintenance organization (DSMO) means an organization designated by the Secretary under Sec. 162.910(a).

Direct data entry means the direct entry of data (for example, using dumb terminals or web browsers) that is immediately transmitted into a health plan's computer.

Electronic media means the mode of electronic transmission. It includes the Internet (wide-open), Extranet (using Internet technology to link a business with information only accessible to collaborating parties), leased lines, dial-up lines, private networks, and those transmissions that are physically moved from one location to another using magnetic tape, disk, or compact disk media.

Format refers to those data elements that provide or control the enveloping or hierarchical structure, or assist in identifying data content of, a transaction.

HCPCS stands for the Health [Care Financing Administration] Common Procedure Coding System.

Maintain or maintenance refers to activities necessary to support the use of a standard adopted by the Secretary, including technical corrections to an implementation specification, and enhancements or expansion of a code set. This term excludes the activities related to the adoption of a new standard or implementation specification, or modification to an adopted standard or implementation specification.

Maximum defined data set means all of the required data elements for a particular standard based on a specific implementation specification.

Segment means a group of related data elements in a transaction.

Standard transaction means a transaction that complies with the applicable standard adopted under this part.

45 CFR 164.501 Definitions [from the Final Privacy Rule]

As used in this subpart, the following terms have the following meanings:

Correctional institution means any penal or correctional facility, jail, reformatory, detention center, work farm, halfway house, or residential community program center operated by, or under contract to, the United States, a State, a territory, a political subdivision of a State or territory, or an Indian tribe, for the confinement or rehabilitation of persons charged with or convicted of a criminal offense or other persons held in lawful custody.

Other persons held in lawful custody includes juvenile offenders adjudicated delinquent, aliens detained awaiting deportation, persons committed to mental institutions through the criminal justice system, witnesses, or others awaiting charges or trial.

Covered functions means those functions of a covered entity the performance of which makes the entity a health plan, health care provider, or health care clearinghouse.

Data aggregation means, with respect to protected health information created or received by a business associate in its capacity as the business associate of a covered entity, the combining of such protected health information by the business associate with the protected health information received by the business associate in its capacity as a business associate of another covered entity, to permit data analyses that relate to the health care operations of the respective covered entities.

Designated record set means:

(1) A group of records maintained by or for a covered entity that is:
    (i) The medical records and billing records about individuals maintained by or for a covered health care provider;
    (ii) The enrollment, payment, claims adjudication, and case or medical management record systems maintained by or for a health plan; or
    (iii) Used, in whole or in part, by or for the covered entity to make decisions about individuals.

(2) For purposes of this paragraph, the term record means any item, collection, or grouping of information that includes protected health information and is maintained, collected, used, or disseminated by or for a covered entity.

Direct treatment relationship means a treatment relationship between an individual and a health care provider that is not an indirect treatment relationship.

Disclosure means the release, transfer, provision of access to, or divulging in any other manner of information outside the entity holding the information.

Health care operations means any of the following activities of the covered entity to the extent that the activities are related to covered functions, and any of the following activities of an organized health care arrangement in which the covered entity participates:

(1) Conducting quality assessment and improvement activities, including outcomes evaluation and development of clinical guidelines, provided that the obtaining of generalizable knowledge is not the primary purpose of any studies resulting from such activities; population-based activities relating to improving health or reducing health care costs, protocol development, case management and care coordination, contacting of health care providers and patients with information about treatment alternatives; and related functions that do not include treatment;

(2) Reviewing the competence or qualifications of health care professionals, evaluating practitioner and provider performance, health plan performance, conducting training programs in which students, trainees, or practitioners in areas of health care learn under supervision to practice or improve their skills as health care providers, training of non-health care professionals, accreditation, certification, licensing, or credentialing activities;

(3) Underwriting, premium rating, and other activities relating to the creation, renewal or replacement of a contract of health insurance or health benefits, and ceding, securing, or placing a contract for reinsurance of risk relating to claims for health care (including stop-loss insurance and excess of loss insurance), provided that the requirements of § 164.514(g) are met, if applicable;

(4) Conducting or arranging for medical review, legal services, and auditing functions, including fraud and abuse detection and compliance programs;

(5) Business planning and development, such as conducting cost-management and planning-related analyses related to managing and

operating the entity, including formulary development and administration, development or improvement of methods of payment or coverage policies; and

(6) Business management and general administrative activities of the entity, including, but not limited to:

(i) Management activities relating to implementation of and compliance with the requirements of this subchapter;

(ii) Customer service, including the provision of data analyses for policy holders, plan sponsors, or other customers, provided that protected health information is not disclosed to such policy holder, plan sponsor, or customer;

(iii) Resolution of internal grievances;

(iv) Due diligence in connection with the sale or transfer of assets to a potential successor in interest, if the potential successor in interest is a covered entity or, following completion of the sale or transfer, will become a covered entity; and

(v) Consistent with the applicable requirements of § 164.514, creating de-identified health information, fundraising for the benefit of the covered entity, and marketing for which an individual authorization is not required as described in §164.514(e)(2).

Health oversight agency means an agency or authority of the United States, a State, a territory, a political subdivision of a State or territory, or an Indian tribe, or a person or entity acting under a grant of authority from or contract with such public agency, including the employees or agents of such public agency or its contractors or persons or entities to whom it has granted authority, that is authorized by law to oversee the health care system (whether public or private) or government programs in which health information is necessary to determine eligibility or compliance, or to enforce civil rights laws for which health information is relevant.

Indirect treatment relationship means a relationship between an individual and a health care provider in which:

(1) The health care provider delivers health care to the individual based on the orders of another health care provider; and

(2) The health care provider typically provides services or products, or reports the diagnosis or results associated with the health care, directly to another health care provider, who provides the services or products or reports to the individual.

Individual means the person who is the subject of protected health information.

Individually identifiable health information is information that is a subset of health information, including demographic information collected from an individual, and:

(1) Is created or received by a health care provider, health plan, employer, or health care clearinghouse; and
(2) Relates to the past, present, or future physical or mental health or condition of an individual; the provision of health care to an individual; or the past, present, or future payment for the provision of health care to an individual; and
    (i) That identifies the individual; or
    (ii) With respect to which there is a reasonable basis to believe the information can be used to identify the individual.

Inmate means a person incarcerated in or otherwise confined to a correctional institution.

Law enforcement official means an officer or employee of any agency or authority of the United States, a State, a territory, a political subdivision of a State or territory, or an Indian tribe, who is empowered by law to:

(1) Investigate or conduct an official inquiry into a potential violation of law; or
(2) Prosecute or otherwise conduct a criminal, civil, or administrative proceeding arising from an alleged violation of law.

Marketing means to make a communication about a product or service a purpose of which is to encourage recipients of the communication to purchase or use the product or service.

(1) Marketing does not include communications that meet the requirements of paragraph (2) of this definition and that are made by a covered entity:
    (i) For the purpose of describing the entities participating in a health care provider network or health plan network, or for the purpose of describing if and the extent to which a product or service (or payment for such product or service) is provided by a covered entity or included in a plan of benefits; or
    (ii) That are tailored to the circumstances of a particular individual and the communications are:
        (A) Made by a health care provider to an individual as part of the treatment of the individual, and for the purpose of furthering the treatment of that individual; or

  (B) Made by a health care provider or health plan to an individual in the course of managing the treatment of that individual, or for the purpose of directing or recommending to that individual alternative treatments, therapies, health care providers, or settings of care.

(2) A communication described in paragraph (1) of this definition is not included in marketing if:

  (i) The communication is made orally; or

  (ii) The communication is in writing and the covered entity does not receive direct or indirect remuneration from a third party for making the communication.

Organized health care arrangement means:

(1) A clinically integrated care setting in which individuals typically receive health care from more than one health care provider;

(2) An organized system of health care in which more than one covered entity participates, and in which the participating covered entities:

  (i) Hold themselves out to the public as participating in a joint arrangement; and

  (ii) Participate in joint activities that include at least one of the following:

    (A) Utilization review, in which health care decisions by participating covered entities are reviewed by other participating covered entities or by a third party on their behalf;

    (B) Quality assessment and improvement activities, in which treatment provided by participating covered entities is assessed by other participating covered entities or by a third party on their behalf; or

    (C) Payment activities, if the financial risk for delivering health care is shared, in part or in whole, by participating covered entities through the joint arrangement and if protected health information created or received by a covered entity is reviewed by other participating covered entities or by a third party on their behalf for the purpose of administering the sharing of financial risk.

(3) A group health plan and a health insurance issuer or HMO with respect to such group health plan, but only with respect to protected health information created or received by such health insurance issuer or HMO that relates to individuals who are or who have been participants or beneficiaries in such group health plan;

(4) A group health plan and one or more other group health plans each of which are maintained by the same plan sponsor; or

(5) The group health plans described in paragraph (4) of this definition and health insurance issuers or HMOs with respect to such group health plans, but only with respect to protected health information created or received by such health insurance issuers or HMOs that relates to individuals who are or have been participants or beneficiaries in any of such group health plans.

Payment means:

(1) The activities undertaken by:
  (i) A health plan to obtain premiums or to determine or fulfill its responsibility for coverage and provision of benefits under the health plan; or
  (ii) A covered health care provider or health plan to obtain or provide reimbursement for the provision of health care; and

(2) The activities in paragraph (1) of this definition relate to the individual to whom health care is provided and include, but are not limited to:
  (i) Determinations of eligibility or coverage (including coordination of benefits or the determination of cost sharing amounts), and adjudication or subrogation of health benefit claims;
  (ii) Risk adjusting amounts due based on enrollee health status and demographic characteristics;
  (iii) Billing, claims management, collection activities, obtaining payment under a contract for reinsurance (including stop-loss insurance and excess of loss insurance), and related health care data processing;
  (iv) Review of health care services with respect to medical necessity, coverage under a health plan, appropriateness of care, or justification of charges;
  (v) Utilization review activities, including pre-certification and preauthorization of services, concurrent and retrospective review of services; and
  (vi) Disclosure to consumer reporting agencies of any of the following protected health information relating to collection of premiums or reimbursement:
    (A) Name and address;
    (B) Date of birth;
    (C) Social security number;
    (D) Payment history;

(E) Account number; and

(F) Name and address of the health care provider and/or health plan.

Plan sponsor is defined as defined at section 3(16)(B) of ERISA, 29 U.S.C. 1002(16)(B). [Note: Section 3(16)(B) of ERISA defines *plan sponsor* as "(i) the employer in the case of an employee benefit plan established or maintained by a single employer, (ii) the employee organization in the case of a plan established or maintained by an employee organization, or (iii) in the case of a plan established or maintained by two or more employers or jointly by one or more employers and one or more employee organizations, the association, committee, joint board of trustees, or other similar group of representatives of the parties who establish or maintain the plan."]

Protected health information means individually identifiable health information:

(1) Except as provided in paragraph (2) of this definition, that is:
   (i) Transmitted by electronic media;
   (ii) Maintained in any medium described in the definition of electronic media at § 162.103 of this subchapter; or
   (iii) Transmitted or maintained in any other form or medium.

(2) *Protected health information* excludes individually identifiable health information in:
   (i) Education records covered by the Family Educational Right and Privacy Act, as amended, 20 U.S.C. 1232g; and
   (ii) Records described at 20 U.S.C. 1232g(a)(4)(B)(iv).

Psychotherapy notes means notes recorded (in any medium) by a health care provider who is a mental health professional documenting or analyzing the contents of conversation during a private counseling session or a group, joint, or family counseling session and that are separated from the rest of the individual's medical record.

Psychotherapy notes excludes medication prescription and monitoring, counseling session start and stop times, the modalities and frequencies of treatment furnished, results of clinical tests, and any summary of the following items: diagnosis, functional status, the treatment plan, symptoms, prognosis, and progress to date.

Public health authority means an agency or authority of the United States, a State, a territory, a political subdivision of a State or territory, or an Indian tribe, or a person or entity acting under a grant of authority from or contract with such public agency, including the employees or agents of such public agency or its contractors or persons or entities to whom it has granted authority, that is responsible for public health matters as part of its official mandate.

Required by law means a mandate contained in law that compels a covered entity to make a use or disclosure of protected health information and that is enforceable in a court of law. *Required by law* includes, but is not limited to, court orders and court-ordered warrants; subpoenas or summons issued by a court, grand jury, a governmental or tribal inspector general, or an administrative body authorized to require the production of information; a civil or an authorized investigative demand; Medicare conditions of participation with respect to health care providers participating in the program; and statutes or regulations that require the production of information, including statutes or regulations that require such information if payment is sought under a government program providing public benefits.

Research means a systematic investigation, including research development, testing, and evaluation, designed to develop or contribute to generalizable knowledge.

Treatment means the provision, coordination, or management of health care and related services by one or more health care providers, including the coordination or management of health care by a health care provider with a third party; consultation between health care providers relating to a patient; or the referral of a patient for health care from one health care provider to another.

Use means, with respect to individually identifiable health information, the sharing, employment, application, utilization, examination, or analysis of such information within an entity that maintains such information.

45 CFR 164.504 Uses and Disclosures: Organizational Requirements

Common control exists if an entity has the power, directly or indirectly, significantly to influence or direct the actions or policies of another entity.

Common ownership exists if an entity or entities possess an ownership or equity interest of 5 percent or more in another entity.

Health care component has the following meaning:

(1) Components of a covered entity that perform covered functions are part of the health care component.
(2) Another component of the covered entity is part of the entity's health care component to the extent that:
   (i) It performs, with respect to a component that performs covered functions, activities that would make such other component a business associate of the component that performs covered functions if the two components were separate legal entities; and

(ii) The activities involve the use or disclosure of protected health information that such other component creates or receives from or on behalf of the component that performs covered functions.

Hybrid entity means a single legal entity that is a covered entity and whose covered functions are not its primary functions.

Plan administration functions means administration functions performed by the plan sponsor of a group health plan on behalf of the group health plan and excludes functions performed by the plan sponsor in connection with any other benefit or benefit plan of the plan sponsor.

Summary health information means information that may be individually identifiable health information, and:

(1) That summarizes the claims history, claims expenses, or type of claims experienced by individuals for whom a plan sponsor has provided health benefits under a group health plan; and

(2) From which the information described at § 164.514(b)(2)(i) has been deleted, except that the geographic information described in § 164.514(b)(2)(i)(B) need only be aggregated to the level of a five digit zip code.

PART III: PURPOSE AND MAINTENANCE

Purpose

Part I provides a general glossary of terms and acronyms likely to be encountered by anyone dealing with the Administrative Simplification portions of HIPAA, or with any of the organizations, standards, and processes involved in developing, maintaining, and using HIPAA-related standards.

It evolved from a glossary developed in the Summer of 1998 to support the development of the MOU covering the DSMO process within X12N/TG3/WG3. That MOU explains how the ADA, HHS, HL7, the NCPDP, the NUBC, the NUCC, and X12N will coordinate their efforts to develop and maintain the HIPAA-related standards and implementation guides. In such a setting it is possible to talk for several days without using a word of English, and this document was an attempt to compensate for that.

Part II provides a single source for all definitions included in the body of the final HIPAA Administrative Simplification rules, and should reflect the cumulative effects of all related rules and correction notices. Including the complete text of those definitions in this part keeps the Part I entries comparatively short and informal. Related definitions in Part I reference the associated Part II definitions.

Part III explains the purposes of Parts I and II, and provides you with a way to complain whenever you feel that your favorite organization or subject has been abused or neglected in those parts.

Maintenance

The contents are necessarily limited by the maintainers' knowledge of and experience with the subjects and organizations included, and by the need to keep it finite. We have avoided including technical security-related terms beyond those needed to understand the rules themselves because there are so many of them, and because they are already fairly well documented by various industry and professional groups. When identifying organizations, we have tried to note when they have special responsibilities under HIPAA, such as the maintenance of a transaction standard or code set, or via the sponsorship of special educational programs.

Appendix
B

HIPAA Security Rule Standards, Implementation Specifications, and NIST Resource Guide for Implementing HIPAA

Administrative Safeguards

Standards	CFR Sections	Implementation Specifications (R)=Required (A)=Addressable		NIST Publication	Publication Title	Web Address/URL
Security management process	164.308(a)(1)	Risk analysis	(R)	NIST SP 800-14	Generally Accepted Principles and Practices for Securing Information Technology Systems	http://csrc.nist.gov/publications/nistpubs/800-14/800-14.pdf
		Risk management	(R)	NIST SP 800-18	Guide for Developing Security Plans for Information Technology Systems	http://csrc.nist.gov/publications/nistpubs/800-18/Planguide.PDF
		Sanction Policy	(R)	NIST SP 800-26	Security Self-Assessment Guide for Information Technology Systems	http://csrc.nist.gov/publications/nistpubs/800-26/sp800-26.pdf
		Information system activity review	(R)	NIST SP 800-27	Engineering Principles for Information Technology Security (Baseline for Achieving Security)	http://csrc.nist.gov/publications/nistpubs/800-27/sp800-27.pdf
				NIST SP 800-30	Risk Management Guide for Information Technology Systems	http://csrc.nist.gov/publications/nistpubs/800-30/sp800-30.pdf
				NIST SP 800-37	Guide for the Security Certification and Accreditation of Federal Information Systems	http://csrc.nist.gov/publications/nistpubs/800-37/SP800-37-final.pdf

				Standard	Title	URL
				NIST SP 800-53	Recommended Security Controls for Federal Information Systems	http://csrc.nist.gov/publications/drafts/draft-SP800-53.pdf
				NIST SP 800-60	Guide for Mapping Types of Information and Information Systems to Security Categories	http://csrc.nist.gov/publications/drafts/800-60v1f.pdf (Vol. 1) http://csrc.nist.gov/publications/drafts/sp800-60V2f.pdf (Vol. 2)
				FIPS 199	Standards for Security Categorization of Federal Information and Information Systems	http://csrc.nist.gov/publications/fips199/FIPS-PUB-199-final.pdf
				NIST SP 800-12 chapter 5	An Introduction to Computer Security: The NIST Handbook	http://csrc.nist.gov/publications/nistpubs/800-12/handbook.pdf
Assigned security responsibility	164.308(a)(2)	None	(R)	NIST SP 800-14	Generally Accepted Principles and Practices for Securing Information Technology Systems	http://csrc.nist.gov/publications/nistpubs/800-14/800-14.pdf
				NIST SP 800-26	Security Self-Assessment Guide for Information Technology Systems	http://csrc.nist.gov/publications/nistpubs/800-26/sp800-26.pdf
				NIST SP 800-53	Recommended Security Controls for Federal Information Systems	http://csrc.nist.gov/publications/drafts/draft-SP800-53.pdf

HIPAA Security Rule Standards, Implementation Specifications, and NIST Resource Guide for Implementing HIPAA

Administrative Safeguards

Standards	CFR Sections	Implementation Specifications (R)=Required (A)=Addressable		NIST Publication	Publication Title	Web Address/URL
				NIST SP 800-12 chapter 3	An Introduction to Computer Security: The NIST Handbook	http://csrc.nist.gov/publications/nistpubs/800-12/handbook.pdf
Workforce security	164.308(a)(3)	Authorization and/or supervision	(A)	NIST SP 800-14	Generally Accepted Principles and Practices for Securing Information Technology Systems	http://csrc.nist.gov/publications/nistpubs/800-14/800-14.pdf
		Workforce clearance procedure	(A)	NIST SP 800-26	Security Self-Assessment Guide for Information Technology Systems	http://csrc.nist.gov/publications/nistpubs/800-26/sp800-26.pdf
		Termination procedures	(A)	NIST SP 800-53	Recommended Security Controls for Federal Information Systems	http://csrc.nist.gov/publications/drafts/draft-SP800-53.pdf
				NIST SP 800-12 chapter 17	An Introduction to Computer Security: The NIST Handbook	http://csrc.nist.gov/publications/nistpubs/800-12/handbook.pdf
Information access management	164.308(a)(4)	Isolating healthcare clearinghouse function	(R)	NIST SP 800-14	Generally Accepted Principles and Practices for Securing Information Technology Systems	http://csrc.nist.gov/publications/nistpubs/800-14/800-14.pdf

	Access authorization	(A)	NIST SP 800-18	Guide for Developing Security Plans for Information Technology Systems	http://csrc.nist.gov/publications/nistpubs/800-18/Planguide.PDF
	Access establishment and modification	(A)	NIST SP 800-53	Recommended Security Controls for Federal Information Systems	http://csrc.nist.gov/publications/drafts/draft-SP800-53.pdf
			NIST SP 800-63	Recommendation for Electronic Authentication	http://csrc.nist.gov/publications/drafts/draft-sp800-63.pdf
			NIST SP 800-12 chapter 17	An Introduction to Computer Security: The NIST Handbook	http://csrc.nist.gov/publications/nistpubs/800-12/handbook.pdf
Security awareness and training	164.308(a)(5)	Security reminders	(A)	NIST SP 800-14	Generally Accepted Principles and Practices for Securing Information Technology Systems	http://csrc.nist.gov/publications/nistpubs/800-14/800-14.pdf
		Protection from malicious software	(A)	NIST SP 800-16	IT Security Training Requirements: Role and Performance Based Model	http://csrc.nist.gov/publications/nistpubs/800-16/800-16.pdf (part 1)
		Log-in monitoring	(A)			http://csrc.nist.gov/publications/nistpubs/800-16/AppendixA-D.pdf (part 2)
		Password management	(A)			http://csrc.nist.gov/publications/nistpubs/800-16/Appendix_E.pdf (part 3)

HIPAA Security Rule Standards, Implementation Specifications, and NIST Resource Guide for Implementing HIPAA

Administrative Safeguards

Standards	CFR Sections	Implementation Specifications (R)=Required (A)=Addressable		NIST Publication	Publication Title	Web Address/URL
				NIST SP 800-53	Recommended Security Controls for Federal Information Systems	http://csrc.nist.gov/publications/drafts/draft-SP800-53.pdf
				NIST SP 800-12 chapter 13	An Introduction to Computer Security: The NIST Handbook	http://csrc.nist.gov/publications/nistpubs/800-12/handbook.pdf
Security incident procedures	164.308(a)(6)	Response and reporting	(R)	NIST SP 800-14	Generally Accepted Principles and Practices for Securing Information Technology Systems	http://csrc.nist.gov/publications/nistpubs/800-14/800-14.pdf
				NIST SP 800-53	Recommended Security Controls for Federal Information Systems	http://csrc.nist.gov/publications/drafts/draft-SP800-53.pdf
				NIST SP 800-12 chapter 12	An Introduction to Computer Security: The NIST Handbook	http://csrc.nist.gov/publications/nistpubs/800-12/handbook.pdf
Contingency plan	164.308(a)(7)	Data backup plan	(R)	NIST SP 800-14	Generally Accepted Principles and Practices for Securing Information Technology Systems	http://csrc.nist.gov/publications/nistpubs/800-14/800-14.pdf

		Disaster recovery plan	(R)	NIST SP 800-18	Guide for Developing Security Plans for Information Technology Systems	http://csrc.nist.gov/publications/nistpubs/800-18/Planguide.PDF
		Emergency mode operation plan	(R)	NIST SP 800-26	Security Self-Assessment Guide for Information Technology Systems	http://csrc.nist.gov/publications/nistpubs/800-26/sp800-26.pdf
		Testing and revision procedure	(A)	NIST SP 800-30	Risk Management Guide for Information Technology Systems	http://csrc.nist.gov/publications/nistpubs/800-30/sp800-30.pdf
		Applications and data criticality analysis	(A)	NIST SP 800-53	Recommended Security Controls for Federal Information Systems	http://csrc.nist.gov/publications/drafts/draft-SP800-53.pdf
				NIST SP 800-34	Contingency Planning Guide for Information Technology Systems	http://csrc.nist.gov/publications/nistpubs/800-34/sp800-34.pdf
				NIST SP 800-12 chapter 11	An Introduction to Computer Security: The NIST Handbook	http://csrc.nist.gov/publications/nistpubs/800-12/handbook.pdf
Evaluation	164.308(a)(8)	None	(R)	NIST SP 800-14	Generally Accepted Principles and Practices for Securing Information Technology Systems	http://csrc.nist.gov/publications/nistpubs/800-14/800-14.pdf
				NIST SP 800-37	Guide for the Security Certification and Accreditation of Federal Information Systems	http://csrc.nist.gov/publications/nistpubs/800-37/SP800-37-final.pdf

HIPAA Security Rule Standards, Implementation Specifications, and NIST Resource Guide for Implementing HIPAA

Administrative Safeguards

Standards	CFR Sections	Implementation Specifications (R)=Required (A)=Addressable		NIST Publication	Publication Title	Web Address/URL
				NIST SP 800-55	Security Metrics Guide for Information Technology Systems	http://csrc.nist.gov/publications/nistpubs/800-55/sp800-55.pdf
				NIST SP 800-12 chapter 9	An Introduction to Computer Security: The NIST Handbook	http://csrc.nist.gov/publications/nistpubs/800-12/handbook.pdf
Business associate contracts	164.308(b)(1)	Written contract or other arrangement	(R)	NIST SP 800-14	Generally Accepted Principles and Practices for Securing Information Technology Systems	http://csrc.nist.gov/publications/nistpubs/800-14/800-14.pdf
				NIST SP 800-36	Guide to Selecting Information Security Products	http://csrc.nist.gov/publications/nistpubs/800-36/NIST-SP800-36.pdf
				NIST SP 800-53	Recommended Security Controls for Federal Information Systems	http://csrc.nist.gov/publications/drafts/draft-SP800-53.pdf
				NIST SP 800-64	Security Considerations in the Information Systems Development Life Cycle	http://csrc.nist.gov/publications/nistpubs/800-64/NIST-SP800-64.pdf
				NIST SP 800-12 chapter 8	An Introduction to Computer Security: The NIST Handbook	http://csrc.nist.gov/publications/nistpubs/800-12/handbook.pdf

Physical Safeguards

Standards	CFR Sections	Implementation Specifications (R)=Required (A)=Addressable		NIST Publication #	Publication Title	Web Address/URL
Facility access controls	164.310(a)(1)	Contingency operations	(A)	NIST SP 800-14	Generally Accepted Principles and Practices for Securing Information Technology Systems	http://csrc.nist.gov/publications/nistpubs/800-14/800-14.pdf
		Facility security plan	(A)	NIST SP 800-18	Guide for Developing Security Plans for Information Technology Systems	http://csrc.nist.gov/publications/nistpubs/800-18/Planguide.PDF
		Access control and validation procedures	(A)	NIST SP 800-26	Security Self-Assessment Guide for Information Technology Systems	http://csrc.nist.gov/publications/nistpubs/800-26/sp800-26.pdf
		Maintenance records	(A)	NIST SP 800-30	Risk Management Guide for Information Technology Systems	http://csrc.nist.gov/publications/nistpubs/800-30/sp800-30.pdf
				NIST SP 800-34	Contingency Planning Guide for Information Technology Systems	http://csrc.nist.gov/publications/nistpubs/800-34/sp800-34.pdf
				NIST SP 800-53	Recommended Security Controls for Federal Information Systems	http://csrc.nist.gov/publications/drafts/draft-SP800-53.pdf
				NIST SP 800-12 chapter 15	An Introduction to Computer Security: The NIST Handbook	http://csrc.nist.gov/publications/nistpubs/800-12/handbook.pdf

HIPAA Security Rule Standards, Implementation Specifications, and NIST Resource Guide for Implementing HIPAA

Physical Safeguards

Standards	CFR Sections	Implementation Specifications (R)=Required (A)=Addressable		NIST Publication	Publication Title	Web Address/URL
Workstation use	164.310(b)	None	(R)	NIST SP 800-14	Generally Accepted Principles and Practices for Securing Information Technology Systems	http://csrc.nist.gov/publications/nistpubs/800-14/800-14.pdf
				NIST SP 800-53	Recommended Security Controls for Federal Information Systems	http://csrc.nist.gov/publications/drafts/draft-SP800-53.pdf
				NIST SP 800-12 chapter 15 & 16	An Introduction to Computer Security: The NIST Handbook	http://csrc.nist.gov/publications/nistpubs/800-12/handbook.pdf
Workstation security	164.310(c)	None	(R)	NIST SP 800-14	Generally Accepted Principles and Practices for Securing Information Technology Systems	http://csrc.nist.gov/publications/nistpubs/800-14/800-14.pdf
				NIST SP 800-53	Recommended Security Controls for Federal Information Systems	http://csrc.nist.gov/publications/drafts/draft-SP800-53.pdf
				NIST SP 800-12 chapter 15	An Introduction to Computer Security: The NIST Handbook	http://csrc.nist.gov/publications/nistpubs/800-12/handbook.pdf

Standards	CFR Sections	Implementation Specifications		NIST Publication	Publication Title	Web Address/URL
Device and media controls	164.310(d)(1)	Media disposal	(R)	NIST SP 800-14	Generally Accepted Principles and Practices for Securing Information Technology Systems	http://csrc.nist.gov/publications/nistpubs/800-14/800-14.pdf
		Media reuse	(R)	NIST SP 800-34	Contingency Planning Guide for Information Technology Systems	http://csrc.nist.gov/publications/nistpubs/800-34/sp800-34.pdf
		Media accountability	(A)	NIST SP 800-53	Recommended Security Controls for Federal Information Systems	http://csrc.nist.gov/publications/drafts/draft-SP800-53.pdf
		Data backup and storage (during transfer)	(A)	NIST SP 800-12 chapter 14	An Introduction to Computer Security: The NIST Handbook	http://csrc.nist.gov/publications/nistpubs/800-12/handbook.pdf

Technical Safeguards

Standards	CFR Sections	Implementation Specifications		NIST Publication	Publication Title	Web Address/URL
Access control	164.312(a)(1)	Unique user identification	(R)	NIST SP 800-14	Generally Accepted Principles and Practices for Securing Information Technology Systems	http://csrc.nist.gov/publications/nistpubs/800-14/800-14.pdf
		Emergency access procedure	(R)	NIST SP 800-53	Recommended Security Controls for Federal Information Systems	http://csrc.nist.gov/publications/drafts/draft-SP800-53.pdf
		Automatic log-off	(A)	NIST SP 800-56	Recommendation on Key Establishment Schemes	http://csrc.nist.gov/CryptoToolkit/tkkeymgmt.html
		Encryption and decryption (data at rest)	(A)	NIST SP 800-57	Recommendation on Key Management	http://csrc.nist.gov/CryptoToolkit/tkkeymgmt.html

				HIPAA Security Rule Standards, Implementation Specifications, and NIST Resource Guide for Implementing HIPAA	
				Technical Safeguards	
Standards	**CFR Sections**	**Implementation Specifications**		**NIST Publication**	**Publication Title**	**Web Address/URL**
				NIST SP 800-63	Recommendation for Electronic Authentication	http://csrc.nist.gov/publications/drafts/draft-sp800-63.pdf
				FIPS 140-2	Security Requirements for Cryptographic Modules	http://csrc.nist.gov/cryptval/140-2.htm
				NIST SP 800-12 chapter 17	An Introduction to Computer Security: The NIST Handbook	http://csrc.nist.gov/publications/nistpubs/800-12/handbook.pdf
Audit controls	164.312(b)	None	(R)	NIST SP 800-14	Generally Accepted Principles and Practices for Securing Information Technology Systems	http://csrc.nist.gov/publications/nistpubs/800-14/800-14.pdf
				NIST SP 800-53	Recommended Security Controls for Federal Information Systems	http://csrc.nist.gov/publications/drafts/draft-SP800-53.pdf
				NIST SP 800-12 chapter 18	An Introduction to Computer Security: The NIST Handbook	http://csrc.nist.gov/publications/nistpubs/800-12/handbook.pdf
Integrity	164.312(c)(1)	Protection against improper alteration or destruction of data	(A)	NIST SP 800-42	Guideline on Network Security Testing	http://csrc.nist.gov/publications/nistpubs/800-42/NIST-SP800-42.pdf

				NIST SP 800-44	Guidelines on Securing Public Web Servers	http://csrc.nist.gov/publications/nistpubs/800-44/sp800-44.pdf
				NIST SP 800-53	Recommended Security Controls for Federal Information Systems	http://csrc.nist.gov/publications/drafts/draft-SP800-53.pdf
				NIST SP 800-12 chapter 5	An Introduction to Computer Security: The NIST Handbook	http://csrc.nist.gov/publications/nistpubs/800-12/handbook.pdf
Person or entity authentication	164.312(d)	None	(R)	NIST SP 800-14	Generally Accepted Principles and Practices for Securing Information Technology Systems	http://csrc.nist.gov/publications/nistpubs/800-14/800-14.pdf
				NIST SP 800-53	Recommended Security Controls for Federal Information Systems	http://csrc.nist.gov/publications/drafts/draft-SP800-53.pdf
				NIST SP 800-63	Recommendation for Electronic Authentication	http://csrc.nist.gov/publications/drafts/draft-sp800-63.pdf
				NIST SP 800-12 chapter 16	An Introduction to Computer Security: The NIST Handbook	http://csrc.nist.gov/publications/nistpubs/800-12/handbook.pdf
Transmission security	164.312(e)(1)	Integrity controls	(A)	NIST SP 800-14	Generally Accepted Principles and Practices for Securing Information Technology Systems	http://csrc.nist.gov/publications/nistpubs/800-14/800-14.pdf
		Encryption (FTP and e-mail over Internet)	(A)	NIST SP 800-42	Guideline on Network Security Testing	http://csrc.nist.gov/publications/nistpubs/800-42/NIST-SP800-42.pdf

HIPAA Security Rule Standards, Implementation Specifications, and NIST Resource Guide for Implementing HIPAA

Technical Safeguards

Standards	CFR Sections	Implementation Specifications	NIST Publication	Publication Title	Web Address/URL
			NIST SP 800-53	Recommended Security Controls for Federal Information Systems	http://csrc.nist.gov/publications/drafts/draft-SP800-53.pdf
			NIST SP 800-63	Recommendation for Electronic Authentication	http://csrc.nist.gov/publications/drafts/draft-sp800-63.pdf
			FIPS 140-2	Security Requirements for Cryptographic Modules	http://csrc.nist.gov/cryptval/140-2.htm
			NIST SP 800-12 chapter 16 & 19	An Introduction to Computer Security: The NIST Handbook	http://csrc.nist.gov/publications/nistpubs/800-12/handbook.pdf

Appendix
C

POLICY EXAMPLES

APPENDIX C.1

Electronic Mail Usage Policy

POLICY NO.: XXX-XXXX.XX
SUBJECT: Electronic Mail Usage Policy
ISSUED BY: <Name of Issuing Authority>
DATE ISSUED: January 1, 2004
DATE DELETED: N/A
SUPERCEDES: None
AFFECTS: All Organization staff

PURPOSE

The purpose of this policy is to define appropriate standards for secure and effective use of <ORGANIZATION NAME> electronic mail system.

POLICY

Electronic mail has become an integrated tool in <ORGANIZATION NAME> business processes. This policy applies to all usage of <ORGANIZATION NAME> electronic mail systems where the mail either originated from or is received into a <ORGANIZATION NAME> computer or network. It applies to all users including, but not limited to, employees, medical staff, contractors, students, and volunteers.

User Responsibilities

The user is any person who has been authorized to read, enter, or update information created or transmitted via <ORGANIZATION NAME> electronic mail system. Electronic mail is intended to be used as a business tool to facilitate communications and the exchange of information needed to perform an employee s job. Incidental personal use is permissible so long as it:

- Does not consume more than a trivial amount of resources
- Does not interfere with worker productivity
- Does not preempt any business activity

Users have an obligation to use e-mail appropriately, effectively, and efficiently. Users must be aware that electronic communications can, depending on the technology, be forwarded, intercepted, printed, and stored by others. Therefore, users must utilize discretion and confidentiality protection equal to or exceeding that which is applied to written documents. E-mail should not be used for urgent or time-sensitive communications. Business e-mail accounts and passwords should not be shared or revealed to anyone else besides the authorized user(s).

Prohibited Uses

Use of electronic mail is to be in compliance with all applicable state and federal statutes and <ORGANIZATION NAME> policies and procedures. Prohibited usage of <ORGANIZATION NAME> electronic mail system includes, but is not limited to:

- Copying or transmission of any document, software, or other information protected by copyright or patent law, without proper authorization by the copyright or patent owner
- Engaging in any communication that is threatening, defamatory, obscene, offensive, or harassing
- Use of e-mail system for solicitation of funds, political messages, gambling, commercial, or illegal activities
- Disclosure of an individual's personal information without appropriate authorization
- Transmission of information to individuals inside or outside the company without a legitimate business need for the information
- Use of e-mail addresses for marketing purposes without explicit permission from the target recipient
- Transmission of highly confidential or sensitive information, e.g., HIV status, mental illness, chemical dependency, and workers compensation claims

- Forwarding of e-mail from in-house or outside legal counsel, or the contents of that mail, to individuals outside of the company without the express authorization of counsel
- Misrepresenting, obscuring, suppressing, or replacing a user's identity on an electronic communication
- Obtaining access to the files or communications of others with no substantial company business purpose
- Attempting unauthorized access to data or attempting to breach any security measure on any electronic communication system, or attempting to intercept any electronic communication transmissions without proper authorization

This list is not considered all-inclusive. Further questions regarding appropriate use of electronic mail should be directed to the employee's supervisor or <TITLE OF THE INFORMATION SECURITY ADMINISTRATOR>.

Ownership and User Privacy of E-Mail

Use of electronic mail is a part of <ORGANIZATION NAME> business processes. All messages originated or transported within or received into <ORGANIZATION NAME> electronic mail system are considered to be the property of <ORGANIZATION NAME>. All users of e-mail systems do so with the understanding that they have no expectation of privacy relating to that use. <ORGANIZATION NAME> reserves the right to access the electronic mail system for the purpose of ensuring the protection of legitimate business interests and proper utilization of its property. Such purposes may include, but are not limited to:

- Locating and retrieving lost messages
- Performing duties when an employee is out of the office or otherwise unavailable
- Maintaining control of the system by analyzing message patterns and implementing revisions as needed
- Collecting or monitoring electronic communications in order to ensure the ongoing availability and reliability of the system
- Recovering from systems failures and other unexpected emergencies
- Investigating suspected breaches of security or violations of policy with probable cause
- Electronic mail information is occasionally visible to IS staff engaged in routine testing, maintenance, and problem resolution. Staff assigned to carry out such assignments will not intentionally seek out and read, or disclose to others, the content of e-mail.

- Supervisors or administrators must advise and receive approval from <TITLE OF THE INFORMATION SECURITY ADMINISTRATOR> of their intent to review an employee's messages prior to accessing employee files.

Confidentiality of Electronic Mail

Users of <ORGANIZATION NAME> electronic mail system may have the capacity to forward, print, and circulate any message transmitted through the system. Therefore:

- Users should utilize discretion and confidentiality protection equal to or exceeding that which is applied to written documents.
- When e-mail is used for communication of confidential or sensitive information, specific measures must be taken to safeguard the confidentiality of the information. These safeguards are as follows:
- Information considered confidential or sensitive must be protected during transmission of the data utilizing encryption or some other system of access controls that ensure the information is not accessed by anyone other than the intended recipient.
- A notation referring to the confidential or sensitive nature of the information should be made in the subject line.
- Confidential or sensitive information may be distributed to multiple recipients; however, the use of distribution lists is prohibited.
- Confidential or sensitive information is to be distributed only to those with a legitimate need to know.

Retention of Electronic Mail

Generally, e-mail messages constitute temporary communications, which are nonvital and may be discarded routinely. However, depending on the content of an e-mail message, it may be considered a more formal record and should be retained pursuant to <ORGANIZATION NAME> record retention schedules. Electronic mail tape backups are performed on a regular basis for the purpose of business recovery. Information stored electronically is subject to the legal discovery process and can be subpoenaed. To manage this risk, consider short retention periods for e-mail backups and execute appropriate third-party retention requirements consistent with organizational needs. Electronic mail tape backups are stored for <retention period>.

Provider/Patient Use of E-mail

Use of provider/patient e-mail can facilitate improved communication between an individual and his or her provider. However, due to the inherent risks involved in e-mail use, the following policy considerations must be clearly addressed prior to using e-mail for provider/patient communications:

- Patient informed consent and agreement to guidelines for use of e-mail must be documented. Informed consent should address the following:
  - E-mail communication is a convenience and not appropriate for emergencies or time-sensitive issues.
  - No one can guarantee the security and privacy of e-mail messages.
  - Employers generally have the right to access any e-mail received or sent by a person at work.
- Highly sensitive or personal information should not be communicated via email.
- Communication guidelines defined, including:
  - How often e-mail will be checked
  - Instructions for when and how to escalate to phone calls and office visits
  - The types of transactions that are appropriate for e-mail
- Staff other than the physician may read and process the mail.
- Clinically relevant messages and responses will be documented in the medical record.
- E-mail message content must include:
  - The category of the communication in the subject line, i.e., prescription refill, appointment request, etc.
  - Clear patient identification including patient name, telephone number, and patient identification number in the body of the message
- Indemnify <ORGANIZATION NAME> for information loss due to technical failures
- Boundaries for clinical and operational staff usage of patient electronic mail must be defined. Considerations include:
  - All employees, including physicians, sign a confidentiality and security agreement that addresses electronic technology
  - Use of a central address for receipt of all e-mail messages
  - Identification of processes to manage triage, routing, response, and filing of e-mail messages

- Process to verify that message is from an established patient before responding
- Reasonable precautions to ensure that e-mail responses to patients are not misdirected or otherwise become available to unintended parties
- Use of discreet subject headers such as personal and confidential communication
- Incorporation of all clinically relevant e-mail messages, including the full text of the patient's query as well as the reply to the sender, in patient's electronic or paper medical record
- Obtaining of patient's express authorization prior to any forwarding of patient identifiable information to a third party such as a consultant or health plan
- Prohibitions on use patient's e-mail addresses for marketing or the supplying of addresses to third parties for advertising or any other use

■ Technical security practices:
- Restriction of access to the professional e-mail account in the same way access to medical records is restricted
- Use of password-protected programs and screen-savers for all workstations
- Firewalls
- Use of the auto-reply feature to notify patients when an e-mail account will not be monitored during a vacation or office closure
- Protection of information considered confidential or sensitive by utilizing encryption or some other system of access controls that ensure the information is not accessed by anyone other than the intended recipient
- Prohibition on use of unsecured wireless e-mail communication when sending patient-identifiable information

Compliance

Employees and users of <ORGANIZATION NAME> electronic mail system(s) who are found to be in violation of any part of this policy are subject to disciplinary action up to and including dismissal.

DEFINITIONS

<Insert list of words or acronyms needing further elaboration or expansion>

REFERENCES/RELATED POLICIES

<Insert bibliographic annotations for references and sources.>

POLICY DEVELOPMENT

DEVELOPER: <PersonOrCommittee>

POLICY APPROVAL

<PersonOrCommittee> <Date>
<PersonOrCommittee> <Date>
<PersonOrCommittee> <Date>

REVIEWS

LAST REVIEW: <Date>
NEXT REVIEW DATE: <Date>

APPENDIX C.2

Information Stewardship Policy

POLICY NO.: XXX-XXXX.XX
SUBJECT: Information Stewardship Policy
ISSUED BY: <Name of Issuing Authority>
DATE ISSUED: January 1, 2004
DATE DELETED: N/A
SUPERCEDES: None
AFFECTS: All Organization staff

PURPOSE

The purpose of this information stewardship policy is to provide a system for protecting information. Information is no longer simply something that supports the provision of a product or service. Information itself has become an asset. The establishment of new roles and responsibilities is needed to properly manage and protect the information assets. To this end, this policy defines the information security roles and responsibilities of Stewards, Custodians, and Users. Information security can no longer be a concern of technical specialists alone—it must instead be addressed by a large team of individuals, each of whom makes his or her own unique contribution.

POLICY

Roles and Responsibilities of Stewards: Information Stewards are senior business unit managers with the authority for acquiring, creating, and maintaining information systems within their assigned area of control. Stewards are responsible for:

- Categorizing the information for which they have been designated a Steward using classifications defined in the Data Classification Policy
- Authorizing User access to information based on the need-to-know
- Defining the validation rules used to verify the correctness and acceptability of input data
- Insuring a sufficient level of training takes place for people entering or modifying data in the system
- Assisting with contingency planning efforts and categorizing information (or specific application systems) according to a criticality scale
- Making decisions about the permissible uses of information
- Understanding the uses and risks associated with the information for which they are accountable. This means that they are responsible for the consequences associated with improper disclosure, insufficient maintenance, inaccurate classification labeling, and other security-related control deficiencies pertaining to the information for which they are the designated Stewards.

Roles and Responsibilities of Custodians: Information Custodians are individuals (often staff within the Information Systems Department or departmental systems administrators) in physical or logical possession of information from Stewards. Custodians are responsible for:

- Protecting the information in their possession from unauthorized access, alteration, destruction, or usage
- Providing and administering general controls such as backup and recovery systems consistent with company policies and standards
- Establishing, monitoring, and operating information systems in a manner consistent with policies and standards
- Providing Stewards with reports about the resources consumed on their behalf (often via a charge-back system), as well as reports indicating User activities
- Changing the production information in their possession only after receiving explicit and temporary permission from either the Steward or an authorized User

Roles and Responsibilities of Users: Information Users are individuals who have been granted explicit authorization to access, modify, delete, and/or utilize information by the relevant Steward. Users must:

- Use the information only for the purposes specifically approved by the Steward.
- Comply with all security measures defined by the Steward, implemented by the Custodian, and/or defined by policies and standards.
- Refrain from disclosing information in their possession (unless it has been designated as Public) without first obtaining permission from the Steward.
- Report all situations where they believe an information security vulnerability or violation may exist.
- Local management must also provide Users with sufficient time to receive periodic information security training. Users of personal computers have special responsibilities (for example, relating to backup and virus screening) which are defined in the Personal Computer Security Policy.

Designating Stewards: If there are several potential information Stewards, higher-level management must assign Stewardship responsibility to the senior manager of the business unit that makes the greatest use of the information. When acting in his or her capacity of Steward, this individual must take into consideration the needs and interests of other stakeholders who rely upon or have an interest in the information. With the exception of operational computer and network information, managers in the Information Systems Department may not be a Steward for any information.

A Steward's roles and responsibilities may be delegated to any manager in the Steward's business unit. A Steward's roles and responsibilities may not be assigned or delegated to contractors, consultants, or individuals in outsourcing firms or external service bureaus.

Designating Custodians: Management must specifically assign responsibility for the control measures protecting every major production type of information. Stewards are responsible for identifying all those individuals who are in possession of the information for which they are the designated Stewards. These individuals by default become Custodians. Although special care must be taken to clearly specify security-related roles and responsibilities when outsiders are involved, it is permissible for Custodians to be contractors, consultants, or individuals at outsourcing firms or external service bureaus.

Designating Users: Users may be employees, temporaries, contractors, consultants, or third parties with whom special arrangements (such as nondisclosure agreements) have been made. All Users must be known to and authorized by Stewards. The security-relevant activities of all Users must be tracked and logged by Custodians. To allow proper privilege assignment and activity logging, Users must always be specific individuals; Users must not be defined as departments, project teams, or other groups.

Changes in Status: Due to promotions, transfers, retirements, etc., the individuals who play the roles of information Stewards, Custodians, and Users will change on a regular basis. It is the responsibility of the local manager of all individuals to promptly report status changes. Custodians must maintain access control systems so that previously provided User privileges are no longer provided whenever there has been a User status change. When a Custodian has a change in status, it is the responsibility of the Steward to promptly assign a new Custodian. When a Steward has a change in status, it is the Chief Information Officer's responsibility to promptly designate a new Steward.

Handling of Information following Status Changes: Users who change their status must leave all production information with their immediate manager. Soon after a User has a change of status, both computer-resident files and paper files must be reviewed by the User's immediate manager to determine who should be given possession of the files, and/or the appropriate methods to be used for file disposal or destruction. The manager must then promptly reassign the User's duties as well as specifically delegate responsibility for information formerly in the User's possession.

DEFINITIONS

<Glossary of specific terms used in this document>

REFERENCES/RELATED POLICIES

<List of related internal policies, guidelines, etc., and any legal sources required>

POLICY DEVELOPMENT

DEVELOPER: Internal Policy Committee December 1, 2003

POLICY APPROVAL

<Name of direct executive approval authority>

REVIEWS

LAST REVIEW:
NEXT REVIEW DATE:

APPENDIX C.3

Information Systems Access Policy

POLICY NO.: XXX-XXXX.XX

SUBJECT: Information Systems Access Policy

ISSUED BY: <Name of Issuing Authority>

DATE ISSUED: January 1, 2004

DATE DELETED: N/A

SUPERCEDES: None

AFFECTS: All Organization staff

PURPOSE

The purpose of this policy is to maintain an adequate level of security to protect <COMPANY NAME> data and information systems from unauthorized access. This policy defines the rules necessary to achieve this protection and to ensure a secure and reliable operation of <COMPANY NAME> information systems.

POLICY

Only authorized users are granted access to information systems, and users are limited to specific defined, documented, and approved applications and levels of access rights. Computer and communication system access control is to be achieved via user IDs that are unique to each individual user to provide individual accountability.

Who Is Affected: This policy affects all employees of <COMPANY NAME> and its subsidiaries, and all contractors, consultants, temporary employees, and business partners. Employees who deliberately violate this policy will be subject disciplinary action up to and including termination.

Affected Systems: This policy applies to all computer and communication systems owned or operated by <COMPANY NAME> and its subsidiaries. Similarly, this policy applies to all platforms (operating systems) and all application systems.

Entity Authentication: Any user (remote or internal), accessing <COMPANY NAME> networks and systems, must be authenticated. The level of authentication must be appropriate to the data classification and transport medium. Entity authentication includes but is not limited to:

- Automatic log-off
- A unique user identifier
- At least one of the following:
  - Biometric identification
  - Password
  - Personal identification number
  - A telephone callback procedure
  - Token

Workstation Access Control System: All workstations used for this <COMPANY NAME> business activity, no matter where they are located, must use an access control system approved by <COMPANY NAME>. In most cases this will involve password-enabled screen-savers with a time-out-after-no-activity feature and a power on password for the CPU and BIOs. Active workstations are not to be left unattended for prolonged periods of time, where appropriate. When a user leaves a workstation, that user is expected to properly log out of all applications and networks. Users will be held responsible for all actions taken under their sign-on. Where appropriate, inactive workstations will be reset after a period of inactivity (typically 30 minutes). Users will then be required to re-log on to continue usage. This minimizes the opportunity for unauthorized users to assume the privileges of the intended user during the authorized user's absence.

Disclosure Notice: A notice warning that those should only access the system with proper authority will be displayed initially before signing on to the system. The warning message will make clear that the system is a private network or application and those unauthorized users should disconnect or log off immediately.

System Access Controls: Access controls will be applied to all computer-resident information based on its Data Classification to ensure that it is not improperly disclosed, modified, deleted, or rendered unavailable.

Access Approval: System access will not be granted to any user without appropriate approval. Management is to immediately notify the Security Administrator and report all significant changes in end-user duties or employment status. User access is to be immediately revoked if the individual has been terminated. In addition, user privileges are to be appropriately changed if the user is transferred to a different job.

Limiting User Access: <COMPANY NAME> approved access controls, such as user log-on scripts, menus, session managers, and other access controls will be used to limit user access to only those network applications and functions for which they have been authorized.

Need-to-Know: Users will be granted access to information on a "need-to-know" basis. That is, users will only receive access to the minimum applications and privileges required performing their jobs.

Compliance Statements: Users who access to this <COMPANY NAME>'s information systems must sign a compliance statement prior to issuance of a user ID. A signature on this compliance statement indicates the user understands and agrees to abide by these <COMPANY NAME> policies and procedures related to computers and information systems. Annual confirmations will be required of all system users.

Audit Trails and Logging: Logging and auditing trails are based on the Data Classification of the systems.

Confidential Systems: Access to confidential systems will be logged and audited in a manner that allows the following information to be deduced:

- Access time
- User account
- Method of access
- All privileged commands must be traceable to specific user accounts

In addition, logs of all inbound access into <COMPANY NAME>'s internal network by systems outside of its defined network perimeter must be maintained. Audit trails for confidential systems should be backed up and stored in accordance with <COMPANY NAME>'s backup and disaster recovery plans. All system and application logs must be maintained in a form that cannot readily be viewed by unauthorized persons. All logs must be audited on a periodic basis. Audit results should be included in periodic management reports.

Access for Nonemployees: Individuals who are not employees, contractors, consultants, or business partners must not be granted a user ID or otherwise be given privileges to use the <COMPANY NAME> computers or information systems unless the written approval of the Department Head has first been obtained. Before any third party or business partner is given access to the <COMPANY NAME> computers or information systems, a chain of trust agreement defining the terms and conditions of such access must have been signed by a responsible manager at the third-party organization.

Unauthorized Access: Employees are prohibited from gaining unauthorized access to any other information systems or in any way damaging, altering, or disrupting the operations of these systems. System privileges allowing the modification of "production data" must be restricted to "production" applications.

Remote Access: Remote access must conform at least minimally to all statutory requirements, including but not limited to HCFA, HRS-323C, and HIPAA.

Password Policy

PURPOSE

The purpose of this policy is to ensure that only authorized users gain access to <COMPANY NAME>'s information systems.

POLICY

To gain access to <COMPANY NAME>'s information systems, authorized users, as a means of authentication, must supply individual user passwords. These passwords must conform to certain rules contained in this document. Who is affected: This policy affects all employees of <COMPANY NAME> and it's subsidiaries, and all contractors, consultants, temporary employees, and business partners. Employees who deliberately violate this policy will be subject to disciplinary action up to and including termination.

Affected Systems: This policy applies to all computer and communication systems owned or operated by <COMPANY NAME> and its subsidiaries. Similarly, this policy applies to all platforms (operating systems) and all application systems.

User Authentication: All systems will require a valid user ID and password. All unnecessary operating system or application user IDs not assigned to an individual user will be deleted or disabled.

Password Storage: Passwords will not be stored in readable form without access control or in other locations where unauthorized persons might discover them. All such passwords are to be strictly controlled using either physical security or computer security controls.

Application Passwords Required: All programs, including third-party purchased software and applications developed internally by <COMPANY NAME>, must be password protected.

Choosing Passwords: All user-chosen passwords must contain at least one alphabetic and one nonalphabetic character. The use of control characters and other nonprinting characters are prohibited. All users must be automatically forced to change their passwords appropriate to the classification level of information. To obtain a new password, a user must present suitable identification.

Changing Passwords: All passwords must be promptly changed if they are suspected of being disclosed, or known to have been disclosed to unauthorized parties. All users must be forced to change their passwords at least once every sixty (60) days.

Password Constraints: The display and printing of passwords should be masked, suppressed, or otherwise obscured so that unauthorized parties will not be able to observe or subsequently recover them. After three unsuccessful attempts to enter a password, the involved user ID must be: (a) suspended until reset by a system administrator, (b) temporarily disabled for no less than three minutes, or (c) if dial-up or other external network connections are involved, disconnected.

APPENDIX C.4
eHealth Code of Ethics

©eHealth Ethics Initiative 2000
Permission is granted to use with acknowledgment of source.

Vision Statement

The goal of the ***eHealth Code of Ethics*** is to ensure that people worldwide can confidently and with full understanding of known risks realize the potential of the Internet in managing their own health and the health of those in their care.

Introduction

The Internet is changing how people give and receive health information and health care. All people who use the Internet for health-related purposes—patients, health care professionals and administrators, researchers, those who create or sell health products or services, and other stakeholders—must join together to create a safe environment and enhance the value of the Internet for meeting health care needs. Because health information, products, and services have the potential both to improve health and to do harm, organizations and individuals that provide health information on the Internet have obligations to be trustworthy, provide high quality content, protect users' privacy, and adhere to standards of best practices for online commerce and online professional services in health care.

People who use Internet health sites and services share a responsibility to help assure the value and integrity of the health Internet by exercising judgment in using sites, products, and services, and by providing meaningful feedback about online health information, products, and services.

Definitions

Health information includes information for staying well, preventing and managing disease, and making other decisions related to health and health care. It includes information for making decisions about health products and health services. It may be in the form of data, text, audio, and/or video. It may involve enhancements through programming and interactivity.

Health products include drugs, medical devices, and other goods used to diagnose and treat illnesses or injuries or to maintain health. Health products include both drugs and medical devices subject to regulatory approval by agencies such as the U.S. Food and Drug Administration or U.K. Medicines Control Agency *and* vitamin, herbal, or other nutritional supplements and other products not subject to such regulatory oversight.

Health services include specific, personal medical care or advice; management of medical records; communication between health care providers and/or patients and health plans or insurers, or health care facilities regarding treatment decisions, claims, billing for services, etc.; and other services provided to support health care. Health services also include listserves, bulletin boards, chat rooms, and other online venues for the exchange of health information. Like health information, health services may be in the form of data, text, audio, and/or video, and may involve enhancements through programming and interactivity.

Anyone who uses the Internet for health-related reasons has a right to expect that organizations and individuals who provide health information, products or services online will uphold the following guiding principles: Disclose information that if known by consumers would likely affect consumers' understanding or use of the site or purchase or use of a product or service, and follow these principles:

> **Candor:** *People who use the Internet for health-related purposes need to be able to judge for themselves that the sites they visit and services they use are credible and trustworthy.* Sites should clearly indicate:

- Who owns or has a significant financial interest in the site or service
- What the purpose of the site or service is. *For example,* whether it is solely educational, sells health products or services, or offers personal medical care or advice
- Any relationship (financial, professional, personal, or other) that a reasonable person would believe would likely influence his or her perception of the information, products, or services offered by the site
- *For example,* if the site has commercial sponsors or partners, who those sponsors/partners are and whether they provide content for the site. "Be truthful and not deceptive."

Honesty: *People who seek health information on the Internet need to know that products or services are described truthfully and that information they receive is not presented in a misleading way.* They should clearly distinguish content intended to promote or sell a product, service, or organization from educational or scientific content. Provide health information that is accurate, easy to understand, and up to date. Sites should be forthright:
- In all content used to promote the sale of health products or services
- In any claims about the efficacy, performance, or benefits of products or services

Quality: *To make wise decisions about their health care, people need and have the right to expect that sites will provide accurate, well-supported information and products and services of high quality.* To assure that the health information they provide is accurate, eHealth sites and services should make good faith efforts to:
- Evaluate information rigorously and fairly, including information used to describe products or services
- Provide information that is consistent with the best available evidence
- Assure that when personalized medical care or advice is provided that care or advice is given by a qualified practitioner
- Indicate clearly whether information is based on scientific studies, expert consensus, or professional or personal experience or opinion
- Acknowledge that some issues are controversial and when that is the case make good faith efforts to present all reasonable sides in a fair and balanced way

- *For example,* advise users that there are alternative treatments for a particular health condition, such as surgery or radiation for prostate cancer

Clarity: *Information and services must be easy for consumers to understand and use.* Sites should present information and describe products or services in language that is clear, easy to read, and appropriate for intended users.

- *For example,* in culturally appropriate ways in the primary language (or languages) of the site's expected audience *and* in a way that accommodates special needs users may have
- *For example,* in large type or through audio channels for users whose vision is impaired. Sites that provide information primarily for educational or scientific purposes should guarantee the independence of their editorial policy and practices by assuring that only the site's content editors determine editorial content and have the authority to reject advertising that they believe is inappropriate.

Timeliness: *Consumers have a right to expect that the information they receive is up to date. Sites should clearly indicate:*

- When the site published the information it provides (and what version of the information users are seeing if it has been revised since it was first published)
- When the site most recently reviewed the information
- Whether the site has made substantive changes in the information and if so, when the information was most recently updated

Respect for users' right to self-determine: *Provide the information users need to make their own judgments about the health information, products, or services provided by the site.* Individuals need to be able to judge for themselves the quality of the health information they find on the Internet. Sites should describe clearly and accurately how content is developed for the site by telling users:

- What sources the site or content provider has used, with references or links to those sources
- How the site evaluates content and what criteria are used to evaluate content, including on what basis the site decides to provide specific links to other sites or services
- *For example,* by describing the site's editorial board and policies when health products or services are subject to government regulation, sites should tell users whether those products (such as drugs or medical devices) have been approved by appropriate

regulatory agencies, such as the U.S. Food and Drug Administration or U.K. Medicines Control Agency

Informed Consent: *People who use the Internet for health-related reasons have the right to be informed* that personal data may be gathered, and to choose whether they will allow their personal data to be shared or how their personal data may be collected, used, or shared (collected and whether they will allow it to be used or shared). They also have a right to be able to choose, consent, and control when and how they actively engage in a commercial relationship. Sites should clearly disclose:

- That there are potential risks to users' privacy on the Internet
- *For example,* that other organizations or individuals may be able to collect personal data when someone visits a site, without that site's knowledge; or that some jurisdictions (such as the European Union) protect privacy more stringently than others

Sites should not collect, use, or share personal data without the user's *specific affirmative consent.* To assure that users understand and make informed decisions about providing personal data, sites should indicate clearly and accurately

- What data is being collected when users visit the site
- Who is collecting that data
- *For example,* data about which parts of the site the user visited, or the user's name and e-mail address, or specific data about the user's health or online purchases
- *For example,* the site itself, or a third party how the site will use that data
- *For example,* to help the site provide better services to users, as part of a scientific study, or to provide personalized medical care or advice
- Whether the site knowingly shares data with other organizations or individuals and if so, what data it shares
- Which organizations or individuals the site shares data with and how it expects its affiliates to use that data
- Obtain users' affirmative consent to collect, use, or share personal data in the ways described
- What consequences there may be when a visitor refuses to give personal data
- *For example,* whether the site will share users' personal data with other organizations or individuals and for what purposes, and note when personal data will be shared with organizations or individuals in other countries

– *For example,* to collect and use the visitor's personal data in scientific research, or for commercial reasons such as sending information about new products or services to the user, or to share his or her personal data with other organizations or individuals

– *For example,* that the site may not be able to tailor the information it provides to the visitor's particular needs, or that the visitor may not have access to all areas of the site. "E-commerce" sites have an obligation to make clear to users when they are about to engage in a commercial transaction and to obtain users' specific affirmative consent to participate in that commercial transaction.

Privacy: *People who use the Internet for health-related reasons have the right to expect that personal data they provide will be kept confidential.* Personal health data in particular may be very sensitive, and the consequences of inappropriate disclosure can be grave. To protect users, sites that collect personal data should:

– Take reasonable steps to prevent unauthorized access to or use of personal data

– Make it easy for users to review personal data they have given and to update it or correct it when appropriate

– Adopt reasonable mechanisms to trace how personal data is used

– Tell how the site stores users' personal data and for how long it stores that data

– Assure that when personal data is "de-identified" (that is, when the user's name, e-mail address, or other data that might identify him or her has been removed from the file) it cannot be linked back to the user

– *For example,* by using "audit trails" that show who viewed the data and when

– *For example,* by "encrypting" data, protecting files with passwords, or using appropriate security software for all transactions involving users' personal medical or financial data

Professionalism in Online Health Care: Respect fundamental ethical obligations to patients; physicians, nurses, pharmacists, therapists, and all other health care professionals who provide specific, personal medical care or advice online should:

– Abide by the ethical codes that govern their professions as clients *and* practitioners in face-to-face relationships

– Do no harm

– Put patients' and clients' interests first

- Protect patients' confidentiality
- Clearly disclose any sponsorships, financial incentives, or other information that would likely affect the patient's or client's perception of professional's role or the services offered
- Clearly disclose what fees, if any, will be charged for the online consultation and how payment for services is to be made
- Obey the laws and regulations of relevant jurisdiction(s), including applicable laws governing professional licensing and prescribing. Inform and educate patients and clients about the limitations of online health care.

The Internet can be a powerful tool for helping to meet patients' health care needs, but users need to understand that it also has limitations. Health care professionals who practice on the Internet should clearly and accurately:

- Identify themselves and tell patients or clients where they practice and what their professional credentials are
- Describe the terms and conditions of the particular online interaction
- Make good faith efforts to understand the patient's or client's particular circumstances and to help him or her identify health care resources that are available locally
- Give clear instructions for follow-up care when appropriate or necessary
- *For example,* whether the health care professional will provide general advice about a particular health condition or will make specific recommendations and or referrals for the patient or client, or whether the health care professional can and will or cannot and will not prescribe medications in the particular situation
- *For example,* to help the patient or client determine whether particular treatment is available in his or her home community or only from providers outside his or her community

Health care professionals who offer personal medical services or advice online should:

- Clearly and accurately describe the constraints of online diagnosis and treatment recommendations
- Help "e-patients" understand when online consultation can and when it cannot and should not take the place of a face-to-face interaction with a health care provider. Ensure that organizations and sites with which they affiliate are trustworthy.
- *For example,* providers should stress that because the online health care professional cannot examine the patient, it is impor-

tant for patients to describe their health care needs as clearly they can.

Responsible Partnering

People need to be confident that organizations and individuals who operate on the Internet undertake to partner only with trustworthy individuals or organizations. Whether they are for profit or nonprofit, sites should make reasonable efforts to ensure that sponsors, partners, or other affiliates abide by applicable law and uphold the same ethical standards as the sites themselves insist that current or prospective sponsors not influence the way search results are displayed for specific information on key words or topics And they should indicate clearly to users:

- Whether links to other sites are provided for information only or are endorsements of those other sites when they are leaving the site
- *For example,* by use of transition screens provide meaningful opportunity for users to give feedback to the site

Accountability

People need to be confident that organizations and individuals that provide health information, products, or services on the Internet take users' concerns seriously and that sites make good faith efforts to ensure that their practices are ethically sound. eHealth sites should indicate clearly to users how they can:

- Contact the owner of the site or service or the party responsible for managing the site or service
- Provide easy-to-use tools for visitors to give feedback about the site and the quality of its information, products, or services
- Review complaints from users promptly and respond in a timely and appropriate manner
- *For example,* how to contact specific manager(s) or customer service representatives with authority to address problems and monitor their compliance with the eHealth Code of Ethics

Sites should encourage users to notify the site's manager(s) or customer service representatives if they believe that a site's commercial or noncommercial partners or affiliates, including sites to which links are provided, may violate law or ethical principles. eHealth sites should describe their policies for self-monitoring clearly for users, and should encourage creative problem solving among site staff and affiliates.

APPENDIX C.5

Chain of Trust Agreement

This Chain of Trust Agreement is made the _____ day of _____, 2004, at _____, by and between HEALTH CARE ORGANIZATION (the "ORGANIZATION") and BUSINESS PARTNER (the "RECIPIENT").

WHEREAS, ORGANIZATION maintains and operates _____, Honolulu, Hawaii;

WHEREAS, RECIPIENT performs _____ work which requires it to have access to information regarding ORGANIZATION's confidential and proprietary health information that is considered protected pursuant to federal, state and/or local laws or regulations ("INFORMATION");

WHEREAS, ORGANIZATION desires to protect the confidentiality and integrity of the INFORMATION and to prevent inappropriate disclosure of the information;

NOW THEREFORE, the parties agree as follows:

1. CONFIDENTIALITY

Any and all INFORMATION shall be kept confidential by RECIPIENT, and shall not, without legal basis to do so and the prior written approval of ORGANIZATION, be made available to any individual or organization by RECIPIENT or used by RECIPIENT for any purpose other than the performance hereunder. RECIPIENT shall require its employees, contractors and agents to comply with the obligations set forth in this section.

In addition, RECIPIENT shall maintain, and shall require that its employees, contractors and agents maintain the confidentiality of all INFORMATION. RECIPIENT shall comply, and shall require its employees, contractor and agents to comply, with all federal and state statutes and regulations concerning confidentiality of INFORMATION, including without limitations, Chapter 323C of the Hawaii Revised Statutes and any regulations promulgated pursuant thereto, as such statutes and regulations currently exist and as they may be amended from time to time. This provision shall survive the termination or expiration of this agreement.

2. TERM

This Agreement shall be effective _____, 2000, and shall continue _____. This Agreement shall automatically renew itself for an additional twelve-month period unless otherwise terminated by either party. In the event that this Agreement is automatically renewed, RECIP-IENT agrees to be bound by the Terms and Conditions currently in effect. The confidentiality provisions of this Agreement shall survive indefinitely, even beyond the termination of this Agreement.

3. DISCLOSURES REQUIRED BY LAW

In the event that RECIPIENT is required by law to disclose INFORMATION, RECIPIENT will provide ORGANIZATION with written notice immediately and in advance of the disclosure, so that ORGANIZATION may take whatever action is deemed appropriate.

4. STATE AND FEDERAL STATUTE COMPLIANCE

RECIPIENT shall maintain all licenses, accreditations and approvals customary to its business, and shall observe and comply with all laws, ordinances, rules, and regulations of the federal, state, county or municipal governments, now in force or which may hereinafter be in force. Further, RECIPIENT understands and acknowledges that RECIPIENT has an affirmative duty to be knowledgeable about and regarding existing laws, rules and regulations that are applicable to the goods and services covered by this Agreement, and how these laws, rules and regulation apply to RECIPIENT s business.

5. POLICY AND PROCEDURE REVIEW

Upon request, RECIPIENT shall make available to ORGANIZATION any and all documentation relevant to the safeguarding of INFORMATION including but not limited to current policies and procedures, operational manuals and/or instructions, and/or employment and/or third party agreements.

6. REPORT OF IMPROPER DISCLOSURE or SYSTEMS COMPROMISE

ORGANIZATION and RECIPIENT agree to immediately notify all parties within their Chain of Trust of any improper or unauthorized access and disclosure of the INFORMATION, or any misuse of the INFORMATION, including but not limited to systems compromises. ORGANIZATION and RECIPIENT will take all necessary steps to prevent and limit any further improper or unauthorized disclosure and misuse of information. RECIPIENT shall also maintain an incident log of all improper or unauthorized disclosures. At the request of ORGANIZATION, RECIPIENT will make available to ORGANIZATION a copy of incident log.

7. RETURN OF MATERIALS

Unless otherwise specifically required by statute or rule, RECIPIENT shall upon request, or at the conclusion of the agreement, return or destroy all material containing or reflecting any ORGANIZATION INFORMATION whether prepared by ORGANIZATION or as a result of providing services for which the RECIPIENT has been specifically authorized by ORGANIZATION. In the case of destruction of the material, the RECIPIENT shall exercise due diligence to destroy the INFORMATION in a manner that will render non-retrievable all documents, memoranda, notes or other writings prepared by RECIPIENT, or its representatives, which are based on the INFORMATION.

8. SUB-CONTRACTORS

RECIPIENT shall obtain written consent from ORGANIZATION prior to disclosure of INFORMATION to any third party. In addition RECIPIENT shall require any third party to execute a CHAIN of TRUST AGREEMENT that upholds the standards contained within this Agreement.

9. AGENCY RELATIONSHIP

The parties acknowledge and agree that solely for the purposes of Hawaii Revised Statutes Chapter 323C, in providing the services required by the Agreement, RECIPIENT is acting as ORGANIZATION's agent under an agency relationship. As such, RECIPIENT agrees that it shall be bound by Chapter 323C of the Hawaii Revised Statutes and any regulations promulgated pursuant thereto, as such statute and regulations currently exist and as they may be amended from time to time.

10. TERMINATION

If, for any reason, RECIPIENT fails to satisfactorily fulfill in a timely or proper manner RECIPIENT's obligations under this Agreement or breaches any of the promises, terms or conditions of this Agreement, and having been given notice of and opportunity of up to 5 days to cure any such default and not having taken satisfactory corrective action within the time specified by ORGANIZATION, ORGANIZATION hall have the right to terminate this Agreement by giving written notice to RECIPIENT of such termination at least seven calendar days before the effective calendar date of such termination. ORGANIZATION may terminate this agreement immediately upon written notice to RECIPIENT if RECIPIENT fails to comply with section 4 of this Agreement. Without cause, either party to this Agreement shall have the right to terminate this Agreement by giving written notice to the other party of such termination at least thirty calendar days before the effective date of such termination.

11. GOVERNMENT ACCESS TO RECORDS

In Accordance with 42 U.S.C. section 1395x(v)(1)(I), RECIPIENT agrees that until the expiration of four (4) years after the completion of services pursuant to this Agreement, RECIPIENT shall make available, upon written request to the Secretary of Health and Human Services, (for Comptroller General of the United States or any of their duly authorized representatives) its contract and books, its documents, and records which are necessary to certify the nature and extent of the cost for services agreed herein to be provided.

Further, if RECIPIENT carries out its duties hereunder through a subcontract with a value or cost of $10,000.00 or more over a twelve-month period, such subcontractor shall make available, until the expiration of four (4) years after completion of services pursuant to this Agreement, upon written request to the Secretary of Health and Human Services, (for Comptroller General of the United States, or any of their duly authorized representatives) its subcontract, books, documents, and records which are necessary to certify the nature and extent of the cost for the services agreed herein to be provided.

12. ADDITIONAL ACCESS TO INFORMATION

If RECIPIENT significantly alters the INFORMATION provided by ORGA-NIZATION, ORGANIZATION shall have the right to access the altered information upon written request to RECIPIENT. Such access shall be provided to ORGANIZATION within a reasonable period after receipt of the request and shall be during the normal business hours of RECIPIENT. RECIPIENT shall incorporate changes or amendments to the INFORMA-TION if requested by the ORGANIZATION.

13. INJUNCTIVE RELIEF

RECIPIENT acknowledges that the remedy at law for any breach by it or the terms of this Agreement shall be inadequate and that the damages resulting from such breach are not readily susceptible to being measured in monetary terms. Accordingly, in the event of a breach or threatened breach by RECIPIENT of the terms of this Agreement, ORGANIZATION shall be entitled to immediate injunctive relief and may obtain a temporary order restraining any threatened or further breach. Nothing herein shall be construed as prohibiting ORGANIZATION from pursuing any other remedies available to ORGANIZATION for such breach or threatened breach, including recovery of damages from RECIPIENT. RECIPIENT further represents that it understands and agrees that the provisions of this agreement shall be strictly enforced and construed against it.

14. THIRD PARTY BENEFICIARIES

Both parties understand and agree that other parties (individuals or entities) who are the subject of the INFORMATION provided to RECIPIENT are intended to be third party beneficiaries of this Agreement.

15. SEVERABILITY

In the event that any provision of this Agreement violates any applicable statute, ordinance or rule of law in any jurisdiction that governs this Agreement, such provision shall be ineffective to the extent of such violation without invalidating any other provision of this Agreement.

16. CONSTRUCTION OF AGREEMENT

The language in all parts of this Agreement shall in all cases be simply construed according to its fair meaning and not strictly for or against the RECIPIENT or ORGANIZATION. The headings preceding each paragraph are for convenience only and shall not in any way be construed to effect the meaning of the paragraphs themselves.

17. HOLD HARMLESS

RECIPIENT agrees to indemnify, defend and hold harmless ORGANIZATION, its directors, officers, agents, shareholders, and employees against all claims, demands, or causes of action that may arise from RECIPIENT's employees, agents, or independent contractors improper disclosure of the INFORMATION and from any intentional or negligent acts or omissions.

18. GOVERNMENT HEALTHCARE PROGRAM REPRESENTATIONS

RECIPIENT hereby represents and warrants to ORGANIZATION that neither RECIPIENT, its shareholders, members, directors, officers, agents, or employees have been excluded or served a notice of exclusion or have been served with a notice of proposed exclusion, or have committed any acts which are cause for exclusion, from participation in, or had any sanctions, or civil or criminal penalties imposed under, any federal or state healthcare program, including but not limited to Medicare or Medicaid, or have been convicted, under federal or state law (including without limitation a plea of nolo contendere or participation in a first offender deterred adjudication or other arrangement whereby a judgment of conviction has been withheld), of a criminal offense related to (a) the neglect or abuse of a patient, (b) the delivery of an item or service, including the performance of management or administrative services related to the delivery of an item or service, under a federal or state healthcare program, (c) fraud, theft, embezzlement, breach of fiduciary responsibility, or other financial misconduct in connection with the delivery of a healthcare item or service or with respect to any act or omission in any program operated by or financed in whole or in part by any federal, state or local government agency, (d) the unlawful, manufacture, distribution, prescription or dispensing of a controlled substance, or (e) interference with or obstruction of any investigation into any criminal offense described in (a) through (d) above. RECIPIENT further agrees to notify ORGANIZATION immediately after RECIPIENT becomes aware that the foregoing representation and warranty may be inaccurate or may be incorrect.

19. ENTIRE AGREEMENT; AMENDMENTS; NO WAIVER

This Agreement contains the entire agreement between the parties with respect to the matters covered by this Agreement and supersedes all prior negotiations, agreements and employment contracts between the parties, whether oral or in writing. This Agreement may not be amended, altered or modified except by written agreement signed by all parties of this Agreement. No provision of this agreement may be waived except by an agreement in writing signed by the waiving party. A waiver of any term or provision shall not be construed as a waiver of any other term or provision.

20. AUTHORITY

The persons signing below have the right and authority to execute this Agreement for their respective entities and no further approvals are necessary to create a binding Agreement.

21. GOVERNING LAW

This Agreement shall be governed by the laws of the State of Hawaii and shall be construed in accordance therewith.

IN WITNESS WHEREOF, the parties have executed this CHAIN OF TRUST AGREEMENT the day and year first written above.

Appendix
D

GUIDE TO HIPAA SECURITY ASSESSMENT

Prepared by WorkSmart MD, A Meyer Technologies, Inc. Company

Extracted from the HIPAA Rx™ Instruction Guides

HIPAA mandates the adoption of **new** security standards to protect an individual's health information while permitting the appropriate access and use of that information by providers, clearinghouses, and health plans. The law also mandates that a new electronic signature standard be used where an electronic signature is employed in the transmission of a HIPAA standard transaction. The proposed standard for **security of health information and electronic signatures** was published in 1998. The proposed standard requires healthcare entities that engage in electronic maintenance or transmission of health information to **assess** their own security needs and risks and **devise, implement, and maintain** appropriate security to address their business requirements. These required measures, which must be documented and maintained regularly, are:

- Administrative procedures
- Physical safeguards
- Technical security services

It is also recommend that you review the HIPAA Security Summary document located in the regulations module. This short document highlights the key elements of HIPAA Security within a healthcare provider location. Please Note: (1) While we have attempted to categorize security requirements for ease of understanding and reading clarity, there are overlapping areas on the matrix in which the same requirements are restated in a slightly different context. (2) To ensure that no Requirement or Implementation feature is considered more important than another is, this matrix has been presented, within each subject area, in alphabetical order.

Administrative Procedures to Protect Data Confidentiality, Integrity, and Availability	
Requirement	**Implementation**
Certification	
Contingency plan (all listed features must be implemented)	Applications and data criticality analysis
	Data backup plan
	Disaster recovery plan
	Emergency mode operation plan
	Testing and revision
Formal mechanism for processing records	
Information access control (all listed features must be implemented)	Access authorization
	Access establishment
	Access modification
Internal audit	
Personnel security (all listed features must be implemented)	Assure supervision of maintenance personnel by authorized knowledgeable personnel
	Personnel security policy/procedure
	Maintenance of access authorizations records
	Operating, and in some cases, maintenance personnel have proper access authorization
	System users, including maintenance personnel, trained in security

Administrative Procedures to Protect Data Confidentiality, Integrity, and Availability	
Requirement	Implementation
	Personnel clearance procedure
Security configuration mgmt. (all listed features must be implemented)	Documentation
	Hardware/software installation and maintenance review and testing for security features
	Inventory
	Security testing
	Virus checking
Security incident procedures (all listed features must be implemented)	Report procedures
	Response procedures
Security management process (all listed features must be implemented)	Risk analysis
	Risk management
	Sanction policy
	Security policy
Termination procedures (all listed features must be implemented)	Combination locks changed
	Removal from access lists
	Removal of user accounts
	Turn in keys, token, or cards that allow access
Training (all listed features must be implemented)	Awareness training for all personnel (including management)
	Periodic security reminders
	User education concerning virus protection
	User education in importance of monitoring log-in success/failure, and how to report discrepancies
	User education in password management

Physical Safeguards to Protect Data Confidentiality, Integrity, and Availability	
Requirement	Implementation
Assigned security responsibility	
Media controls (all listed features must be implemented)	Access control
	Accountability (tracking mechanism)
	Data backup
	Data storage
	Disposal
Physical access controls (limited access)(all listed implementation must be implemented)	Disaster recovery
	Emergency mode operation
	Equipment control (into and out of site)
	Facility security plan
	Procedures for verifying access authorizations prior to physical access
	Maintenance records
	Need-to-know procedures for personnel access
	Sign-in for visitors and escort, if appropriate
	Testing and revision
Policy/guideline on workstation use	
Secure workstation location	
Security awareness training	

Technical Security Services to Protect Data Confidentiality, Integrity, and Availability	
Requirement	**Implementation**
Access control (The following feature must be implemented: procedure for emergency access. In addition, at least one of the following three features must be implemented: context-based access, role-based access, user-based access. The use of encryption is optional)	Context-based access
	Encryption
	Procedure for emergency access
	Role-based access
	User-based access
Audit controls	
Authorization control (at least one of the listed features must be implemented)	Role-based access
	User-based access
Data authentication	
Entity authentication (The following features must be implemented: automatic log-off, unique user identification. In addition, at least one of the other listed features must be implemented)	Automatic log-off
	Biometric
	Password
	PIN
	Telephone callback
	Token
	Unique user identification

Technical Security Mechanisms to Guard against Unauthorized Access to Data that Is Transmitted over a Communications Network	
Requirement	**Implementation**
Communications/network controls (The following features must be implemented: integrity controls, message authentication. If communications or networking is employed, one of the following features must be implemented: access controls, encryption. In addition, if using a network, the following four features must be implemented: alarm, audit trail, entity authentication, event reporting)	Access controls
	Alarm
	Audit trail
	Encryption
	Entity authentication
	Event reporting
	Integrity controls
	Message authentication
Electronic Signature	
Requirement	**Implementation**
Digital signature (If digital signature is employed, the following three implementation features must be implemented: message integrity, nonrepudiation, user authentication. Other features are optional)	Ability to add attributes
	Continuity of signature capability
	Countersignatures
	Independent verifiability
	Interoperability
	Message integrity
	Multiple signatures
	Nonrepudiation
	Transportability
	User authentication

THE SECURITY REQUIREMENTS OF HIPAA

Requirements for Security Administration

SEC.01 Certification §.308(a)(1)

HIPAA Requirement

(The technical evaluation performed as part of, and in support of, the accreditation process that establishes the extent to which a particular computer system or network design and implementation meet a pre-specified set of security requirements. This evaluation may be performed internally or by an external accrediting agency.)

Explanation of HIPAA Regulation

Certification is the process of determining whether technical security controls are implemented and comply with specified criteria. Each covered entity is required to establish a certification process that demonstrates and documents that its computer systems and networks meet these criteria. Either internal staff or external persons may perform certifications. The process should consider risks identified in the risk assessment process.

Key Issues

- What systems and services require certification?
- How often should certification occur?
- Who or what organization is the certifying authority? Is it internal or external? How will the certifying authority be selected?
- Do reference documents exist to describe the covered entity's secure configuration of network components, servers, databases, and applications?
- Is there a periodic comparison of the actual configuration against the reference documents to confirm compliance or reveal non-compliance? If there are differences, is there a process for correction?
- Do routine testing, auditing, and change management procedures support the certification process?
- What is the relationship between auditors and certifiers?
- With what frequency or upon what event(s) should certification be done?

Actions required to address these

- Implement a certification process to determine the extent to which systems and networks meet established security criteria.

Actions highly recommended to address these

- Document the network configuration.
- Ensure that individuals performing certifications are knowledgeable about security requirements and best practices.
- Ensure that conflicts of interest do not exist in the certification process — specifically that certifiers are not responsible for the system or network's administration or maintenance.
- Perform certification a minimum of once every three years due to the changing nature of computer systems and accelerating rate of change of IT-related security risks.
- Prepare a formal "Certification and Accreditation Report" upon the completion of certification and forward it, along with any recommendations on accreditation, to the accrediting official. Maintain records and reports of certification and accreditation activities for the last two certification efforts to provide for an adequate history of certification information and an audit trail of certification. Establish routine testing, auditing, and change management procedures to support the certification process.
- Consider certification for system changes prior to placing such systems into production.
- Consider a phased approach to certification in order to encourage continuity of the process.
- Consider linking the certification process to JCAHO Information Management requirements.
- Consider requiring formal security credentials for those conducting the certification process.

Roadblocks

In complex institutions, it may be difficult to establish the necessary credibility and authority for the certifier.

Comments

Although the evaluation of the program or one of its parts may be done by outside entities, the certification is a statement by senior management of the institution. State law on record keeping may mandate additional retention requirements. Covered entities should be prepared to budget for remedial action as necessary if deficiencies are discovered during the certification process.

SEC.02 *Chain of Trust Partner Agreement §.308(a)(2)*

HIPAA Requirement

A chain of trust partner agreement (a contract entered into by two business partners in which the partners agree to electronically exchange data and protect the integrity and confidentiality of the data exchanged).

Explanation of HIPAA Regulation

A Chain of Trust Agreement is required between two business partners whenever data is electronically exchanged. The Agreement requires that the sender and the receiver of the protected health information work with each other to maintain the information's integrity and confidentiality. Such contracts provide a legal basis for maintaining consistent levels of data integrity and confidentiality.

Key Issues

- With which persons or organizations is the health care provider, health plan, or health care clearinghouse required to execute a Chain of Trust Agreement (COT)?
- Is there a documented process for identifying all partners with which a COT is required? Does the COT identify a process or processes to ensure the integrity and confidentiality of the data transmitted?
- How will security responsibilities and accountabilities be determined, drafted, and monitored?
- Does more than one unit have the authority to contract with a business partner?
- Is there a process in place to assure that all AMC contracts have the required and appropriate language? Is there a process that will identify the data rights of the trading partners and incorporate such rights in the COT language?
- Does the agreement identify appropriate sanctions for failure to abide by its terms?
- Is the duration of the agreement appropriate?
- Is there a process in place to assure that all AMC contracting officers are aware of the need for, and know the requisites of, an effective COT?
- What organizational unit will be responsible for managing the COT policy implementation?

- Does the COT propagate with any further transfers of information between partners and their other partners?
- Does the COT survive other agreements with the partner?
- How do COTs relate to the business associate contractual terms in the Privacy rule?

Actions required to address these

- Develop a Chain of Trust Agreement with each party with which protected health information is shared, including language that states that:
  - The parties agree to electronically exchange data and protect the transmitted data.
  - Each party will maintain the integrity and confidentiality of the transmitted information.
- Develop a plan to update all current agreements to ensure that the terms and conditions do not contain any provisions, including data content and format definitions, which conflict with the standards outlined in the security regulations
- Develop a plan to ensure that all future agreements have appropriate provisions.

Actions highly recommended to address these

- Engage legal counsel to develop and review contract language for the COT.
- Establish monitors to ensure compliance by all parties subject to the agreement.
- Train all contracting officials about the nature and intent of the COT.
- Devise and promulgate a COT template for all Contracting Officers to use.
- Establish a process to determine when/how to activate the sanctions for nonperformance with regard to COT.
- Periodically review all current partnerships for COT need.
- Develop process to review partners' COTs for adequacy and fairness.

Roadblocks

It will likely be difficult to get approval for COTs which are inconsistent between partners, or which are perceived as unbalanced in responsibility. Contracts are frequently negotiated and approved by various departments within the University or AMC. Each area within the University and AMC must be trained as to when and with whom this required language should be used.

Comments

Since the originator of information bears the responsibility for improper disclosure or other security failures regarding that information, a COT is the only protection most providers will have once information is turned over to their partners in healthcare provision. As part of a compliance program, business associates should warrant, and the AMC department responsible for negotiating and signing the Agreement should verify, that the trading partner is not excluded from participation in any government program. Contracts should also include a statement that the trading partner warrants that any subcontractors or agents are not excluded from participation in any government program. The Chain of Trust Agreement in the Supplement contains language that can be used to satisfy both the proposed security regulation (discussed in this point) and the final privacy regulation (discussed in PRIV.03).

SEC.03 Contingency Planning §.380 (a)(3)

HIPAA Requirement

...a routinely updated plan for responding to a system emergency, that includes performing backups, preparing critical facilities that can be used to facilitate continuity of operations in the event of an emergency, and recovering from a disaster. The plan must include all of the following implementation features:

1. An applications and data criticality analysis (an entity's formal assessment of the sensitivity, vulnerabilities, and security of its programs and information it receives, manipulates, stores, or transmits).
2. A data backup plan (a documented and routinely updated plan to create and maintain, for a specific period of time, retrievable exact copies of information).
3. A disaster recovery plan (the part of an overall contingency plan that contains a process enabling an enterprise to restore any loss of data in the event of fire, vandalism, natural disaster, or system failure).
4. An emergency mode operation plan (the part of an overall contingency plan that contains a process enabling an enterprise to continue to operate in the event of fire, vandalism, natural disaster, or system failure).

5. Testing and revision procedures (the documented process of periodic testing of written contingency plans to discover weaknesses and the subsequent process of revising the documentation, if necessary).

Explanation of HIPAA Regulation

Each covered entity is required to maintain a contingency plan for responding to system emergencies involving systems that contain protected health information. The covered entity is required to perform periodic backups of data, have critical facilities for continuing operations in the event of an emergency, and have disaster recovery procedures in place for such systems. Systems that do not involve protected health information are not required to have contingency plans.

Key Issues

- What will be needed to recreate each data element in the event of an emergency? Has an assessment been performed?
- What is the appropriate frequency and depth of backups?
- Where should backup data be located?
- How easy is restoration of backup data?
- How timely would such a restoration be?
- How is security of data assured at the backup location?
- What is the mechanism for testing the plans and procedures?
- How long will backups be retained?
- How is overall integrity of data assured?
- How often will various levels or types of tests be performed?

Actions required to address these

- Assess all systems with protected health information for reasonably anticipated risks, focusing on the potential impact of the lack of availability of specific applications and data on the secure operation of the covered entity.
- Prepare a data backup plan that details how data will be maintained and duplicated in order to prevent its loss during a natural or man-made disaster.
- Prepare a disaster recovery plan that details how data and operations would be restored in a timely fashion following a catastrophic event or unanticipated interruption of operations. Prepare a plan

to use for emergency operations following a catastrophic event until normal operations can be restored.

■ Test these procedures periodically and revise them accordingly to address any weaknesses discovered during testing.

Actions highly recommended to address these

■ Develop a data storage plan that ensures that the medium and location of backup storage are secure from physical damage and that backup storage is separated in some way from the main site.

■ Dispose of information in a manner that maintains its security. Shred paper and wipe magnetic or optical media.

■ Make backups at regular intervals.

■ Develop a procedure covering the scope (full, incremental, and differential) of backups.

■ Provide adequate facilities to support recovery operations.

■ Test contingency and disaster recovery plans regularly, specifically including restoration of data.

■ Protect backup information at the same level as the original data.

Roadblocks

Identifying and testing critical components may be more realistic and cost effective than testing plans sufficiently often to ensure that they are viable. Formal disaster recovery/contingency plans usually occur at the level of central IT within an AMC. The distributed nature of support and systems within an AMC may serve as a roadblock to ensuring consistent planning.

Comments

The security regulations (unlike the privacy regulations) supersede conflicting state laws. Non-conflicting state laws, however, still apply and may affect various aspects of this plan. Also see: AMC.09 Stricter State Law, SEC.14 Media Controls.

SEC.04 Formal Mechanism for Processing Records §.308(a)(4)

HIPAA Requirement

Formal mechanism for processing record (documented policies and procedures for the routine and non-routine receipt, manipulation, storage, dissemination, transmission, or disposal of health information).

Explanation of HIPAA Regulation

Covered entities are required to maintain documented policies and procedures for the routine and non-routine receipt, manipulation, storage, dissemination, transmission, or disposal of protected health information.

Key Issues

- Do clear lines of authority and responsibilities exist that fit the structure and function of entities (Hospital, Departments, Sections)?
- Are there provisions for evaluating and improving policies and procedures at all levels?

Actions required to address these

- Develop and document processes to govern the creation of protected health information.
- Establish policies and procedures on storage of data, including administrative policies governing the length of time various types of data are to be stored and policies for the archiving and destruction of data.
- Establish policies for data dissemination within and external to the covered entity. (See Comments.)
- Develop policies for secure disposal of protected health information, including information contained on media and systems that are replaced.

Actions highly recommended to address these

- Protect records to a degree commensurate with the risk associated with them.
- Consider standardizing record management policies across the enterprise.

Roadblocks

The presence of already existing unofficial systems may act as a barrier to change, as these will need to be brought under the umbrella of protection. If staff members do not accept needed changes, then implementation may be delayed. Redundancy of records in multiple systems presents a challenge, with updates in one system not always filing or updating correctly in other systems downstream.

Comments

Policies external to the covered entity may be problematic in terms of generality or specificity. Standards such as message types (HL7, XML, etc.) may help in this regard.

SEC.05 Information Access and Control §.308(a)(5)

HIPAA Requirement

(Formal, documented policies and procedures for granting different levels of access to health care information) that includes all of the following implementation features:

1. Access authorization (information-use policies and procedures that establish the rules for granting access, for example, to a terminal, transaction, program, process, or some other user)
2. Access establishment (security policies and rules that determine an entity's initial right of access to a terminal, transaction, program, process, or some other user)
3. Access modification (security policies and rules that determine the types of, and reasons for, modification to an entity's established right of access, to a terminal, transaction, program, process, or some other user)

Explanation of HIPAA Regulation

Each covered entity is required to establish and maintain formal, documented policies and procedures for granting different levels of access to protected health information. These policies and procedures must, at a minimum, include:

- Access authorization policies and procedures
- Access establishment policies and procedures
- Access modification policies and procedures

Key Issues

- Does the covered entity currently have a documented access control policy?
- Is there a process to establish an individual right-to-know or need-to-know?
- Does the access control policy consider all means of access?

- Do procedures define the authorization requirements for various forms of protected health information, and is special authorization required for more sensitive information (e.g., psychiatry, infectious diseases, or genetic disorders)?
- Is access authorization documented and maintained?
- Is there a documented process for revoking access?
- How does the covered entity authorize, implement, and revoke emergency access?

Actions required to address these

- Establish documented policies and procedures to assign, implement, revoke, and modify access to protected health information.

Actions highly recommended to address these

- Create a process for determining access needs for individuals and other entities such as law enforcement and public health.
- Grant access based on need-to-know or right-to-know.
- Provide a means to review the effectiveness of access management and control. Assign responsibility for implementing the policy to specific individuals or organizations within the covered entity.
- Enact a process to modify access, taking into account the types of, and reasons for, previously established access.
- Require implementation of technical means to control information access. Require execution of a grantor-grantee agreement to honor information security requirements before access is granted.
- Establish a process to ensure that system access is available at appropriate times for repair and other maintenance purposes.
- Establish a documented plan to ensure that all workforce members can demonstrate knowledge of access control responsibilities and how to obtain access authorization.
- Establish a process whereby termination of a workforce member or other entity's need for data access will trigger timely revocation of access.
- Require data owners or stewards to list functions that will require access to data for which they are responsible.

Roadblocks

Any part of the access control process can be rendered ineffective if those with access do not respect the process — if the users do not understand their responsibilities and buy in to the program, it will not work.

Comments

Also see: SEC.19 Access Control.

Access control requirements appear throughout the security regulations in a number of different contexts relating to personnel security requirements, physical safeguards, technical security services, and technical security mechanisms. Access control is an integral part of almost every element of information security. Vulnerabilities in this area include *ad hoc* practices or incomplete policies and procedures for authorizing and establishing access to organizational systems, failure to include smaller departmental systems in access control policies and practices, and broken processes to address the modification and revocation of user access following job changes or termination.

SEC.06 Internal Audit §.308(a)(6)

HIPAA Requirement

...in-house review of the records of system activity (such as logins, file accesses, and security incidents) maintained by an organization.

Explanation of HIPAA Regulation

This requirement calls for periodic reviews of a covered entity's internal security controls, including records of logins, file accesses, and security incidents.

Key Issues

■ At what level in data structures should audits be maintained? Table? Record? Field?
■ How will this degrade system performance?
■ For what data will logs be maintained, and for how long?
■ Who will review the records? (The log itself may have protected health information in it.)
■ How much of the review can be done by software?
■ How often will audits occur?
■ What logged activity will be considered suspicious?
■ What actions will be taken in response to suspicious audit information?

Actions required to address these

Maintain, and periodically review, audit trails or activity logs for critical application systems, including user-written applications.

Actions highly recommended to address these

- Follow up on suspicious entries such as unauthorized accesses and access attempts.
- Identify and resolve inappropriate activity.
- Ensure that audit procedures validate the necessity for data input, processing, and output.
- Ensure that audit requirements and activities do not disrupt important business processes.
- Agree to and control the scope of the checks.
- Explicitly identify resources for performing the checks and ensure that they are available. Identify and agree to requirements for special or additional processing, such as prospective audits of user activity.
- Document all procedures, requirements, and responsibilities.
- Consider making logs of access to individuals' health information available to the subjects of the records via a "patient portal."
- Develop an audit process to ensure that users comply with access control procedures.

Roadblocks

Users, in carrying out their respective duties, should never feel threatened by an audit. In most cases, information systems personnel are checking a system for problem-solving purposes and it remains transparent to the user. If the user is made aware, it is usually for the purpose of problem solving or procedure correction.

Comments

The logs themselves may contain protected health information and should be appropriately secure. Additional controls may be required for systems that process or have an impact on sensitive, valuable, or critical organizational assets. Such controls should be determined by the security requirements and a formal risk assessment. Audit trails may become evidence in legal proceedings, so care should be taken to protect their integrity in order to preserve their usefulness for such purposes. Take the possibility of using audit trails as evidence into account when deciding how long they should be retained. Prospective audits are onerous and usually require clinician input to resolve need-to-know issues; they should be performed sparingly and only with good cause as determined through the risk analysis process. Audits can be a significant cost consideration and logging records could have an unreasonable cost impact. A cost/benefit and risk analysis would be in order to determine what systems should employ logging and how long the records should be stored. Formal audit log retention standards are prudent. Destruction of log data should not appear to be an attempt to destroy evidence in the case of legal action. Also see: SEC.20 Audit Controls.

SEC.07 Personnel Security §.308(a)(7)

HIPAA Requirement

(All personnel who have access to any sensitive information have the required authorities as well as all appropriate clearances) that includes all of the following implementation features:

1. Assuring supervision of maintenance personnel by an authorized, knowledgeable person. These procedures are documented formal procedures and instructions for the oversight of maintenance personnel when the personnel are near health information pertaining to an individual.
2. Maintaining a record of access authorizations (ongoing documentation and review of the levels of access granted to a user, program, or procedure accessing health information).
3. Assuring that operating and maintenance personnel have proper access authorization (formal documented policies and procedures for determining the access level to be granted to individuals working on, or near, health information).
4. Establishing personnel clearance procedures (a protective measure applied to determine that unclassified automated information is admissible).
5. Establishing and maintaining personnel security policies and procedures (formal documentation of procedures to ensure that all personnel who have access to sensitive information have the required authority as well as appropriate clearances).
6. Assuring that system users, including maintenance personnel, receive security awareness training.

Explanation of HIPAA Regulation

Each covered entity must establish a personnel security clearance process to determine administratively that persons and computers are trustworthy before giving them access to protected health information. This process must account for, and document, levels of access granted to individuals, programs, and procedures. The process must also address persons who fill roles where incidental access to protected health information may occur, such as system and network support and maintenance personnel. Supervision of uncleared or unauthorized personnel, such as support and maintenance personnel, is necessary unless their access to protected health information can be precluded. Awareness training on these policies and procedures is required for both those who are cleared for and given access and those who have incidental access.

Key Issues

- How closely must maintenance personnel be supervised?
- How often should procedures, instructions, and levels of access be reviewed?
- How broad, or how specific, should security training be? What should it cover?
- How often should security training be repeated for employees? For vendors and other contracting personnel?

Actions required to address these

- Establish written personnel clearance procedures for determining the appropriateness of access to protected health information or systems.
- Maintain documentation regarding the levels of access granted to each individual, program, and procedure.
- Review access levels periodically.
- Review access levels when the status of the workforce member changes.
- Ensure that system users and technical maintenance staff receive security awareness training. Ensure that maintenance and vendor personnel are supervised when working on or near protected health information.

Actions highly recommended to address these

- Conduct records checks on applicants for employment, including residence, employment, criminal history, and education, when job requires access to protected health information. (See Comments.)
- Require staff and maintenance/vendor employees to sign non-disclosure statements before being given access to protected health information.

Roadblocks

Workforce member status changes can be difficult to track in a large covered entity. Consistent application of personnel access policies may be problematic when protected health information is shared between institutions.

Comments

The personnel clearance process is an administrative determination of trustworthiness. Human Resources normally performs this function in AMCs. A nominal records check should ascertain that an individual is not falsifying identity, previous employment or education, or any professional certifications. Additionally, any potentially disqualifying criminal activity should be discovered. Federal criminal records are centralized in the FBI database, but state and local records are largely unlinked. It is therefore necessary to determine where individuals have resided in order to check state and local criminal records in disparate jurisdictions. Arrest and conviction data is public information and available on request.

SEC.08 Security Configuration Management §.308(a)(8)

HIPAA Requirement

(Measures, practices, and procedures for the security of information systems that must be coordinated and integrated with each other and other measures, practices, and procedures of the organization established in order to create a coherent system of security) that includes all of the following implementation features:

1. Documentation (written security plans, rules, procedures, and instructions concerning all components of an entity's security).
2. Hardware and software installation and maintenance review and testing for security features (formal, documented procedures for connecting and loading new equipment and programs, periodic review of the maintenance occurring on that equipment and programs, and periodic security testing of the security attributes of that hardware/software).
3. Inventory (the formal, documented identification of hardware and software assets).
4. Security testing (process used to determine that the security features of a system are implemented as designed and that they are adequate for a proposed applications environment; this process includes hands-on functional testing, penetration testing, and verification).

5. Virus checking. (The act of running a computer program that identifies and disables:

Another "virus" computer program, typically hidden, that attaches itself to other programs and has the ability to replicate.

A code fragment (not an independent program) that reproduces by attaching to another program.

A code embedded within a program that causes a copy of itself to be inserted in one or more other programs.)

Explanation of HIPAA Requirement

A covered entity is required to have written security plans and procedures guiding its security efforts so as to create a comprehensive security program. The security program must include an inventory of system assets, formal procedures for installing and testing new systems, a regular security testing schedule, and virus checking.

Key Issues

■ How can a covered entity identify all components of its security features?
■ How should inventory be reviewed and updated — when assets are added and removed or on a routine schedule?
■ At what levels should virus scans be run? Servers? Mail hubs?
■ How often should virus scans be run?
■ How often should virus detection programs be updated?
■ How frequently should security testing, such as penetration testing, occur?

Actions required to address these

■ Develop written security plans, procedures, and instructions to cover all areas of the covered entity's information security needs.
■ Create and document procedures for installing and maintaining software and hardware and periodic testing of that software or hardware's security attributes.
■ Develop a written inventory of hardware and software assets and keep the inventory current.
■ Conduct security testing to ensure that the covered entity's security features are adequate; security testing must include a manual or automated process of identifying vulnerabilities, functional and penetration testing, and verification.
■ Ensure that virus scans are run on a regular schedule.

Actions highly recommended to address these

- Establish a team representing diverse perspectives to plan security controls.
- Have written procedures to report equipment malfunctions and any remedial actions taken. Require departmental systems not managed centrally to comply with the same security configuration requirements as centrally managed systems.
- Employ anti-virus countermeasures at multiple levels, for example on servers, e-mail hosts, and desktops. Maintain a separate test environment and test system changes for security integrity there before moving them to the production systems.

Roadblocks

A single, well-integrated security plan is difficult to establish in an institution with hundreds of distributed, heterogeneous systems using a wide range of technologies. The plan should be multi-tiered and well coordinated. Even identifying all departmental systems with patient information may be difficult in a decentralized AMC.

Comments

AMCs may want to consider coordinating their inventory reviews with accreditation agency standards and reviews.

SEC.09 Security Incident Procedures §.308(a)(9)

HIPAA Requirement

(Formal documented instructions for reporting security breaches) that include all of the following implementation features:

1. Report procedures (documented formal mechanism employed to document security incidents).
2. Response procedures (documented formal rules or instructions for actions to be taken as a result of the receipt of a security incident report).

Explanation of HIPAA Regulation

The covered entity must have written procedures for reporting security breaches to ensure that security violations are handled promptly and appropriately. These must include:

1. Procedures for reporting security incidents
2. Procedures describing response, i.e., actions to take when a security incident is reported

Key Issues

- What constitutes a security incident?
- How should the covered entity define levels of incidents and sanctions for each (e.g., accessing protected health information as opposed to sharing protected health information)?
- How can security awareness be kept "hot?"
- How can a covered entity determine when access to protected health information is inappropriate?

Actions required to address these

- Implement an incident reporting and response procedure and document it.

Actions highly recommended to address these

- Tell workforce members when, how, and to whom to report a security incident.
- Require workforce members to acknowledge that they have received security incident training. Require workforce members to report the incident if they inadvertently access protected health information they should not have accessed.
- Ensure that workforce members know that they should report security violations to a supervisor, system administrator, security, internal audit, or others as appropriate.
- Require workforce members to report instances of noncompliance.
- Ensure that the teams of people who are typically involved in responding to a security incident have a well understood working arrangement that ensures that the incident is handled efficiently, expeditiously, and with respect for law and individual rights.

Roadblocks

Communications between different organizational units within an AMC can be poor. Covered entities should make sure that their IT organizations share information about security incidents with each other in a timely manner, and may need to set up mechanisms to ensure that this happens. Determining where potential security breaches may occur is challenging. For instance, physicians may download medical data onto personal digital assistants. They often purchase such devices themselves, and Security Management has no way of knowing about the purchase or whether the physicians are adhering to security standards.

Comments

Also see: PRIV.53 Sanctions.

SEC.10 Security Management Process §.308(a)(10)

HIPAA Requirement

(Creation, administration, and oversight of policies to ensure the prevention, detection, containment, and correction of security breaches involving risk analysis and risk management). It includes the establishment of accountability, management controls (policies and education), electronic controls, physical security, and penalties for the abuse and misuse of its assets (both physical and electronic) that includes all of the following implementation features:

1. Risk analysis (a process whereby cost-effective security/control measures may be selected by balancing the costs of various security/control measures against the losses that would be expected if these measures were not in place).
2. Risk management (process of assessing risk, taking steps to reduce risk to an acceptable level, and maintaining that level of risk).
3. Sanction policies and procedures (statements regarding disciplinary actions that are communicated to all employees, agents, and contractors; for example, verbal warning, notice of disciplinary action placed in personnel files, removal of system privileges, termination of employment, and contract penalties). They must include employee, agent, and contractor notice of civil or criminal penalties for misuse or misappropriation of health information and must make employees, agents, and contractors aware that violations may result in notification to law enforcement officials and regulatory, accreditation, and licensure organizations.
4. Security policy (statement(s) of information values, protection responsibilities, and organization commitment for a system). This is the framework within which an entity establishes needed levels of information security to achieve the desired confidentiality goals.

Explanation of HIPAA Regulation

An overall information security management process is necessary to establish policy, provide oversight, and administer operational aspects of the program. The process must function in a proactive, risk-appropriate manner and establish the framework for safeguarding protected health information within the AMC. An over-arching information security policy that commits the AMC to safeguard protected health information, to establish goals, and to assign responsibility is necessary.

Supporting policy statements and procedures are required to facilitate the prevention, detection, containment, and correction of security breaches. Specific areas that the security management process must cover are: risk analysis process, risk management process, sanctions process, and security policy.

Key Issues

- What are the covered entity's values with regard to protecting information?
- What are the covered entity's security goals?
- How does the covered entity's security policy demonstrate commitment to these goals?
- How will values, policy, and process be effectively communicated to those covered by them?
- What activities cannot be managed in a secure way?

Actions required to address these

- Establish a management structure that identifies roles and responsibilities for security oversight and operational aspects.
- Establish an overall information security policy that articulates the organization's priorities and expectations with respect to safeguarding protected health information.
- Identify and communicate security responsibilities of workforce member who access or manage access to protected health information.
- Employ risk analysis to identify information assets, threats, and the likelihood and costs of adverse occurrences.
- Manage risk by applying cost-effective security solutions to reduce likelihood and extent of losses due to adverse occurrences.
- Develop a sanctioning process for violators and communicate it to all workforce members. In addition to institutional corrective action, the policy must include notices of civil or criminal penalties and

notices that violations may result in notification of law enforcement, or regulatory, accreditation, and licensure organizations.

Actions highly recommended to address these

- Develop and apply a data criticality/sensitivity classification scheme.
- Make risk analysis and risk management ongoing.
- Consider establishing progressive sanctions, such as verbal warning, written warning, suspension, and employment termination.
- Ensure that the sanction policy provides for swift and strong action when appropriate.
- Establish a process to document and evaluate trends in breaches and sanctions in order to identify potential improvements in security, e.g., changes to policy, procedures, training, or technical measures.
- Require all who have, or may have, access to protected health information to sign security, confidentiality, and computer usage agreements.

Roadblocks

Developing and implementing consistent policies and procedures for sanctions and security policy may be hindered by the typical AMC's decentralized structure and culture of autonomy (academic freedom). At some AMCs, these policies may also have to be coordinated with the associated university's central administration, especially its legal counsel's office and human resources department.

Comments

The reader is referred to the following additional references:

- Carnegie Mellon University
- Software Engineering Institute
- Computer Emergency Response Team Coordination Center (Cert/CC) http://www.cert.org/octave/

SEC.11 Termination Procedures §.308(a)(11)

HIPAA Requirement

(Formal documented instructions, which include appropriate security measures, for the ending of an employee's employment or an internal/external user's access) that include procedures for all of the following implementation features:

1. Changing locks (a documented procedure for changing combinations of locking mechanisms, both on a recurring basis and when personnel knowledgeable of combinations no longer have a need to know or require access to the protected facility or system).
2. Removal from access lists (physical eradication of an entity's access privileges).
3. Removal of user account(s) (termination or deletion of an individual's access privileges to the information, services, and resources for which they currently have clearance, authorization, and need-to-know when such clearance, authorization and need-to-know no longer exists).
4. Turning in of keys, tokens, or cards that allow access (formal, documented procedure to ensure all physical items that allow a terminated employee to access a property, building, or equipment are retrieved from that employee, preferably before termination).

Explanation of HIPAA Regulation

Entities must revoke physical access to controlled areas and remove user accounts when employees terminate employment or when others, such as contractors and vendors, no longer require access. Academic medical centers can reduce risk by implementing procedures to ensure prompt collection of the items that enable access (e.g., identification cards, keys, and physical tokens) by changing locks or lock combinations, and by revoking computer accounts. Although this point is entitled "termination," the text includes provisions for other occasions in which removal of access rights is called for.

Key Issues

- Is access disabled in a timely and consistent manner for terminated users?
- Is there timely notification to: human resources, central security administration, decentralized security administrators, when an employee is terminated?
- Is there a way to deal with terminations of individuals who are not employees, e.g., physicians, contractors, vendors, volunteers? Are there provisions to modify/remove access when workforce members change roles in ways that imply change in access privileges?

Actions required to address these

- When workforce members either terminate employment or lose clearance, or their authorization or need-to-know no longer exists, take the following actions:
- Recover keys, identification cards, physical tokens, and any other objects that facilitate physical access to property, buildings, and equipment.
- Change locks or combinations that control physical access to areas and equipment (this must also be done on a recurring basis).
- Revoke user accounts that provide access to information, services, and resources.
- Remove them from lists that document authorized access to controlled areas and information, services, and resources.
- Document these processes as formal instructions.

Actions highly recommended to address these

- Establish a policy and process to promptly report all terminations and ensure that the revocation process works promptly.
- Document explicit maximum time intervals that are permissible for:
  - Reporting terminations
  - Communicating terminations to security administrators
  - Disabling access
- Develop and document a process to ensure that, in instances of involuntary termination, the action is immediately reported to security administrators and that items that enable access are collected or inactivated immediately.
- Consider revoking access prior to employment termination, particularly in instances of involuntary termination.
- Consider conditions in which people put on administrative leave (e.g., pending an investigation of misuse of access) should have their access privileges altered.
- Revise access when roles change.
- Disable access privileges for any user account that shows no activity for a pre-determined period of time (i.e., three months).
- Review all suspended accounts for activity or attempted activity and report any such activity for investigation as a potential breach.
- Periodically audit the effectiveness of the process for disabling access in the event of a termination to ensure that procedures and guidelines are being followed.
- Record the completion of inactivation activities.

■ Perform exit interviews for any termination in which a potential security concern has been identified. Maintain a record of any changes made to an individual's access privileges, and retain it long enough so it is possible to determine the extent of an individual's historic access in case it is relevant to an investigation.

Roadblocks

AMCs often have a decentralized structure and culture, and thus have many computer systems with decentralized management. Take into consideration that AMCs often have many sites with controlled physical access.

Comments

Linkage of HR, Payroll, and IT systems is a major step in resolving this difficult issue. Education, procedures, and checklists for managers on terminating staff are essential for a successful termination process.

SEC.12 Security Training §.308(a)(12)

HIPAA Requirement

(Education concerning the vulnerabilities of the health information in an entity's possession and ways to ensure the protection of that information) that includes all of the following implementation features:

1. Awareness training for all personnel, including management personnel (in security awareness, including, but not limited to, password maintenance, incident reporting, and viruses and other forms of malicious software)
2. Periodic security reminders (employees, agents, and contractors are made aware of security concerns on an ongoing basis)
3. User education concerning virus protection (training relative to user awareness of the potential harm that can be caused by a virus, how to prevent the introduction of a virus to a computer system, and what to do if a virus is detected)
4. User education in importance of monitoring log-in success or failure and how to report discrepancies (training in the user's responsibility to ensure the security of health care information)
5. User education in password management (type of user training in the rules to be followed in creating and changing passwords and the need to keep them confidential)

Explanation of HIPAA Regulation

Security training is necessary for all workforce members who access protected health information. This training must include overall security awareness, periodic reminders, virus awareness, password management, and user-specific topics necessary for individual workstation security.

Key Issues

- How will the security training program be updated to reflect changes in the security environment and security responsibilities of workforce members?
- How is the training program tailored to support the various classes of system users and the level of information sensitivity to which each class of user has access?
- Are all system users included in the training program, including those accessing organizational systems from remote sites?
- How is training documented?
- How is training effectiveness evaluated?
- Does the training content meet all of the HIPAA training requirements?
- How often should reminders or refresher courses be provided?

Actions required to address these

- Establish a formal, documented security awareness training program for all workforce members that addresses, at a minimum, the following topics:
  - Protection against, and reporting of, viruses
  - Reporting security incidents
  - Managing individual passwords
- Establish a formal, documented security awareness program tailored to system users that addresses, at a minimum:
  - Virus protection
  - Potential harm viruses can cause
  - How to prevent the introduction of viruses into a computer system
  - What to do if a virus is detected
  - The importance of monitoring log-in success or failure
  - How to report discrepancies in the log-in process
  - Rules for creating and changing passwords
  - Safeguarding passwords

- Provide periodic security awareness reminders to all workforce members.

Actions highly recommended to address these

- Make training role- or job-specific.
- Assign responsibility for security training.
- Document the training that has been provided to each individual.
- Develop a training program that demonstrates mastery of the material presented.
- Evaluate the effectiveness of training.

Roadblocks

Security training is generally not given a high priority in orientation and training for new hires, so the time available may be inadequate. It is also often difficult to arrange security training for third-party agents and subcontractors with access to health information. Without centralized responsibility for the development of content for the security program, it will be difficult to ensure consistent training across the AMC.

Comments

Using experts in this field will enhance the content of security training programs. Some AMCs reduce the costs of security training by weaving training into ongoing training activities. Consider including a security training curriculum for residents, as well as for medical and nursing students. Also see: SEC.18 Security Awareness Training.

Requirements for Physical Safeguards

SEC.13 Assigned Security Responsibility §.308(b)(1)

HIPAA Requirement

(Practices established by management to manage and supervise the execution and use of security measures to protect data and to manage and supervise the conduct of personnel in relation to the protection of data).

Explanation of HIPAA Regulation

The governing body of each covered entity must designate a security officer or group to oversee the safeguarding of protected health information and assign the necessary responsibility and accountability to that role.

This person or group will manage the execution and use of security measures and supervise the conduct of personnel in relation to data protection.

Key Issues

- Will the covered entity instill this responsibility in an individual role or charge a committee?
- How will the covered entity empower the security officer or group to accomplish effectively the security goals?
- How will multiple facility entities assign oversight?
- How will multiple entity systems assign oversight?

Actions required to address these

- Assign overall responsibility for securing protected health information to an individual security officer or a group specifically charged to do so.
- Make this person or group accountable for the information security program to include:
  - Processes employed to safeguard protected health information
  - Technologies and architectures employed to safeguard protected health information
  - Conduct of personnel in relation to the safeguarding of protected health information

Actions highly recommended to address these

- Have the organization's governing body assign this responsibility and instill the authority to accomplish the task effectively.
- Ensure that the security officer possesses the necessary body of knowledge, skill set, and experience to oversee the security program effectively.
- Extend the security officer's responsibility to the entire entity.
- If the organization has multiple security officers, coordinate their efforts. Avoid combining the responsibilities of the security officer and the privacy official, as the knowledge bases and skill sets required for each differ.

Roadblocks

Security officers with the knowledge, skills, and experience necessary to manage effectively an information security program in an AMC are few and difficult to recruit. On the other hand, training a person with a general or non-healthcare information security background on the job takes a good deal of time.

SEC.14 Media Controls §.308(b)(2)

HIPAA Requirement

(Formal, documented policies and procedures that govern the receipt and removal of hardware/software (such as diskettes and tapes) into and out of a facility) that include all of the following implementation features:

- Access control
- Accountability (the property that ensures that the actions of an entity can be traced uniquely to that entity)
- Data backup (a retrievable, exact copy of information)
- Data storage (the retention of healthcare information pertaining to an individual in an electronic format)
- Disposal (final disposition of electronic data, or the hardware on which electronic data is stored)

Explanation of HIPAA Regulation

While this item states that it is focused upon the transfer of hardware and software media into and out of a facility, it also requires consideration of the larger issue of how to handle record copies of protected media from creation to destruction. Each entity will need to decide how to categorize, annotate, account for, store, and dispose of protected health information in record form.

Key Issues

- How and by whom is new media introduced into the record environment?
- How are working materials created, marked, controlled, and destroyed?
- How are media and computer equipment controlled when entering and leaving the facility?
- Is equipment properly inventoried?
- Is media disposed of properly?
- Do the use of unofficial and "shadow" record systems undermine accountability and controls and, if so, how can they be brought into line with media controls?

Actions required to address these

- Establish accountability and access controls for media containing protected health information, including equipment with media installed and hardcopies containing protected health information, from creation to disposition.
- Ensure that policies and procedures address access control, accountability, data backup, data storage, and data disposal.

Actions highly recommended to address these

- Establish uniform terminology and guidelines for classifying and marking materials as "confidential," "proprietary," "patient-confidential," etc.
- Establish procedures for assigning accountability for newly created media, including hardcopy when created and recording/removing the media from accountability when properly destroyed.
- Establish guidelines to restrict the use of "unofficial" or "shadow" records to ensure the integrity and protection of protected health information.
- Mark temporary working materials, whether on computer media or hardcopy, that contain protected health information appropriately when created and establish a date for either destroying the working materials or bringing them under control as record documents.
- Ensure that appropriate secure storage and destruction facilities, such as shredders, are readily available, clearly marked, and used.
- Ensure that protected health information in hardcopy format is disposed of properly. Responsible personnel should authorize the shipping and receiving of protected media and maintain appropriate records. Establish a formal system for shipping and transporting materials containing protected health information with receipts to ensure that shipped materials have been properly received and accountability has been transferred to the receiving office. Establish standards for wrapping and marking shipped media that both minimize the likelihood of its being identified as containing protected health information and prevent tampering.
- Set a standard for purging protected health information from magnetic media, and adhere to it. Degaussing and overwriting are acceptable methods. (See Comments.)
- Before releasing any magnetic media that may contain protected health information outside the entity, process it to purge any information residing on it.

- If media is left unattended, secure it and use reasonable care.
- Do not leave printed versions (hardcopy) of protected health information unattended and open to compromise, and do not copy it indiscriminately.
- Establish and maintain accountability for all equipment used to process protected health information, including requirements for regular inventory and resolving any loss of accountability.
- Ensure that essential patient care information is properly backed up in a secure location.
- Periodically check to ensure that data can be restored from backup media.
- Consider periodic audits by outside agencies to ensure that appropriate media controls are maintained.

Roadblocks

Unlike many business environments, there is no real control over movement of people and equipment on and off campus. While establishing controls for centrally managed data is relatively straightforward, the issue of enforcing media controls for "shadows" and other unofficial systems is a significant one.

Comments

A reasonable standard for purging magnetic media containing protected health information by overwriting is a one-time bit-by-bit method that wipes the entire piece of media. The government standard for declassifying media is a three-time overwrite: First, overwrite with a character or character string, second, overwrite with the binary compliment of the first, and third, overwrite with any character or character string.

SEC.15 Physical access controls §.308(b)(3)

HIPAA Requirement

(Limited access) (Formal, documented policies and procedures to be followed to limit physical access to an entity while ensuring that properly authorized access is allowed) that include all of the following implementation features:

1. Disaster recovery (the process enabling an entity to restore any loss of data in the event of fire, vandalism, natural disaster, or system failure).

2. An emergency mode operation (access controls in place that enable an entity to continue to operate in the event of fire, vandalism, natural disaster, or system failure).

3. Equipment control (into and out of site) (documented security procedures for bringing hardware and software into and out of a facility and for maintaining a record of that equipment. This includes, but is not limited to, the marking, handling, and disposal of hardware and storage media).

4. A facility security plan (a plan to safeguard the premises and building (exterior and interior) from unauthorized physical access and to safeguard the equipment therein from unauthorized physical access, tampering, and theft).

5. Procedures for verifying access authorizations before granting physical access (formal, documented policies and instructions for validating the access privileges of an entity before granting those privileges)

6. Maintenance records (documentation of repairs and modifications to the physical components of a facility, such as hardware, software, walls, doors, and locks).

7. Need-to-know procedures for personnel access (a security principle stating that a user should have access only to the data he or she needs to perform a particular function).

8. Procedures to sign in visitors and provide escorts, if appropriate (formal documented procedure governing the reception and hosting of visitors).

9. Testing and revision (the restriction of program testing and revision to formally authorized personnel).

Explanation of HIPAA Regulation

Each covered entity is required to establish formal, documented policies and procedures for limiting physical access while ensuring that properly authorized access is allowed. Mandatory implementation features also include plans for emergency operation and disaster recovery as well as for testing and revision.

Actions required to address these

■ House critical or sensitive protected health information processing facilities in secure areas, protected by a defined security perimeter, with appropriate security barriers and entry controls. Physically protect them from unauthorized access, damage, and interference.

- Establish and maintain a specific disaster recovery plan.
- Supervise or clear contractors and other visitors to secure areas, and record their date and time of entry and departure.
- Control access to protected health information and information processing facilities, and restrict it to authorized persons only.
- Provide security for off-site equipment that is equivalent to that provided for on-site equipment used for the same purpose, taking into account the risks of working outside the covered entity's premises. Keep records of maintenance of equipment.
- Restrict testing and revision to authorized personnel.

Actions highly recommended to address these

- Provide protection commensurate with the identified risks.
- Regularly review and update access rights to secure areas.
- Grant contractors and visitors access only for specific, authorized purposes and issue them with instructions on the security requirements of the area and on emergency procedures.
- Require all workforce members to wear some form of visible identification and encourage them to challenge unescorted strangers and anyone not wearing visible identification.
- Physically protect equipment from security threats and environmental hazards.
- Maintain equipment in accordance with the supplier's recommended service intervals and specifications.
- Use authentication controls, e.g., swipe card plus PIN, to authorize and validate all access.
- Maintain a secure audit trail of all access.
- Require management authorization for the use of any equipment outside a covered entity's premises for processing of protected health information.
- Ensure that only authorized maintenance personnel carry out repairs and service equipment.
- Maintain records of all suspected or actual faults and all preventative and corrective maintenance.
- Establish appropriate controls when sending equipment off premises for maintenance.
- Comply with all requirements imposed by insurance policies.
- Check all items of equipment containing storage media, e.g., fixed hard disks, to ensure that any protected health information and licensed software has been removed or overwritten prior to disposal.

- Require authorization in order to take any equipment, protected health information, or software off site.
- Where necessary and appropriate, require equipment to be logged out and logged back in when returned.
- Perform spot checks to detect unauthorized removal of property, and make individuals aware that spot checks will take place.
- Forbid users to connect unauthorized devices to the enterprise network.
- Escort and supervise maintenance personnel; assign knowledgeable persons to this task.

Roadblocks

Those responsible for implementation and enforcement may be slow to accept the need for new policies. Also see: SEC.14 Media Controls.

SEC.16 Policy/guideline on workstation use §.308(b)(4)

HIPAA Requirement

(Documented instructions/procedures delineating the proper functions to be performed, the manner in which those functions are to be performed, and the physical attributes of the surroundings of a specific computer terminal site or type of site, dependent upon the sensitivity of the information accessed from that site).

Explanation of HIPAA Regulation

Each covered entity is required to establish a policy/guideline on secure workstation use. These documents will establish the rules for minimizing the risk of exposing protected health information to unauthorized access. They will include technical measures (automatic log-off) as well as behavioral rules (no sharing of passwords).

Key Issues

- Is there a documented procedure for positioning workstations (including both printers and data entry/display terminals) in such a way as to minimize shoulder surfing?
- Is there a process for determining automatic log-off intervals for each site?

■ Is there a process for activating and deactivating passwords?
■ Is there a documented process to train users about their responsibilities in maintaining workstation security?

Actions required to address these

■ Develop a Workstation Use Policy.
■ Position workstations to minimize unauthorized viewing of protected health information either by shoulder surfing or by other direct physical means of obtaining access to data present on the workstation.
■ Grant workstation access only to those who need it in order to perform their job function.

Actions highly recommended to address these

■ Develop a policy/guideline to protect the workstations from exposure to physical threats including theft.
■ Consider establishing automatic log-off to minimize opportunities for unauthorized use of a workstation.
■ Educate users about their responsibilities for workstation security.
■ Monitor workstation sites for good user practice including log-off and password usage.
■ Consider two-factor log-in for user authentication.
■ Avoid log-in methods that may require the use of multiple passwords by an individual.

Roadblocks

In many institutions, guarding passwords and workstations is of secondary importance to the need to accomplish the goal of providing healthcare. Procedures that substantially impede the use of data entry and data retrieval will meet resistance.

Comments

When interpreting this rule, consider that a workstation may include any or all of several devices such as data terminals, printers, and fax machines. Printouts may contain the most sensitive information in a patient's file and are as great a security risk as any other source of information. Because turnover may be high among those who have broad access to protected health information, it is important to have a facile and flexible way to manage granting and revocation of access privileges. Training users about their security responsibilities as well as functional aspects is vital.

SEC.17 Secure work station location §.308(b)(5)

HIPAA Requirement

(Physical safeguards to eliminate or minimize the possibility of unauthorized access to information; example, locating a terminal used to access sensitive information in a locked room and restricting access to that room authorized personnel, not placing terminal used to access patient information in any area of a doctor's office where the screen contents can viewed from the reception area).

Explanation of HIPAA Regulation

Each covered entity is required to implement physical safeguards to eliminate or minimize the possibility of unauthorized access to protected health information. This is especially important in public buildings, provider locations, and other areas where there is heavy pedestrian traffic.

Key Issues

- What are the trade-offs between workstation accessibility and protection of protected health information?
- How will potential workstation location changes affect workflow?

Actions required to address these

- Establish workstation location criteria to eliminate or minimize the possibility of unauthorized access to protected health information.
- Employ physical safeguards as determined by risk analysis, such as locating workstations in controlled access areas or installing covers or enclosures to preclude passerby access to protected health information.

Actions highly recommended to address these

- When practical, locate workstations used to access protected health information in areas that are continuously monitored by cleared personnel when open for business and otherwise securely locked and alarmed with a 24-hour security monitoring service.

- Locate workstations to minimize the possibility of unauthorized personnel viewing screens or data.
- Establish workstation inactivity timeouts and use timed, password-protected screen savers.
- Consider the use of proximity detectors to reduce exposure at unattended workstations.

Comments

Ideally, workstations used to access protected health information would be located only in controlled areas — but this may unacceptably restrict access to and use of electronic patient records. In these cases, consider additional controls such physical devices to limit viewing, timeout/lockout of individual sessions, use of password-protected screensavers, and other procedures to provide adequate confidentiality.

SEC.18 Security Awareness training §.308(b)(6)

HIPAA Requirement

(Information security awareness training programs in which all employees, agents, and contractors must participate, including, based on job responsibilities, customized education programs that focus on issues regarding use of health information and responsibilities regarding confidentiality and security).

Explanation of HIPAA Regulation

Covered entities are required to establish security awareness training programs customized to individual job responsibilities. Training for all workforce members in the use of protected health information and its confidentiality and security is required.

Key Issues

- How will the covered entity tailor security awareness training to hundreds of separate roles?
- How will the covered entity merge privacy training (use of information) with security training to address this requirement?

Actions required to address these

- Provide job-specific security awareness training to all workforce members.

■ Focus the training on use of protected health information (privacy) and security.

Actions highly recommended to address these

■ Make this aspect of training a supervisory or departmental responsibility, as appropriate.
■ Consider the security guidelines in this document and determine which pertain to each job class.
■ Develop a training program to communicate them.

Roadblocks

Developing meaningful job-specific training programs in large organizations is difficult. Making supervisors responsible and accountable for training at this level is an approach that should maximize the likelihood of success.

Comments

Also see: SEC.12, as covered in §.308(a)(12). SEC.12 Security Training is general in nature, establishing high-level expectations for all staff and somewhat more focused expectations for the system user community. This Security Awareness Training point focuses on customized education tailored to individual job responsibilities.

Requirements for Technical Security Services and Mechanisms

SEC.19 Access Control §.308©(1)(i)

HIPAA Requirement

The technical security services must include…Access control that includes:

1. A procedure for emergency access (documented instructions for obtaining necessary information during a crisis)
2. At least one of the following implementation features:
   a. Context-based access (an access control procedure based on the context of a transaction as opposed to being based on attributes of the initiator or target)
   b. Role-based access
   c. User-based access
3. The optional use of encryption

Explanation of HIPAA Regulation

Each covered entity is required to maintain a mechanism for access control that restricts access to resources and allows access only by privileged entities, providing access only to those workforce members with a business need for it. Possible types of access control include mandatory access control, discretionary access control, time-of-day, classification, and subject/object separation. In addition, a mechanism to enable emergency access is required.

Key Issues

- Is there a documented procedure for emergency access?
- Is there a process for screening unwarranted demands for access?
- Do systems and applications have technical capability to implement user, role, or context-based access?
- Do systems prohibit or allow simultaneous access of the same user ID/concurrent connections? Why or why not?
- Does the organization allow group, shared, trusted, or generic logon?
- How does encryption affect access control?

Actions required to address these

- Define a context-based, role-based, or user-based access policy as appropriate for each of the various situations in the covered entity and adopt implementation procedures to enforce need-to-know accordingly.
- Enact a clearly stated and widely understood "break the glass" procedure for allowing access via alternate or manual methods in the event of an emergency requiring access to protected health information.

Actions highly recommended to address these

- Establish a centrally administered service to define access profiles — context-based, role-based, or user-based — and oversee consistent implementation of access control mechanisms.
- Document and test the emergency access procedure.
- Evaluate information technology projects, proposals, contracts, and existing services for access control features and implementation.
- Consider adopting ASTM-defined healthcare roles.

Roadblocks

Centrally administered access control services are difficult to implement in the diverse IT environments typical of Academic Medical Centers. Take into consideration that reduced log-on solutions, PKI, Kerberos, password-brokering services, and the like are expensive, complicated, and often require expertise not found in the healthcare industry. Testing emergency access procedures in a realistic fashion is often cumbersome. Controlling contractor and business partner access is challenging, particularly when remote network connections are involved and accountability is necessary on the remote end. Modifying access profiles when staff members change roles within the covered entity will require efficient communication between personnel and IT.

Comments

A user-based access model would require the organization to determine appropriate access for each individual user. A role-based access model would require the organization to develop an access profile for each role; for example, nurses, doctors, and desk attendants each have different access needs dependent upon their role in the organization. A context-based access model would, for example, allow all staff working in Endocrinology to access Endocrinology records. Some AMCs may choose to implement combinations of access models.

Also see: SEC.05 Information Access and Control, SEC.10 Security Management Process, and SEC.11 Termination Procedures.

SEC.20 Audit Controls §.308©(1)(ii)

HIPAA Requirement

The technical security services must include…(mechanisms employed to record and examine system activity).

Explanation of HIPAA Regulation

System activity logging is required in order to recreate pertinent system events and actions taken by system users and administrators. An audit process of examining logged information is required in order to identify questionable data access activities, investigate breaches, respond to potential weaknesses, and assess the security program.

Key Issues

- What activities need to be monitored?
- What level of logging detail is necessary?

- How long should covered entities retain audit log data?
- How should covered entities protect audit log data?
- Who may access audit log data?
- How can a covered entity identify inappropriate access?
- How can a covered entity best use audit tools to assess its security program?
- When should prospective audits be used?

Actions required to address these

- Employ event logging on systems that process or store protected health information where warranted by risk analysis.

Actions highly recommended to address these

- Log system administration events
  - Creation and removal of accounts
  - Assigning and changing of privileges
  - Installation, maintenance, and changing of software
  - Changes in hardware configurations
- Log user activities
  - Log-on and log-off, both successful and unsuccessful
  - Read, write, create, and delete actions at the file level
  - Individual user access to individual patient records
  - Attempts to access unauthorized data or services
- Perform prospective audits of user activity where risk levels warrant
- Maintain log data for a specified period of time
- Protect system logs, especially those containing personally identifiable healthcare information, from unauthorized access or alteration
- Employ audit reduction tools or "intelligent" methods of correlating log data to detect unauthorized activity and reduce volumes to manageable size

Roadblocks

Be aware that system audit logs can quickly become voluminous and require additional maintenance time. Prospective auditing and determining appropriateness of access and actions taken is an expensive, time consuming, and difficult process.

Comments

The purpose of system event logging is to be able to recreate pertinent events should a security violation or compromise occur. Log data is typically examined reactively, when indications of unauthorized activity are reported. How entities interpret and respond to findings is a measure of compliance. Because prospective audits are onerous and usually require the input of clinicians to resolve need-to-know issues, they should be performed sparingly and with good cause in accordance with risk and threat levels as determined through the risk analysis process. Enterprise systems are normally subject to audit controls. Departmental systems and those with limited numbers of users and lower functionality, such as laboratory systems or those that feed data up to enterprise systems, are normally not subject to audit controls unless the risk analysis process determines otherwise. The risk analysis process should consider track records of violations. Logging and audit strategies should reflect levels of abuse. Logging to a high level of detail, such as individual keystroke capture, is generally not necessary. The required retention period for audit log data may vary. In general, at least several months of data are necessary to adequately investigate instances of inappropriate access. The National Industrial Security Program, which oversees the protection of U.S. government classified information, requires at least six months of log data. This may be a reasonable and defensible goal for Academic Medical Centers as well.

Also see: SEC.06 Internal Audit, SEC.09 Security Incident Procedures, PRIV.53 Complaints, and PRIV.54 Sanctions.

SEC.21 Authorization Control §.308 ©(3)

HIPAA Requirement

(The mechanism for obtaining consent for the use and disclosure of health information) that includes at least one of the following implementation features:

1. Role-based access
2. User-based access

Explanation of HIPAA Regulation

Covered entities must implement a mechanism to authorize the privileged use of protected health information available via systems and applications.

The mechanism must limit these privileges to the maximum practical extent commensurate with professional needs.

Key Issues

- How can a covered entity determine which type of authorization mechanism — role-based or user-based — is appropriate?

Actions required to address these

- Employ a system or application-based mechanism to authorize activities within system resources in accordance with the Least Privilege Principle. (See Comments.)
- Implement:
  - A role-based mechanism where users with common information needs are provided access and privileges through common security authorization classes, or a user-based mechanism where users' information access and privilege needs are determined and provided on an individual basis.
  - Maintain individual accountability for actions taken by forbidding group (shared, generic, trusted, etc.) log-ons.

Roadblocks

Implementing a data stewardship model is prudent but will likely be difficult in large covered entities. Individuals or groups sometimes perform stewardship functions but may not understand the concept of accountability for usage and disclosure.

Comments

The Least Privilege Principle pertains to one's ability to perform specified system functions. Users should not have system capabilities not required of their positions. For example, a user who requires only read access to medical information should not have the ability to change or delete it. AMCs will almost certainly use the role-based authorization approach given the large numbers of users typical of these organizations. Covered entities are cautioned to avoid developing too many authorization profiles in a role-based model, as management of a large number of profiles is unwieldy.

SEC.22 Data Authentication §.308 ©(4)

HIPAA Requirement

(The corroboration that data has not been altered or destroyed in an unauthorized manner. Examples of how data corroboration may be assured include the use of a checksum, double keying, a message authentication code, or digital signature.)

Explanation of HIPAA Regulation

Each covered entity must be able to provide corroboration that protected health information in its possession has not been altered or destroyed in an unauthorized manner. Data corroboration methods include, but are not limited to, the use of checksums, double keying, message authentication codes, and digital signatures.

Key Issues

- Is the use of digital signatures a cost effective approach?
- Are technical integrity controls a reasonable expectation for more than certain critical functions?
- Can trusted procedures supplant technical controls in some respects?

Actions required to address these

- Employ technical controls such as checksums, digital signatures, double keying, and message authentication codes where feasible and appropriate to the level of risk.

Actions highly recommended to address these

- Employ technical integrity controls for critical automated functions such as physicians' orders and prescriptions.
- Procedural aspects closely related to technical authentication and integrity:
  - Maintain separation of duties. Avoid overlapping responsibilities of application and system programmers, data center operators, data base administrators, network operations, and user functions.
  - Establish and demonstrate change management discipline.

SEC.23 Entity Authentication §.308 ©(5)

HIPAA Requirement

(The corroboration that an entity is the one claimed) that includes:

1. Automatic log-off (a security procedure that causes an electronic session to terminate after a predetermined time of inactivity, such as 15 minutes)
2. Unique user identifier (a combination name/number assigned and maintained in security procedures for identifying and tracking individual user identity)
3. At least one of the following implementation features:
   a. Biometric identification (an identification system that identifies a human from a measurement of a physical feature or repeatable action of the individual (for example, hand geometry, retinal scan, iris scan, fingerprint patterns, facial characteristics, DNA sequence characteristics, voice prints, and handwritten signature))
   b. Password
   c. Personal identification number (PIN) (a number or code assigned to an individual and used to provide verification of identity)
   d. A telephone callback procedure (method of authenticating the identity of the receiver and sender of information through a series of "questions" and "answers" sent back and forth establishing the identity of each). For example, when the communicating systems exchange a series of identification codes as part of the initiation of a session to exchange information, or when a host computer disconnects the initial session before the authentication is complete, and the host calls the user back to establish a session at a predetermined telephone number
   e. Token

Explanation of HIPAA Regulation

Entities (an entity may be a person, system, or process) must be authenticated prior to accessing protected health information. Authentication is the process of corroborating that an entity is who or what it claims to be; it may occur through a trusted process such as the provision of a secret password, a personal identification number, or a token. Dial-up remote access users are subject to stronger, or two-tiered, authentication that may include telephone call-back or other strong authentication methods. Automatic log-offs, or inactivity time-outs, can help enforce authentication by precluding others from accessing unattended sessions.

Key Issues

- Is a unique user ID with password authentication secure enough?
- Should alternative authentication methods such as biometrics be considered?
- What standards are necessary to make a public key infrastructure (PKI) interoperable and truly useful?

Actions required to address these

- Uniquely identify each user and authenticate identity.
- Implement at least one of the following methods to authenticate a user:
  - Password
  - Biometrics
  - Personal Identification Number (PIN)
  - Physical token
  - Call-back or strong authentication for dial-up remote access users
- Implement automatic log-offs to terminate sessions after set periods of inactivity. Determine appropriate periods based on the levels of risk and exposure.

Actions highly recommended to address these

- Include procedures for initiating user access, resetting passwords or tokens, and providing administrative access in the authentication system, and ensure it is fully documented.
- Employ a formal risk management methodology to identify risks and threats to the authentication process. Employ secure architectures, where risk appropriate, to authenticate entities. These may include Kerberos, RADIUS, TACACS, PKI, or similar methods.
- Encrypt hard-coded passwords that reside on client machines or in applications. Securely authenticate contractors. Device-to-device or firewall-to-firewall authentication is acceptable provided the contractor demonstrates individual accountability for access. Change passwords periodically.
- Specify time-out intervals based on business need and levels of risk and exposure.
- Allow users to select and change their own passwords.

Comments

Dial-back has been largely replaced by more robust architectures such as Remote Dial-In User Authentication (RADIUS). Most covered entities will continue to employ user ID and password authentication. Managed properly this is adequate, but processing speeds and wide availability of hacker tools and techniques have made this method obsolete for all but internal authentication. Inactivity time-outs are secondary controls and users should not rely on them to end their sessions. Password standards must be risk appropriate. Covered entities will need to address password length, complexity, change frequency, user selection, etc. This will continue to be a moving target.

SEC.24 Communications/network controls §.308(d)

HIPAA Requirement

(1) If an entity uses communications or network controls, its security standards for technical security mechanisms must include the following:

1. The following implementation features:
   a. Integrity controls (a security mechanism employed to ensure the validity of the information being electronically transmitted or stored)
   b. Message authentication (ensuring, typically with a message authentication code, that a message received (usually via a network) matches the message sent)
2. One of the following implementation features:
   a. Access controls (protection of sensitive communications transmissions over open or private networks so that they cannot be easily intercepted and interpreted by parties other than the intended recipient)
   b. Encryption

(2) If an entity uses network controls (to protect sensitive communication that is transmitted electronically over open networks so that it cannot be easily intercepted and interpreted by parties other than the intended recipient), its technical security mechanisms must include all of the following implementation features:

1. Alarm. (In communication systems, any device that can sense an abnormal condition within the system and provide, either locally or remotely, a signal indicating the presence of the abnormality. The signal may be in any desired form ranging from a simple contact closure (or opening) to a time-phased automatic shutdown and restart cycle.)
2. Audit trail (the data collected and potentially used to facilitate a security audit).

3. Entity authentication (a communications or network mechanism to irrefutably identify authorized users, programs, and processes and to deny access to unauthorized users, programs, and processes).
4. Event reporting (a network message indicating operational irregularities in physical elements of a network or a response to the occurrence of a significant task, typically the completion of a request for information).

Explanation of HIPAA Regulation

Covered entities that use external communication systems, such as the public switched telephone system, or open networks, such as the Internet, are required to safeguard protected health information that traverses them. The specified technical security services address network risks of message interception and interpretation by parties other than the intended recipient. Additionally, these services protect information systems from intruders attempting to exploit external communication points such as Internet host systems and telephone switches. In addition to the other listed precautions, some form of encryption is required when using open networks.

Key Issues

- How is relative risk determined?
- How much encryption is enough?
- When should encryption be used?

Actions required to address these

- If the covered entity employs an internal, private, or value-added network, the covered entity must:
  - Employ alarms to sense abnormal conditions.
  - Enact an audit trail to recreate events in the instance of violations or compromises.
  - Identify and authenticate authorized users, programs, and processes.
  - Deny access to unauthorized users, programs, and processes.
  - Employ event reporting to identify operational irregularities and occurrences of significant tasks.
- If the covered entity employs the public switched telephone system, the covered entity must:
  - Enact integrity controls to ensure the validity of protected health information transmitted.

- Enact message authentication to ensure that content is not altered in transmission.
- Enact access controls or risk appropriate encryption to preclude unauthorized access, interception, or interpretation.
■ If the covered entity employs the public Internet, the covered entity must enact the controls listed for the public switched telephone system as well as using risk appropriate encryption. (See Comments.)

Actions highly recommended to address these

■ Do not store or transmit system passwords in the clear.
■ Control network access through individual identification and authentication.
■ Employ encryption keys of the length specified by the HCFA Internet Security Policy.

Roadblocks

Encryption is often difficult to implement. Hardware-based encryption is generally costly but fast because it does not require CPU cycles, while software-based encryption is generally less costly but tends to be system or application dependent and impedes performance.

Comments

Threats to data transmissions are difficult to quantify and widely misunderstood. Threat levels vary and are sometimes based on factors such as geography. For example, the threat of eavesdropping on the public switched telephone system within the United States is very low, but the threat rises dramatically when international communications are considered. State-sponsored eavesdropping is the norm in some parts of the world — particularly when U.S. interests are involved. In November of 1998, the Healthcare Finance Administration (HCFA) released an Internet Security Policy describing appropriate encryption key lengths for public, private, and elliptical curve algorithms. Required key lengths are, of course, subject to change as technology improves. Academic Medical Centers should use strong encryption with key lengths at least as long as those specified by HCFA for Internet transmissions. AMCs may need further advice from communications experts and national agencies/organizations.

INDEX

INDEX